Clinical Focus on
High-Risk Pregnancy

Clinical Focus on
High-Risk Pregnancy

Series Editors

Neharika Malhotra
MD (Gold Medalist) DRM (Germany) FICMCH
Fellow ICOG (Rep Med) ICOG (USG)
Director and Consultant
ART Rainbow IVF and MNMH (P) Ltd
and Ujala Cygnus Rainbow Hospital
Agra, Uttar Pradesh, India
Joint Secretary, FOGSI
Chair, YTP Committee, FOGSI

Jaideep Malhotra
MD FICMCH FICOG FRCOG FRCPI FMAS
Managing Director
ART Rainbow IVF and MNMH (P) Ltd
and Ujala Cygnus Rainbow Hospital
Agra, Uttar Pradesh, India
President, SAFOM/ISPAT
Past President, IMS/ISAR/FOGSI/ASPIRE

Narendra Malhotra
MD FICMCH FICOG FRCOG FICS FMAS FIAP
Managing Director
Global Rainbow Health Care and MNMH (P) Ltd
and Ujala Cygnus Rainbow Hospital
Agra, Uttar Pradesh, India
Professor, Sarajevo School of Science and Technology, Croatia
Past President, FOGSI/IFUMB/ISPAT/ISAR, INSARG
Vice President, WAPM/SAFOG
Director, International IAN Donald School and SAFOG

Editors

Ashwini Kale
MBBS DGO DNB FICMCH
Chief IVF Consultant
ASHA IVF Centre and Ashakiran Hospitals
Pune, Maharashtra, India

Shreya Prabhoo
MBBS DNB DGO MNAMS
Consultant Obstetrician and Gynecologist
Mukund Hospital and Surya Hospital
Honorary Consultant
Hinduhridaysamrat Balasaheb Thackeray Medical
College and Dr RN Cooper Hospital
Mumbai, Maharashtra, India
Managing Committee Member
Obstetrics and Gynecological Society

Sheeba Marwah
MBBS DNB (Obs/Gyne) FICOG FICMCH
Fellowship Critical Care Obstetrics (ICOG-FOGSI)
Associate Professor
Department of Obstetrics and Gynecology
VMMC and Safdarjung Hospital
New Delhi, India

Foreword
Jaydeep Tank

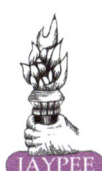

JAYPEE BROTHERS MEDICAL PUBLISHERS
The Health Sciences Publisher
New Delhi | London

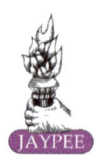 **Jaypee Brothers Medical Publishers (P) Ltd**

Headquarters
Jaypee Brothers Medical Publishers (P) Ltd
EMCA House, 23/23-B
Ansari Road, Daryaganj
New Delhi 110 002, India
Landline: +91-11-23272143, +91-11-23272703
+91-11-23282021, +91-11-23245672
Email: jaypee@jaypeebrothers.com

Corporate Office
Jaypee Brothers Medical Publishers (P) Ltd
4838/24, Ansari Road, Daryaganj
New Delhi 110 002, India
Phone: +91-11-43574357
Fax: +91-11-43574314
Email: jaypee@jaypeebrothers.com

Overseas Office
JP Medical Ltd
83 Victoria Street, London
SW1H 0HW (UK)
Phone: +44 20 3170 8910
Fax: +44 (0)20 3008 6180
Email: info@jpmedpub.com

Website: www.jaypeebrothers.com
Website: www.jaypeedigital.com

© 2023, Jaypee Brothers Medical Publishers

The views and opinions expressed in this book are solely those of the original contributor(s)/author(s) and do not necessarily represent those of editor(s) or publisher of the book.

All rights reserved. No part of this publication may be reproduced, stored or transmitted in any form or by any means, electronic, mechanical, photocopying, recording or otherwise, without the prior permission in writing of the publishers.

All brand names and product names used in this book are trade names, service marks, trademarks or registered trademarks of their respective owners. The publisher is not associated with any product or vendor mentioned in this book.

Medical knowledge and practice change constantly. This book is designed to provide accurate, authoritative information about the subject matter in question. However, readers are advised to check the most current information available on procedures included and check information from the manufacturer of each product to be administered, to verify the recommended dose, formula, method and duration of administration, adverse effects and contraindications. It is the responsibility of the practitioner to take all appropriate safety precautions. Neither the publisher nor the author(s)/editor(s) assume any liability for any injury and/or damage to persons or property arising from or related to use of material in this book.

This book is sold on the understanding that the publisher is not engaged in providing professional medical services. If such advice or services are required, the services of a competent medical professional should be sought.

Every effort has been made where necessary to contact holders of copyright to obtain permission to reproduce copyright material. If any have been inadvertently overlooked, the publisher will be pleased to make the necessary arrangements at the first opportunity.

Inquiries for bulk sales may be solicited at: jaypee@jaypeebrothers.com

Clinical Focus on High-Risk Pregnancy

First Edition: **2023**

ISBN: 978-93-5696-090-9

Dedicated to

Our parents, teachers, and all practicing Obstetricians and Gynecologists

Contributors

Amit Singh MBBS MD (Pulmonary Medicine)
Senior Resident
All India Institute of Medical Sciences
Bhopal, Madhya Pradesh, India

Ankita Jain MBBS DNB (Obs/Gyne)
ICOG fellow (Critical Care Obstetrics)
Assistant Professor
VMMC and Safdarjung Hospital
New Delhi, India

Anshika Rakesh MBBS MS (Obs/Gyne)
Senior Resident
Department of Obstetrics and Gynecology
VMMC and Safdarjung Hospital
New Delhi, India

Aruna Verma MBBS MD (Obs/Gyne) FICOG
Professor
Department of Obstetrics and Gynecology
Lala Lajpat Rai Memorial Medical College
Meerut, Uttar Pradesh, India

Ashwini Kale MBBS DGO DNB FICMCH
Chief IVF Consultant
Asha IVF CENTRE and Ashakiran Hospitals
Pune, Maharashtra, India

Athulya Shajan MBBS MS
Senior Resident
Institute of Kidney Diseases and Research Centre
Ahmedabad, Gujarat, India

Ekta Tiwari MD (Obs/Gyne)
Postgraduate Student
Department of Obstetrics and Gynecology
Aligarh Muslim University
Aligarh, Uttar Pradesh, India

Garima Gupta MD (Obs/Gyne)
Associate Professor
GSVM Medical College
Kanpur, Uttar Pradesh, India

Juhi Deshpande MBBS MS FMAS
Assistant Professor
Department of Obstetrics and Gynecology
Maa Vindhyavasini Autonomous State
Medical College
Mirzapur, Uttar Pradesh, India

Monisha Singh MBBS MD (Obs/Gyne)
Consultant (Obs/Gyne) and
Fertility Specialist
Sarojini Hospital
Varanasi, Uttar Pradesh, India

Neharika Malhotra MD (Gold Medalist) DRM
(Germany) FICMCH Fellow ICOG (Rep Med) ICOG (USG)
Director and Consultant
ART Rainbow IVF and MNMH (P) Ltd and
Ujala Cygnus Rainbow Hospital
Agra, Uttar Pradesh, India
Joint Secretary, FOGSI
Chair, YTP Committee, FOGSI

Nidhi Bansal MBBS MS (Obs/Gyne) (Gold Medalist)
Consultant and Director
SR Hospital
Agra, Uttar Pradesh, India
Secretary
Agra Menopause Society Currently

Parul Sinha MS FICOG
Associate Professor
All India Institute of Medical Sciences
Raebareli, Uttar Pradesh, India

Poonam Goyal MD FICOG FICMCH
Head IVF and Infertility
Max Hospital
Ghaziabad, Uttar Pradesh, India
Medical Director and Head (Obs/Gyne)
Panchsheel Hospital
New Delhi, India

Contributors

Prabhat Agrawal MD (Medicine) FRCP
Professor (Medicine)
Sarojini Naidu Medical College
Agra, Uttar Pradesh, India

Pradnya More MS DNB (Obs/Gyne)
Obstetrician and Gynecologist
Assistant Professor (Obs/Gyne)
Symbiosis Medical College for Women
Pune, Maharashtra, India

Pradnya Supe MS (Obs/Gyne) IBCLC
Fellowship in Laparoscopy
Consultant Obstetrician and Gynecologist
Zen, Surya, Dev Hospitals
Former Assistant Professor
LTMMC and LTMGH
Sion, Maharshtra, India

Priyankur Roy MBBS MS FIRM FAGE
Infertilty Specialist
Consultant Roy's Clinic
Siliguri, West Bengal, India
Assistant Professor
Lord Buddha Koshi Medical College and Hospital
Saharsa, Bihar

Rekha Rajendrakumar MD DNB PGDMLE
FICOG FICMCH
Fellow Reproductive Medicine
IVF Specialist and Medical Director
Chandana Hospital and Miracle IVF Hospital
Bengaluru, Karnataka, India

Riddhi Desai MS FICOG PGDMLS Dip Endoscopy
(Pune, USA) Dip Office Hysteroscopy (Italy)
Consultant Endoscopic Surgeon
Gynaecologist and Obstetrician
Sunflower Clinics
Mumbai, Maharashtra, India

Ruchika Garg MD FICOG FICMCH MRCOG1
FMAS MAMS
Professor
Department of Obstetrics and Gynecology
Sarojini Naidu Medical College
Agra, Uttar Pradesh, India

Sayamstuti Pattanaik MBBS MS (Obs/Gyne)
FRM FMAS
Consultant Obstetrician and Gynecologist
Laparoscopic Surgeon and Infertility Specialist
Shanti Memorial Hospital
Rourkela, Odisha, India

Shaheen Anjum MD (Obs/Gyne)
Professor and In-charge
ART Unit
Department of Obstetrics and Gynecology
Aligarh Muslim University
Aligarh, Uttar Pradesh, India

Shazia Parveen MD (Obs/Gyne)
Assistant Professor
Department of Obstetrics and Gynecology
Aligarh Muslim University
Aligarh, Uttar Pradesh, India

Sheeba Marwah MBBS DNB OBGY FICOG FICMCH
Fellowship CCOB (ICOG-FOGSI)
Associate Professor
Department of Obstetrics and Gynecology
VMMC and Safdarjung Hospital
New Delhi, India

Umme Ruman (Lt Col) (Retd)
MBBS (Gold Medalist) FCPS (Obs/Gyne)
Associate Professor (Obs/Gyne) and
Infertility Specialist
East West Medical College
Dhaka, Bangladesh

Foreword

"The goal of education is the advancement of knowledge and the dissemination of truth."

It gives me great pleasure to write the foreword for this book which is been written by my dear friends Jaideep Malhotra and Narendra Malhotra.

The book is a part of a series on books on various topics.

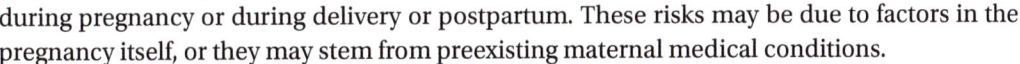

As we know, a high-risk pregnancy is one in which a woman and her fetus face a higher-than-normal chance of experiencing problems during pregnancy or during delivery or postpartum. These risks may be due to factors in the pregnancy itself, or they may stem from preexisting maternal medical conditions.

Medicine is vast and constantly changing and updating and as Obs/Gyne, we also must constantly keep updating ourselves. This handbook will be very helpful to doctors practicing obstetrics.

I would like to congratulate the Editors—Dr Neharika Malhotra, Dr Ashwini Kale, Dr Sheeba Marwah and Dr Shreya Prabhoo for getting in all topics so beautifully done.

Jaydeep Tank MD DGO DNB FCPS FICOG
Consultant at Ashwini Maternity and Surgical Hospital
Centre for Endoscopy and IVF
Program Director and Partner at ProFert IVF PLC
Founding Partner Esperanza Healthcare PLC
Independent Director appointed to the Board of
API Holdings Limited (Pharmacy)
Consultant, Jupiter Hospital
Visiting Consultant for IVF at over a dozen IVF Centre

Preface

The editors and authors of this series on *High-Risk Pregnancy* have worked hard to get a ready reckoner for all practicing Obstetrics and Gynecologists. This book is a compilation of chapters to help the readers manage high-risk pregnancies easily and confidently. Each chapter has been immaculately formulated to present working knowledge of the latest management protocols. We sincerely hope that the readers will find this book very useful.

"Reading is the gateway skill the makes all other learning possible."

Neharika Malhotra
Jaideep Malhotra
Narendra Malhotra

Acknowledgments

We have the pleasure of introducing *Clinical Focus on High-Risk Pregnancy*.

We thank the Almighty God for helping us throughout the journey of completing this task. Our heartfelt gratitude to Dr Jaydeep Tank for accepting to write the foreword for this book and also give his blessings.

It is with utmost pleasure that we thank Dr Narendra Malhotra, Dr Jaideep Malhotra and Dr Neharika Malhotra, our mentors and guide for this clinical series, who lent their considerable clinical and academic prowess. Their enthusiasm and encouragement kept us motivated to accomplish this task.

In constructing a compilation of this breadth, clinicians from several departments and their expertise were needed to add vital, contemporaneous information. We wish to thank all our contributors who responded to our requests with promptness. Our heartfelt thanks to them. We wish to appreciate the efforts of M/s Jaypee Brothers Medical Publishers (P) Ltd, New Delhi, India for bringing out this book in its final shape with their talent of skillfully and expediently coordinating and overseeing composition. We also thank publishing team of Jaypee Brothers Medical Publishers, especially Ms Rajni Chauhan. Without the thoughtful, creative efforts of many, our Focus Series would have been a barren wasteland of words. Their attention to detail and accurate renderings added important academic support to our words.

Our special appreciation and thanks to all our colleagues and friends who supported our idea of bringing out this series and gave us the confidence to finish this book. Lastly, we offer an enthusiastic thanks to our families and friends. Without their patience, generosity and encouragement, this task would have been impossible. We sincerely thank you for your love and support which kept us going to finish this work of ours.

Editors
Ashwini Kale
Shreya Prabhoo
Sheeba Marwah

Contents

SECTION 1: Introduction

1. **Prenatal Screening** 3
   Poonam Goyal, Neharika Malhotra

SECTION 2: Medications

2. **Teratogens** 13
   Ruchika Garg, Prabhat Agrawal

SECTION 3: Endocrine Diseases

3. **Glucose Intolerance in Pregnancy (DM + GDM)** 29
   Pradnya Supe, Pradnya More

4. **Thyroid Disorders** 40
   Aruna Verma

SECTION 4: Systemic Diseases

5. **Cardiac Diseases (Commonly found Disorders be Discussed)** 53
   Sheeba Marwah, Anshika Rakesh

6. **Hepatic Diseases in Pregnancy** 61
   Riddhi Desai

7. **Respiratory and Pulmonary Diseases** 68
   Monisha Singh, Amit Singh, Juhi Deshpande

8. **Renal Disorders** 79
   Ankita Jain

9. **Hematological and Coagulation Disorders (VTE)** 85
   Nidhi Bansal

10. **Neurological Disorders in Pregnancy** 106
    Prabhat Agrawal

11. **Hypertensive Disorders in Pregnancy** 113
    Parul Sinha, Garima Gupta

SECTION 5: General

12. **Multiple Births** 125
    Priyankur Roy, Athulya Shajan

13. **Isoimmunization in Pregnancy** 137
    Rekha Rajendrakumar

14. **Bleeding in Pregnancy** 151
    Sayamstuti Pattanaik

15. **Bad Obstetric History in Pregnancy** 159
    Umme Ruman

16. **Assisted Reproductive Technology Pregnancy—Are They Different?** 167
    Neharika Malhotra

SECTION 6: Infections

17. **Infections in Pregnancy** 173
    Ashwini Kale

18. **Maternal Sepsis and its Management** 195
    Shazia Parveen, Ekta Tiwari, Shaheen Anjum

Appendix *201*

Index *203*

Introduction

- **Prenatal Screening**
  Poonam Goyal, Neharika Malhotra

CHAPTER 1

Prenatal Screening

Poonam Goyal, Neharika Malhotra

INTRODUCTION

Nature created women for the purpose of procreation but did not guarantee success. Not all pregnancies end in a healthy mother and baby. This is where an obstetrician, a fetal medicine specialist and a pediatrician steps in. Aim is to provide prenatal and antenatal care so that each pregnancy can be taken on a judicious path and complications are detected at the earliest possible. High-risk pregnancies are to be identified inverting the pyramid of basic care. Screening is a process of identifying healthy population who are at a risk of any disease or condition. They can then be offered information, further tests and appropriate treatment to reduce their risk and/or any complications arising from the disease or condition prenatally and managed accordingly. Genetic testing refers to the use of specific tests to characterize the genetic status of individual, who is suspected to be at an increased risk for inherited diseases.

Genetic testing is an important tool in screening and diagnosing many conditions and there is a difference between screening and diagnosis **(Table 1)**.

DEFINITION OF HIGH-RISK PREGNANCY

Any pregnancy that carries increased risks for pregnant woman, unborn baby or both. These women need extra care before, during and after confinement. This reduces the risk of complications.

TABLE 1: Basic differences between screening and diagnosis.

Screening	Diagnostic
Testing done on a particular population	Testing done on individuals
Asymptomatic individuals	Often Symptomatic individuals
May lead to diagnostic tests	May lead to treatment options
Identifies individual at higher risk	May have had a positive screening test

PREVALENCE AND INCIDENCE

In India, 20–30% pregnancies are high risk resulting in 70–75% perinatal morbidity and mortality.

PRENATAL SCREENING OF HIGH-RISK FACTORS

Prenatal visit to a doctor should be encouraged by creating public awareness or when woman visits the clinic for any other reason and she is a potential candidate then opportunity should not be missed. High-risk factors are identified and targeted management done for reduction of underlying risk factors responsible for poor maternal and child consequences **(Flowchart 1)**.

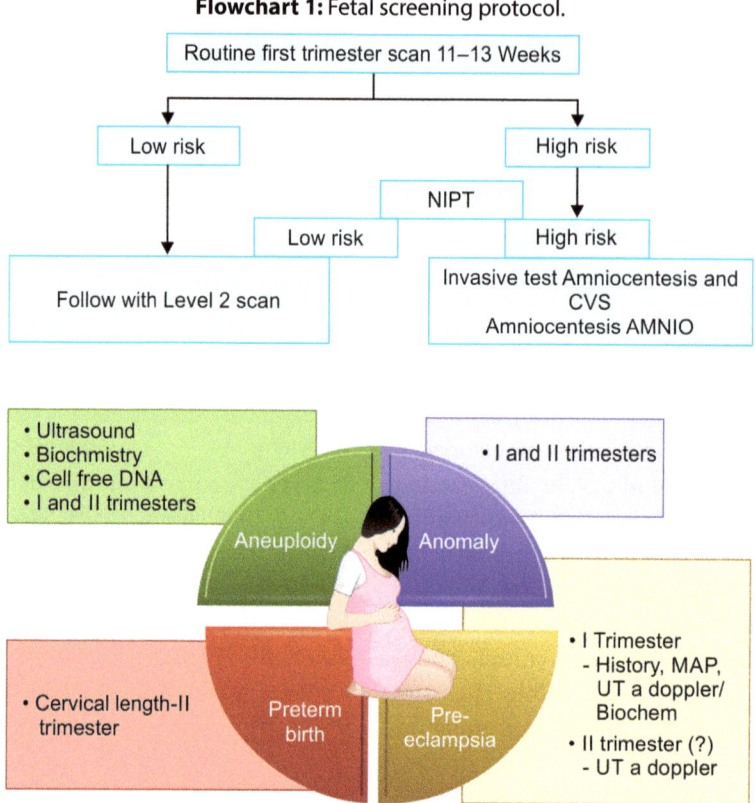

Flowchart 1: Fetal screening protocol.

Fig. 1: Process of prenatal screening. (MAP: mean arterial pressure; UT: uterine)

Figure 1 shows—how prenatal screening should be done.

Maternal Age

Young age: Different age groups have different risk issues such as we know preterm labor incidence increases with advanced age and similarly teenage pregnancies are more prone to anemia and postinflammatory hyperpigmentation (PIH). Teen pregnancies also have higher incidence of sexually transmitted infections (STIs). Some STIs can cause problems with the pregnancy or for the baby.[1] Teens may be less likely to get prenatal care or to keep prenatal appointments as many such pregnancies may be unwanted.

Advanced age: Older women are at higher risk for certain problems than younger women such as PIH, gestational diabetes mellitus (GDM), abortions, ectopic pregnancy,[4] operative delivery and Genetic disorders, such as Down syndrome, in the baby.[2,3]

Preexisting Health Conditions

- High blood pressure has potential bad effect on pregnancy and increase chances of eclampsia,[5] fetal growth restriction (FGR).
- DM can lead to fetal macrosomia and intrauterine death (IUD). Even women whose diabetes is well under control may have changes in their metabolism during

- pregnancy that requires extra care or treatment to promote a healthy birth.[5]
- PCOS can lead to GDM and there are increased chances of abortions before 20 weeks of pregnancy.[6]
- Kidney disease: Women with mild kidney disease usually have minimum issues during pregnancy. But kidney disease can cause difficulties getting in pregnant and also sometimes problems during pregnancy, including preterm labor (PTL), FGR, and preeclampsia and low birth weight babies. Nearly one-fifth of women who develop preeclampsia early in pregnancy are found to have undiagnosed kidney disease.[6,7] Pregnant women with kidney disease require additional changes in diet and medication.[8]
- *Thyroid disease:* Women with overactive or underactive thyroid, have problems for both mother and fetus. The risk of abortion is increased, GDM, PIH, anemia, abruptio placenta and postpartum hemorrhage is increased. Fetal brain development is also hampered. Hyperthyroidism can lead to hypertension, congestive heart failure, thyroid storm with labor, increased abortion rate, premature labor, stillbirth or neonatal death, low birth weight baby, fetal abnormalities.[9,10]
- *Obesity:* In obese females, pregnancy is associated with a number of risks for poor pregnancy outcomes such as GDM, fetal macrosomia. Weight gain should be controlled in obese patients.
- *Autoimmune diseases* such as lupus can cause PTL and stillbirth. Disease may flare up. Certain medicines to treat autoimmune diseases may be harmful to the fetus
- HIV can pass to a fetus during pregnancy, labor and delivery, and breastfeeding. Chances of PTL and FGR.
- Zika infection has shown to risk for pregnancy loss and stillbirth. There is microcephaly in fetus.
- History of (H/O) deep venous thrombosis (DVT) will also require special management.
- H/O epilepsy is also important because antiepileptic drugs require timely modifications to avoid teratogenic effects.
- H/O asthma especially if severe.
- H/O cardiac problem.

Lifestyle Factors

- *Alcohol use:* It can increase the baby's risk for fetal alcohol spectrum disorders (FASDs). There can be sudden infant death and intellectual, developmental disabilities, behavior problems, and abnormal facial features. There is nothing as safe amount of alcohol to drink while pregnant.[11]
- *Tobacco use:* Multiple issues can present in tobacco eaters especially PTL, FGRs and IUDs.[12] One study showed that smoking doubled or even tripled the risk of stillbirth, or fetal death after 20 weeks of pregnancy. Even secondhand smoke[13] also puts a woman and her developing fetus at increased risk for health problems.
- *Drug use:* Research shows that smoking marijuana and taking drugs during pregnancy can also harm the fetus and affect infant health. One study showed that smoking marijuana and using illegal drugs doubled the risk of stillbirth.[14]

HIGH-RISK PREGNANCY SITUATIONS (FLOWCHART 2)

- PIH, PET, eclampsia, GDM, FGR, PTL in previous pregnancy
- IVF conception

SECTION 1: Introduction

Flowchart 2: Prenatal screening and diagnosis for chromosomal abnormalities and neural tube defects.
(Based on ACOG screening re-commendations, 2016; ACOG committee opinion re-commendations, 2015)

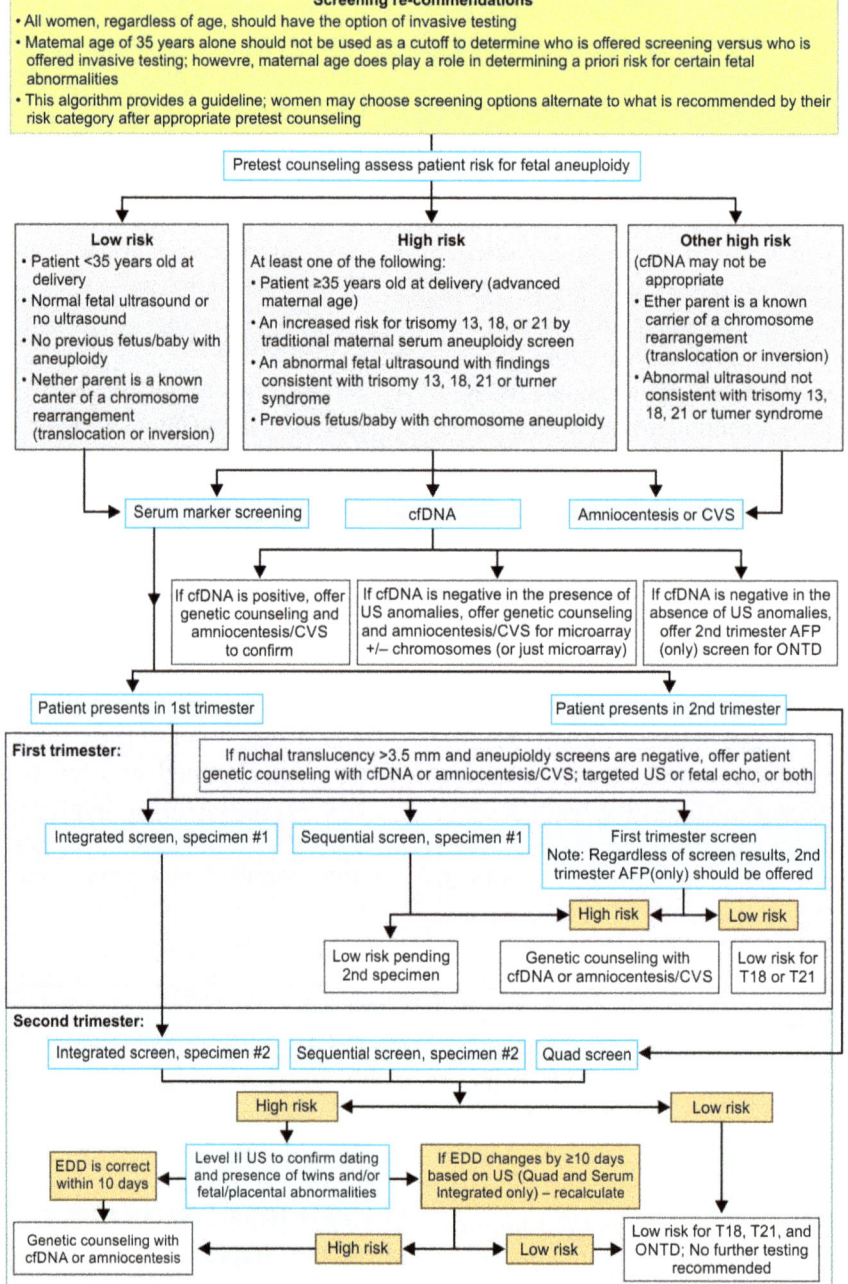

(AFP: alpha fetoprotein; cfDNA: cell-free DNA; CRL: crown rump length; CVS: chorionic villus sampling; DIA: dimeric inhibin A; DR: detection rate; EDD: estimated delivery date; hCG: human chorionic gonadotropin; NT: nuchal translucency; ONTD: open neural tub defects; PAPP-A: pregnancy-associated placental protein A; SPR: screen positive rate; T18: trisomy 18; T21: trisomy 21 (Down syndrome)

- Any genetic issue with parents/previous child
- Higher order pregnancy
- Previous lower segment cesarean section (LSCS)—one or more.

High Risk Factors on Examination at Prenatal Visit

- Anemia
- Any injury to pelvis or any bony defect in pelvis.
- Obese/overweight.

Antenatal High Risk Factors

- Unplanned pregnancy: Patients embarking on pregnancy without modifying drugs such as antiepileptics, antidepressants
- And uncontrolled diabetes and liver and kidney and autoimmune diseases. So as a healthcare provided we should counsel and encourage couples to go for a planned one
- Anemia
- H/O bleeding in early pregnancy
- PIH
- GDM
- Infections, if any
- Thyroid disease
- Short cervix on USG
- Low lying placenta
- Chest pain
- Abdominal pain not settling with routine medications
- PUO
- Leaking P/V
- Extreme fatigue/dizziness/fainting
- Previous LSCS
- APH.

■ CLINICAL EXAMINATION

- Pallor
- Edema pedal or generalized
- Tachycardia
- Respiratory rate fast
- Not maintaining SpO_2
- Mean arterial pressure (MAP)[15,16] should be calculated with formula—
  - MAP = [systolic blood pressure + (2 × diastolic blood pressure)]/3
  - Cut-off is taken as 125. If high chances of PIH/PE are more.
- P/A examination for fundal height and presentation and FHS; any disparity in uterus size is noted it can be AGA, SGA, LGA.
- Weight gain is noted; excessive or very less gain in weight is noted.

■ INVESTIGATIONS

- CBC
- TSH, Free T3, T4
- Anti TPO
- OGTT
- HPLC
- Blood Grouping
- ICT if mother is Rh negative and Rh positive
- Rubella IgG
- Urine R/E and C/S wherever indicated
- LFT and bile acids where ever indicated
- KFT
- PFT
- GTT.

Ultrasonography is really a boon when it comes to diagnosis of pregnancy related complications. We do scans as per requirement but we must do following scans in routine in all cases to mark the high risk patients:

- Dating scan
- NT/NB/DV/TR scan at 45–84 CRL
- Level 2 scan at around 20 weeks
- Growth/Doppler scan at 30–32 weeks
- BPP scan and general well-being scan at 36–37 weeks.

In special situations we need
- Genetic scan
- Scan SOS if bleeding /discharge or any unusual complaint by mother.
- Serial growth Doppler scans in case of FGR to judge the timing of delivery to save the baby
- TVS for short cervix
- NST for fetal well-being and to diagnose fetal hypoxia.

Investigations for Fetal Screening
- Dual marker is done at the time of 11–13 weeks scan and combined risk is calculated to detect trisomy T21, 13, 18. From this we get to know if patient is low risk or high risk for trisomy.
- Dual Marker test includes PaPP A and free beta hCG
- For T21, Low risk is when it is 1: >1,000
  - Intermediate risk for is 1: 251–999
  - High risk is 1: <250
- For T13, 18
  - Low risk is 1: >101
  - High risk 1: <100.

Mid Trimester
- We do quadruple marker that is AFP, unconjugated estriol, free beta hCG and inhibin A.
- Penta marker includes quad plus h-HCG that is hyperglycosylated hCG.
- Important is to do integrated screening for better detection
- Noninvasive prenatal testing (NIPT): It a noninvasive screening which is currently validated for T21, 18, and 1w3, and sex chromosomes. It checks the cell free fetal DNA present in maternal blood. Fraction has to be >4% for the test to be considered valid. It can be done 9 week onward anytime in pregnancy. T21 detection rate is almost 99%. A meta-analysis was done on NIPT and data of >750,000 cases was studied there was 1.211% FP and 0.0079 a FN result.

Invasive/Confirmatory Test
- CVS: It is chorion villous sampling done at 11 weeks. There is placental mosaicism which can give FN or FP result.
- Amniocentesis is test of amniotic fluid for karyotype and CMA done at 15.6 weeks.

■ CONCLUSION
Every pregnancy should reach to a judicious end, which is the main aim of health care provider. For this high-risk pregnancies should be identified as soon as possible and proper timely management done to reduce the perinatal mortality and morbidity. Right from preconception period to delivery we have to be vigilant.

■ REFERENCES
1. American College of Obstetricians and Gynecologists. FAQ 103: Having a baby (especially for teens). Washington DC: ACOG; 2015.
2. Gill SK, Broussard C, Devine O, Green RF, Rasmussen SA, Reefhuis J. The National Birth Defects Prevention Study. Association between maternal age and birth defects of unknown etiology: United States, 1997–2007. Birth Defects Res A Clin Mol Teratol. 2012;94(12):1010-8.
3. Grande M, Borrell A, Garcia-Posada R, Borobio V, Muñoz, M, Creus M, et al. The effect of maternal age on chromosomal anomaly rate and spectrum in recurrent miscarriage. Hum Reprod. 2012;27(10):3109-17.
4. Sivalingam VN, Duncan WC, Kirk E, Shephard LA, Horne AW. (2011). Diagnosis and management of ectopic pregnancy. J Fam Plan Reprod Health Care. 2011;37(4):231-40.

5. American College of Obstetricians and Gynecologists. FAQs: Preeclampsia and high blood pressure during pregnancy Washington DC: ACOG; 2018.
6. Office on Women's Health. (2016). Polycystic ovary syndrome (PCOS) fact sheet. [online] Available from: http://www.womenshealth.gov/publications/our-publications/fact-sheet/polycystic-ovary-syndrome.html. [Last Accessed November, 2022].
7. National Institute of Diabetes and Digestive and Kidney Diseases. (2017). Pregnancy if you have diabetes. [online] Available from: https://www.niddk.nih.gov/health-information/diabetes/diabetes-pregnancy. [Last Accessed November, 2022].
8. Williams D, Daviso J. Chronic kidney disease in pregnancy. BMJ. 2008;336(7637):211-5.
9. Office on Women's Health. (2017). Thyroid disease fact sheet. [online] Available from: https://www.womenshealth.gov/a-z-topics/thyroid-disease. [Last Accessed November, 2022].
10. American College of Obstetricians and Gynecologists. Thyroid disease in pregnancy. Obstet Gynecol. 2002;100:387-96.
11. Eckstrand KL, Ding Z, Dodge NC, Cowan RL, Jacobson JL, Jacobson SW. et al. Persistent dose-dependent changes in brain structure in young adults with low-to-moderate alcohol exposure in utero. Alcoholism: Clinical and Experimental Research, 2012;36(11);1892-902.
12. NICHD. (2013). Tobacco, drug use in pregnancy can double risk of stillbirth. [online] Available from: https://www.nichd.nih.gov/news/releases/Pages/121113-stillbirth-drug-use.aspx. [Last Accessed November, 2022].
13. NICHD. (2016). Cigarette smoking during pregnancy linked to changes in baby's immune system. [online] Available from: https://www.nichd.nih.gov/news/releases/122316-smoking-pregnancy. [Last Accessed November, 2022].
14. Centers for Disease Control and Preventio. Pregnant? Don't smoke. [online] Available from: http://www.cdc.gov/Features/PregnantDontSmoke/. [Last Accessed November, 2022].
15. Zheng L, Sun Z, Li J, Zhang R, Zhang X, Liu S, et al. Pulse pressure and mean arterial pressure in relation to ischemic stroke among patients with uncontrolled hypertension in rural areas of China. Stroke. 2008;39(7):1932-7.
16. DeMers D, Wachs D. Physiology, Mean Arterial Pressure. Treasure Island (FL): StatPearls Publishing; 2022.

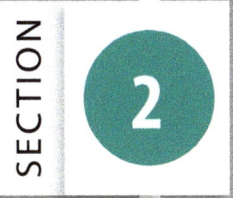

SECTION 2: Medications

- **Teratogens**
  Ruchika Garg, Prabhat Agrawal

CHAPTER 2

Teratogens

Ruchika Garg, Prabhat Agrawal

■ INTRODUCTION

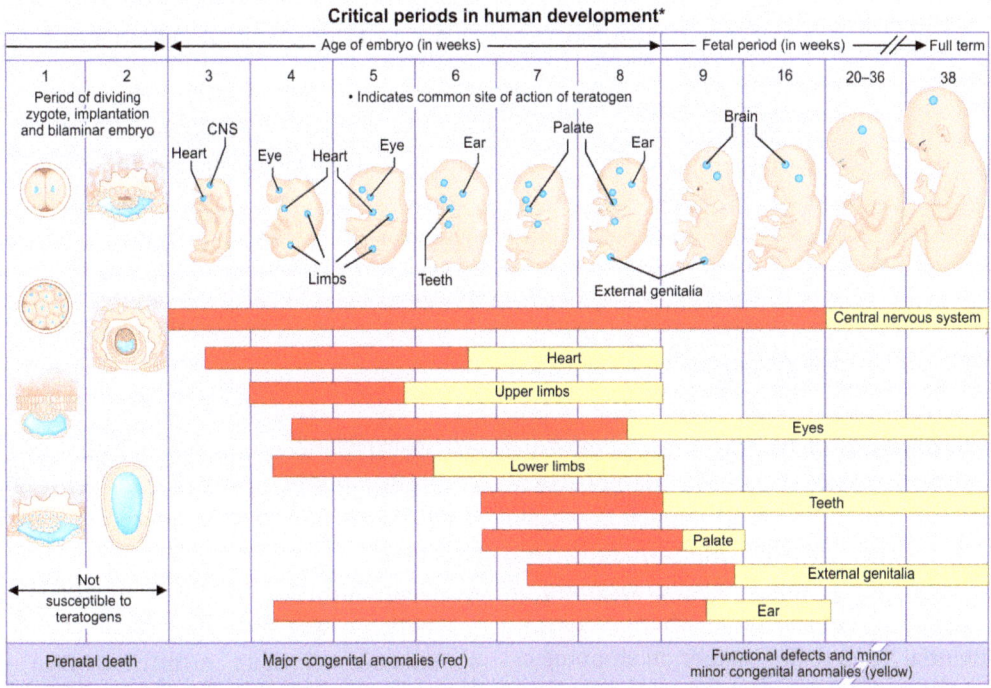

* Read indicates highly sensitive periods when teratogens may induce major anomalies.

In order to simplify the criteria whether a drug can be used during pregnancy or not the United States Food and Drug Administration Drug (US-FDA) has classified all the drugs in to five categories. Categories A and B medications usually are considered safe in humans. Category C drugs have not been definitively shown to be unsafe to human fetuses, but reasons exist to be cautious while prescribing them. Category D drugs are those with evidence of human fetal risk based on previous human studies, but the benefits of treatment prevail over the risks **(Table 1)**.

The decision whether to recommend a drug for a pregnant woman or not, must be made by the physician while considering many factors such as route of administration, gestational age of the fetus or embryo,

TABLE 1: The United States Food and Drug Administration (US-FDA) drug classification system.

FDA category*	Pregnancy category definition
A	• Controlled studies showed no risk to humans • Adequate, well-controlled studies in pregnant women have not shown an increased risk of fetal abnormalities
B	• No evidence of risk in humans • Animal studies have revealed no evidence of harm to the fetus. However, there are no adequate and well-controlled studies in pregnant women • Animal studies have shown an adverse effect, but adequate and well-controlled studies in pregnant women have failed to demonstrate a risk to the fetus
C	• Risks cannot be ruled out in humans • Animal studies have shown an adverse effect, and there are no adequate and well-controlled studies in pregnant women • No animal studies have been conducted, and there are no adequate and well-controlled studies in pregnant women
D	• Clear evidence of risk in humans • Studies, adequate well-controlled or observational, in pregnant women have demonstrated a risk to the fetus. However, the benefits of therapy may outweigh the potential risk
X	• Drugs contraindicated in human pregnancy • Studies, adequate well-controlled or observational, in animals or pregnant women have demonstrated positive evidence of fetal abnormalities. The use of the product is contraindicated in women who are or may become pregnant

*FDA categorization of drugs for use in pregnancy.

absorption rate of the drug, whether the drug crosses the placenta or not, the necessary effective dose of the drug, molecular weight of the drug, whether monotherapy will suffice or if multiple drugs are required to be effective, and also the mother's genotype. Potential harm to the mother on stopping or not prescribing the drug at all is of utmost importance among these factors along with the risk to the fetus. The decision therefore totally depends upon, *"does the benefit of the drug outweigh over its risks?"*

In the Indian setup, most of the pregnancies are complicated by infections and therefore deciding upon which antibiotic to use has always been a dilemma.

What makes antibiotic usage during pregnancy even trickier is the fact that there are marked and progressive physiological changes during pregnancy, and the drug disposition can be altered. Some of these are:

- Gastrointestinal motility is impaired and therefore drug absorption is reduced.
- Volume of drug administration is increased as plasma volume is expanded.
- Due to decrease in serum albumin and increase in α1-acid glycoprotein the unbound fraction of acidic drug increases while that of basic drugs decreases.
- Renal blood flow is markedly increased and hence increased clearance of the drugs.
- Due to induction of the hepatic microenzymes many of the drugs are cleared rapidly.

DRUGS CAN AFFECT THE FETUS AT THREE STAGES

1. *Before day 31:* During this phase drug produces all or none effect. The conceptus either survives without anomalies or does not survive at all. As there are only few cells during this early stage, so any damage at this stage is either irreparable or lethal.
2. *Day 31–ay 31:* This is the most critical period for organ formation and most of the teratogenic effects are therefore precipitated during this phase.
3. *Day 71 onward:* During this phase growth of the organs formed during organogenesis occurs and teratogenic effects can occur but are less common than the second phase.

Although a large number of studies have been conducted by researchers and the pharmaceutical companies till date, the license to market the drug is usually obtained before its long-term effects have been studied. *Therefore, the usage of antibiotics must be individualized depending upon the patient requirements* (Tables 1 and 2).

TABLE 2: Individual drug status and considerations during pregnancy.

Drug	Consideration	Teratogenicity	Category
Cephalosporins			
Cefazolin	Safe	No teratogenicity	B
Cefadroxil			B
Cephalexin			B
Cefuroxime			B
Cefaclor			B
Cefotaxime			B
Ceftazidime			B
Cefixime			B
Ceftriaxone	• Safe • Can interfere with hemostasis due to its hypoprothrombinemic action	• No • Vitamin K should be given to infant if given near to term	B
Cefoperazone	• Safe • Can derange liver enzymes and can interfere with hemostasis by having similar effect as that of ceftriaxone	No	B
Cefpirome	Can derange liver enzymes and can lead to eosinophilia, thrombocytopenia	No	B

Penicillins are considered safe
Can be used with β-lactamase inhibitors such as clavulanic acid and sulbactam

Contd…

Contd…

Drug	Consideration	Teratogenicity	Category
Amoxicillin	Should be avoided in women at risk of preterm delivery due to increased risk of neonatal necrotizing enterocolitis	No	B
Ampicillin	Safe	No	B
Methicillin			B
Piperacillin			B
Mezlocillin			B
Cloxacillin			B
Carbenicillin	Safe to use however can lead to pregnancy-induced hypertension and interferes with platelet function	No	B
Meropenem	Safe	No human data; however, there is no evidence of increased risk of major congenital malformations with other β-lactam antibiotics	B
Ertapenem			B
Sulfonamides	Contraindicated in third trimester as they increase the risk of kernicterus in the fetus	Association with neural tube defects (NTDs), cardiovascular malformations and facial cleft as a result of antifolate effect	C
Tetracyclines	• Contraindicated • Can lead to acute fatty liver of pregnancy	Can lead to yellowish discoloration of teeth and growth retardation due to its deposition in small bones	D
Chloramphenicol	Contraindicated	No	C
Macrolides			
Azithromycin	Can be used	Not expected to increase risk of major congenital malformations	B
Clindamycin			B
Clarithromycin			C
Vancomycin	Should be avoided, associated with maternal nephrotoxicity and ototoxicity		C
Nitrofurantoin	Should be avoided	Papillary adenomas and growth retardation in neonates	C

Contd…

Contd...

Drug	Consideration	Teratogenicity	Category
Tigecycline	• No reports on use during human pregnancy • Tigecycline is structurally related to tetracycline and thus *should be avoided after 15 weeks of gestation*	Use of an alternate agent with a known safety profile would be preferred	D
Aminoglycosides			
Amikacin		Theoretical risk of ototoxicity and nephrotoxicity	D
Gentamicin			D
Tobramycin	Contraindicated		D
Kanamycin			D
Streptomycin			D
Fluoroquinolones			
Levofloxacin		• Teratogenic effects have • Seen in experimental animals such as decreased placental light, cartilage lesions, and embryonic losses	C
Norfloxacin			C
Ofloxacin			C
Ciprofloxacin			C
Moxifloxacin			C
Linezolid	Can be used if benefits outweighs the risk	Not expected to increase risk of major congenital malformations	C
Antifungal agents			
Miconazole	Safe if used topically	Syndactyly, oligodactyly, and dystocia have been seen in animals	C
5-flucytosine	Use only if the potential benefit outweighs the risk	Can lead to encephaloceles, macroglossia, and major skeleton defects	C
Ketoconazole	Should be avoided Local application is safe	Leads to increased placental weight. Has been associated with abortions, supranumerary ribs, renal pelvis dilatation, and delayed ossification	C
Itraconazole	Should be avoided	Associated with increased central nervous system (CNS) and skeletal abnormalities	C
Fluconazole	Inhibits estrogen synthesis in fetus		C

Contd...

Contd...

Drug	Consideration	Teratogenicity	Category
Griseofulvin	As it interferes with mitosis can lead to formation of conjoined twins if used in first trimester		C
Antivirals			
Acyclovir	Contraindicated for systemic administration	Head and tail development in lower animal fetuses	B
Famcyclovir			C
Gancyclovir			C
Amantadine	Use only if clearly indicated	At high doses may lead to cardiac malformations	C
Foscarnet	• No human data in first trimester • Case reports describe treatment in second and third trimester with no adverse effects in the neonates • Should be used only when the benefit outweighs the unknown risk to the fetus • Due to potential for renal toxicity, close follow-up of the fetus and monitoring of amniotic fluid volume is recommended		C
Antitubercular drugs			
Isoniazid	Safe		C
Rifampicin	Safe	When used in last weeks of pregnancy, can lead to postnatal hemorrhage in mothers and infants	C
Rifabutin	Safe		B
Ethambutol	Safe	Optic neuritis has not been shown in infant	C
Pyrazinamide	Should be avoided		C
PAS	Has increased incidence of hepatotoxicity in mothers		C
Ethionamide	Contraindicated	Teratogenic effects have been shown in the animals	D
Cycloserine	Contraindicated Increased risk of psychosis in mothers		C
Streptomycin	Contraindicated		D

Contd...

Contd...

Drug	Consideration	Teratogenicity	Category
Antimalarials			
Chloroquine	Safe	Not expected to increase risk of major congenital malformations	C
Quinine			C
Mefloquine			C
Primaquine	*Contraindicated* Prophylactic administration of this drug should be withheld until after delivery	Associated with hemolysis in newborn	C
Artesunate	• Limited human data, mostly on use in second and third trimester • Should be used only when the benefit outweighs the unknown risk to the fetus	Not expected to increase risk of major congenital malformations	
Drugs used for hyperuricemia			
Allopurinol	Animal studies using high doses have revealed evidence of fetotoxicity and teratogenicity; it is not clear if these effects are a result of direct toxicity or maternal toxicity. There are no controlled data in human pregnancy	Allopurinol should only be given during pregnancy when benefit outweighs risk	C
Febuxostat	Febuxostat was not teratogenic in animal studies at high human doses; however, increased neonatal mortality and a reduction in febuxostat is only recommended for use during pregnancy when benefit outweighs risk		C
	The neonatal body weight gain was observed when pregnant rats were treated with oral doses up to 40 times the human equivalent. There are no adequate and well-controlled studies in pregnant women		

Antiepileptics in pregnancy: No drug has been proven to be completely safe in pregnancy however as the seizure itself is harmful to the mother and fetus, it is advised that any patient on antiepileptic drugs should be continued on the same drugs as prescribed

TABLE 3: Commonly used drugs and safer alternatives.

Condition/drug	Safety uncertain	Safer alternative
Antiemetics	Domperidone*, ondansetron	Promethazine, doxylamine, dicyclomine, metoclopramide
Antacid	Cimetidine, cisapride*, mosapride, lansoprazole	Ranitidine, pantoprazole
Laxatives	Senna, bisacodyl, docusate	Lactulose, isabgol, dietary fibers
Antidiarrheals	Diphenoxylate atropine, loperamide	ORS
Analgesics	Aspirin, Cox-2 inhibitors, morphine*, tramadol	Paracetamol, ibuprofen (low dose)
Cold cough remedies	Codeine, dextromethorphan	Xylometazoline nasal drops, chlorpheniramine can be given safely.
Antiallergics	Cetirizine, fexofenadine, astemizole*	Chlorpheniramine, promethazine
Antiamebic	Metronidazole, tinidazole	Diloxanide furoate, paromomycin
Antihelminthic	Albendazole*, mebendazole*, ivermectin, diethylcarbamazine*	Piperazine, niclosamide, praziquantel
Antiretroviral	Didanosine, abacavir, indinavir, ritonavir, efavirenz	Zidovudine, lamivudine, nevirapine, nelfinavir, saquinavir
Antihypertensives	ACE inhibitors*, ARBs*, thiazides, furosemide, propranolol	Methyldopa, hydralazine, atenolol, metoprolol, nifedipine, prazosin, clonidine
Antidiabetics	Metformin, acarbose*, sulphonylurea*, pioglitazone, gliptins	Preferably insulin to be used, however metformin and glibenclamide has been given successfully in some trials
Antithyroid drugs	Carbimazole, methimazole, radioactive iodine*	Propylthiouracil
Antiasthmatics	Theophylline, montelukast, systemic corticosteroids	Inhaled agents must be preferred.
Antipsychotics	Chlorpromazine, clozapine, olanzapine, resperidone	Haloperidol, trifluoperazine
Antidepressants	Dothiepin*, escitalopram, sertraline, trazodone, venlafaxine	Amitriptyline, imipramine, fluoxetine

(ACE: angiotensin-converting enzyme; ARBs: angiotensin receptor blockers)
*Strictly contraindicated drugs.

before conception. However if possible valproate should be avoided or switched to some other drugs if pregnancy is to be planned. Carbamazepine, lamotrigine, and levetiracetam are relatively safe.

If initiation of antiepileptics is required phenobarbitone is the drug of choice.

DRUGS USED FOR URINARY TRACT INFECTIONS

- Ampicillin and cotrimoxazole can be given.
- Meropenem and piperacillin-tazobactam can be given in resistant cases.

- Nitrofurantoin and fluoroquinolones are better to be avoided.

DRUGS USED FOR UPPER AND LOWER RESPIRATORY TRACT INFECTIONS

- Macrolides like azithromycin and clarithromycin can be given safely.
- Cephalosporins and meropenem can be used if associated with septicemia.

DRUGS USED FOR TUBERCULOSIS

- Isoniazid, rifampicin, and ethambutol can be given safely.
- Safety regarding pyrazinamide (PZA) cannot be assured, but when used for 6 months regimen, the benefits may outweigh the possible risks.
- Streptomycin may cause congenital deafness, as this drug interferes with the development of ear and must be avoided.
- Other injectables such as amikacin, kanamycin, and capreomycin may also cause fetal nephrotoxicity and ototoxicity and should be avoided.
- Ethionamide and prothionamide are contraindicated in pregnancy, as they are found teratogenic in animal studies.
- Cycloserine crosses placenta, and since its safety in pregnancy is not established, it should be avoided and used only if no other suitable alternatives are available.

Important note: Readers may find it surprising that though certain drugs are placed in category C yet the comment reads that they are safe since many infections during pregnancy have to be treated carefully and therefore even they are placed in category C they can be used safely.

TERATOGENIC DRUGS

To date, very few drugs are proven teratogens. However, malformations induced by drugs are important because they are potentially preventable. Proper prescribing of drugs in pregnancy is a challenge and should provide maximal safety to the fetus as well as therapeutic benefit to the mother.

PLACENTAL TRANSFER

The rate of placental transfer is affected by metabolism and gestational age, and the protein binding, ionization, lipid solubility, and molecular weight of the drug. Almost all drugs are able to pass freely through the placenta, with only those with a molecular weight of >1,000 Da being unable to do so, e.g., insulin and heparin.

TERATOGENICITY

If exposure in utero causes structural or functional abnormalities in the fetus or in the child after birth. Neuropsychological and behavioral abnormalities may also occur after drug exposure. Some antiepileptic drugs and drugs of abuse have been associated with learning and behavioral problems following in utero exposure.

TIMING OF EXPOSURE

During the preimplantation stage, in pregnancy, exposure to a drug is unlikely to produce a teratogenic effect due to an inbuilt "recovery process" in the conceptus. If a teratogenic insult occurs and there is damage to only a small number of cells then "compensation" occurs whereby the remaining viable cells continue to divide to replace any that were damaged.

However, if a large number of cells are damaged then implantation will not occur. This is known as the "all or nothing" or totipotent period. The 10 weeks following implantation are the most sensitive as this is the time during which major structural changes and organogenesis are taking place. It is during this period that the neural tube closes and major organs and limbs develop. While the first trimester is the most sensitive period to structural malformations, some drugs may affect the fetus in the later stages of pregnancy, so care should be taken when prescribing throughout pregnancy.

Angiotensin-converting enzyme (ACE) inhibitors in the second and third trimesters can cause serious adverse effects such as oligohydramnios, growth retardation, lung and kidney hypoplasia, and hypocalvaria.

GENERAL PRINCIPLES OF PRESCRIBING IN PREGNANCY

- Involve the woman, and her family where appropriate, in all decisions about treatment.
- Not treating mental illness in pregnancy or the postpartum period may be associated with adverse outcomes.
- Establish a clear indication for drug treatment.
- Choose treatments with the lowest known risk.
- In choosing consider the implications for breastfeeding and the benefits of avoiding the need to switch drugs.
- Use lowest effective dose for the shortest period necessary.
- Be aware of drug interactions, particularly with nonpsychotropics, and aim for monotherapy.
- Where there is no clear evidence-base that one drug is safer than another, the safest option is not to switch. The only drug with a clear indication for switching on safety grounds is valproate.
- Be aware of the potential effects of pregnancy and childbirth on drug pharmacokinetics and pharmacodynamics.
- Long-term neurodevelopmental effects of psychotropic medications in pregnancy and breastfeeding are extremely limited.
- Close monitoring for change in mental state where a woman decides to cease her usual medication.
- Where there is known risk, ensure that women are offered appropriate fetal screening and monitoring of the neonate for adverse effects.
- Premature or ill babies are more at risk of harmful drug effects.
- Monitor the infant for drug side effects, feeding patterns, growth, and development.
- Caution women against sleeping in bed with the infant, particularly if taking sedative drugs.

The risk posed by drug use in pregnancy can be minimized through prepregnancy counseling. When prescribing for a patient planning pregnancy or a patient who has become pregnant, consideration should be given whether drug is absolutely essential. When prescribing it is important to balance the risk of treatment to the fetus against the risk to both mother and fetus from failing to treat the maternal condition. Each case should be individualized.

All drugs in pregnancy should be prescribed in the lowest possible dose for the shortest possible time.

INTERPRETING PREGNANCY OUTCOME DATA

Robust pregnancy outcome data especially for new drugs are lacking. This is partly due to ethical constraints of enrolling pregnant women into clinical trials.

TABLE 4: Selected drugs or substances suspected or proven to be human teratogens.

Alcohol	Methimazole
ACE inhibitors	Methylmercury
Aminopterin	Methotrexate
Androgens	Misoprostol
Bexarotene	Mycophenolate
Carbamazepine	Paroxetine
Chloramphenicol	Penicillamine
Chlorobiphenyls	Phenobarbital
Cocaine	Phenytoin
Corticosteroids	Radioactive iodine
Cyclophosphamide	Ribavirin
Danazol	Streptomycin
DES	Tamoxifen
Efavirenz	Tetracycline
Etretinate	Thalidomide
Leflunomide	Tobacco
Lithium	Tretinoin
Valproate	Warfarin

(DES: diethylstilbestrol)

PROVEN TERATOGENIC DRUGS IN HUMANS

Alcohol

The fetal alcohol syndrome is characterized by intrauterine growth retardation (IUGR), microcephaly, developmental delay, and dysmorphic faces. Cleft palate and cardiac anomalies may also occur. Thus, alcohol is one of the most frequent nongenetic causes of mental retardation as well as the leading cause of preventable birth defects in the United States.

Angiotensin-converting enzyme inhibitors (captopril, enalapril, and lisinopril) and angiotensin receptor blockers:

There use in late pregnancy has been associated with renal insufficiency. IUGR, prematurity and complications of oligohydramnios (fetal limb contractures, lung hypoplasia) have been reported with their use in late pregnancy. Teratogenic risk with first trimester use of them appears to below.

Carbamazepine: Exposure causes 1% risk of neural tube defects (10 times their baseline risk).

Phenytoin: It causes fetal hydantoin syndrome with craniofacial dysmorphology, growth retardation and cardiac defects.

Valproate: First trimester exposure is associated with neural tube defects.

Cocaine: It is associated with abruption placentae, prematurity, fetal loss, decreased birth weight, microcephaly, and limb defects.

Coumarin anticoagulants (warfarin): The critical period of exposure for the *fetal warfarin syndrome* appears to be between 6 and 9 weeks of gestation. Second and third trimester exposure is associated with hemorrhage leading to disharmonic growth and deformation.

DES: Clear cell adenocarcinoma of vagina is associated with first trimester exposure. Hypoplastic, T-shaped uterine cavity, and septa are also reported.

Antineoplastic Agents

Folic acid antagonists: Aminopterin and methotrexate.

Central nervous system (CNS) defects facial anomalies and mental retardation occur following first trimester exposure. After a review of 20 first-trimester exposure, Feldkamp and Carey (1993) calculated that a doses of 10 mg/week is necessary to produce abnormalities.

Cyclophosphamide: First trimester use is associated with missing and hypoplastic digits, cleft palate, and imperforate anus. Nurses who administer cyclophosphamide may be at increased risk for fetal loss, but there are no adequate epidemiological studies.

Isotretinoin: It is prescribed for acne and causes a pattern of anomalies called retinoic acid embryopathy.

Psychiatric Medications

- Lithium: Ebstein's anomaly (a rare malformation of tricuspid value) is caused by it.
- Selective serotonin reuptake inhibitors (SSRIs): Paroxetine exposure is associated with congenital cardiac malformations and persistent pulmonary hypertension in the newborn. *American College of Obstetricians and Gynecologists* (2007) concluded that SSRIs are not major teratogens and treatment must be individualized.

Misoprostol

First-trimester exposure is associated with limb defects with or without *Moebius sequence*.

Prescribing Misoprostol in Obstetrics and Gynecology

Routes of administration: Oral, vaginal, sublingual, buccal, or rectal.

Vaginal misoprostol is associated with slower absorption, lower peak plasma levels, and slower clearance, similar to an extended-release preparation.

Vaginal misoprostol is also associated with a greater overall exposure to the drug [area under the curve (AUC)] and greater effects on the cervix and uterus.5 There is, however, a wide variation in the absorption of misoprostol through the vaginal epithelium among different women. *There is no clinically significant difference between vaginal misoprostol that is administered dry and vaginal misoprostol moistened with water, saline, or acetic acid.*

Misoprostol is considered a teratogen. The absolute risk of congenital malformations is 1%.

Breastfeeding: Misoprostol is excreted into breast milk levels become undetectable within 5 hours of maternal ingestion. Women should be advised that misoprostol may cause infant diarrhea.

Tetracycline: Yellowish brown discoloration of teeth may occur with exposure of drug after 17 weeks of gestation.

Hormones

Androgenic progestins: Norethindrone (a progesterone only contraceptive) causes virilization of 1% of exposed female fetus.

Androgens: Exposure of a female fetus to anabolic steroids results in varying degrees of virilization.

Danazol: Virilization of female fetus.

Corticosteroids

First trimester exposure is associated with increased incidence of facial clefts. However, they are not considered to represent a major teratogenic risk.

Methylmercury

Prenatal exposure is associated with developmental delay and neurological abnormalities. Ingestion of contaminated fish (enters the echosystem through industrial pollution) may expose the fetus to it.

Antivirals

- *Ribavirin:* It is highly teratogenic in all animal species studied.
- *Amantadine:* There is possible association with cardiac defects.

POSSIBLE TERATOGENIC DRUGS IN HUMANS

- *D-penicillamine*—connective tissue disorders (cutis laxa).
- *Methimazole*—scalp defects (aplasia cutis congenita).
- *Diazepam*—first trimester exposure has been associated in small studies with a small increase in the incidence of cleft lip and palate. Larger studies did not confirm the association.

Fluconazole and Itraconazole

There have been several reports of skull abnormalities and limb defects with their exposure. Despite this large cohort studies suggest that neither drug is teratogenic.

Leflunomide: It is used to treat rheumatoid arthritis. In animals, its use is associated with hydrocephalus, skeletal anomalies.

BIBLIOGRAPHY

1. Cunningham F, Leveno KJ, Bloom SL, Spong CY, Dashe JS, Hoffman BL (Eds). Williams Obstetrics, 24th edition. New York: McGraw-Hill Education; 2014.
2. Dutta DC, Konar H. DC Dutta's Textbook of Obstetrics, 6th edition. New Delhi: Jaypee Brothers Medical Publishers (P) Ltd.; 2013.
3. Facts and Comparisons (Firm), Ovid Technologies, Inc. Drug Facts and Comparisons. Saint Louis: Wolters Kluwer health; 2013.
4. KD Tripathi. Essentials of Medical Pharmacology, 7th edition. New Delhi: Jaypee Brothers Medical Publishers (P) Ltd.; 2013.
5. Medscape. Tigecycline (Rx). [online] Available from https://reference.medscape.com/drug/tygacil-tigecycline-342527#:~:text=USES%3A%20Tigecycline%20is%20used%20to,antibiotic%20treats%20only%20bacterial%20infections [Last accessed November, 2022].
6. Perinatology.com. (2002). Drugs in Pregnancy and Breastfeeding. [online] Available from www.perinatology.com/exposures/druglist.htm [Last accessed November, 2022].

SECTION 3

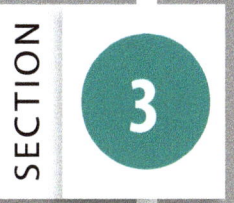

Endocrine Diseases

- **Glucose Intolerance in Pregnancy (DM + GDM)**
  Pradnya Supe, Pradnya More

- **Thyroid Disorders**
  Aruna Verma

CHAPTER 3

Glucose Intolerance in Pregnancy (DM + GDM)

Pradnya Supe, Pradnya More

INTRODUCTION

More than 21 million births are affected by maternal diabetes worldwide each year, this includes pre-existing diabetes and gestational diabetes mellitus (GDM). When it comes to India, it is estimated that about 4 million women are affected by GDM, at any given time point.[1] In 2019, almost three in 10 women were considered obese prior to becoming pregnant. The strong relationship between diabetes and the current obesity epidemic calls for the need to bring in diet and lifestyle interventions to change the trajectory of both. It is essential to screen, diagnose, and treat diabetes in pregnancy, to prevent both maternal and fetal complications caused by diabetes complicating pregnancy.

TYPES OF DIABETES MELLITUS

In a non-pregnant person, diabetes could be either because of absolute deficiency of insulin, known as type 1 diabetes mellitus (DM) or there could be insulin resistance, relative insulin deficiency or elevated glucose production known as type 2 DM. Both type 1 and type 2 DM are generally preceded by a period of abnormal glucose homeostasis, which is called as prediabetes.

Gestational diabetes mellitus is defined as any degree of glucose intolerance with onset or first recognition during pregnancy.

According to CDC, approximately 7% of all pregnancies are complicated by GDM, resulting in >200,000 cases annually. The prevalence may range from 1–14% of all pregnancies, depending on the population studied and the diagnostic tests employed and nearly 50% of women with GDM will become overt diabetes (type-2) over a period of 5–20 years.

HISTORY OF GESTATIONAL DIABETES MELLITUS

Since the 1979 publication on "classification and diagnosis of DM and other categories of glucose intolerance" by the National Diabetes Data Group, gestational diabetes has been defined as *"carbohydrate intolerance of variable severity with onset or recognition during pregnancy"*. The diagnosis and treatment of gestational diabetes focus on the prevention or reduction of adverse outcomes.

Diabetes occurring during pregnancy was recognized early in the 19th century,[2] and in 1882, *J. Matthews Duncan* described what would later be called GDM when he indicated that *"diabetes may occur only during pregnancy being absent at other times or may cease with the termination of pregnancy recurring some time afterwards".*[3] Duncan also concluded that women who develop diabetes during pregnancy might be at higher risk of developing the condition again later in life.

It is essential to screen women in early pregnancy to distinguish GDM from pre-existing diabetes. But many women do not receive screening and this makes it hard to distinguish between GDM and pre-existing DM. Screening methodology shifted away from only obtaining a patient history when, in 1964 in Boston, Massachusetts, John O'Sullivan and Claire Mahan invented the two-step oral glucose tolerance test, which physicians still commonly use as of 2022 to diagnose women with gestational diabetes. Despite many studies there have been disagreements within the medical community on the best ways to screen and diagnose gestational diabetes.

In the 1980s, the World Health Organization (WHO) published recommendations that equated gestational diabetes with diabetes detected during pregnancy and with values used for diagnosis of impaired glucose tolerance in non-pregnant persons.[4,5]

GESTATIONAL DIABETES MELLITUS

Gestational diabetes is defined as carbohydrate intolerance of variable severity with its onset or first recognition during pregnancy.[6] This definition applies whether or not insulin is used for treatment and undoubtedly includes some women with previously unrecognized overt diabetes. The term, gestational diabetes, aims to communicate the need for enhanced surveillance during pregnancy and to stimulate further testing postpartum.

The presence of GDM has serious implications for both the baby and the mother. As for the baby, there is increased risk of macrosomia, shoulder dystocia, birth injuries as well as neonatal hypoglycemia and hypalbuminaemia.[7] GDM also adds an intrauterine environmental risk factor to an increased genetic risk for the development of obesity, diabetes and/or metabolic syndrome in childhood.

In terms of maternal effects of diabetes, there remains a predisposition to the development of metabolic syndrome and type 2 diabetes. Mothers with GDM also have an excess of hypertensive disorders during pregnancy. Maternal obesity as well as cardiovascular disease are also potential long-term consequences of GDM.

There is a growing body of evidence suggesting that the risk of many of these consequences can be significantly reduced or eliminated by screening, prompt diagnosis, and aggressive treatment of GDM.

Pathophysiology: Normal Maternal Glucose Metabolism and Development of Gestational Diabetes

- Early pregnancy is a time of relative glucose sensitivity. This sensitivity decreases sharply in the second and early third trimester. This reduces insulin-dependent glucose uptake in tissues such as muscle and fat and serves as a maternal physiologic adaption to preserve carbohydrate for the rapidly growing fetus.
- Also, impaired insulin mediated suppression of maternal lipolysis and fat oxidation provides fatty acids as an alternative energy source.
- These processes are mediated by a number of factors including an increase in progesterone, estrogen, cortisol, and human placental growth hormone.
- Typically, a two- to three-fold increase in insulin production is sufficient to meet this challenge and studies have confirmed

an increase in pancreatic fractional beta cell area in human pregnancy to meet with the increased requirement.
- As the placenta grows, more of these hormones are produced, and the risk of insulin resistance becomes greater.
- Normally, the pancreas is able to make additional insulin to overcome insulin resistance, but when the production of insulin is not enough to overcome the effect of the placental hormones, gestational diabetes results.

Screening for Gestational Diabetes Mellitus

There have been many developments when it comes to screening for GDM. This has brought about many disagreements, as there are various screening tests and criteria available. The American College of Obstetricians and Gynecologists (ACOG), says that use of historic factors (family or personal history of diabetes, previous adverse pregnancy outcome, glycosuria, and obesity) to identify GDM will fail to identify approximately one half of women with GDM. Moreover, not screening the 10% of women who are low risk would add to unnecessary complexity to the screening process. Therefore, in 2014, the U.S. Preventive Services Task Force made a recommendation to screen all pregnant women for GDM at or beyond 24 weeks of gestation.[9]

According to National Institute for Health and Care Excellence (NICE) guidelines for gestational diabetes, the risk should be assessed in a healthy population. Risk assessment should be done at booking by checking the following factors:
- Body mass index (BMI) above 30 kg/m^2
- Previous macrosomic baby weighing 4.5 kg or more
- Previous gestational diabetes
- Family history of diabetes (first-degree relative with diabetes)
- An ethnicity with a high prevalence of diabetes.

And, testing for gestational diabetes is offered to women with above mentioned risk factors. The 75 g, 2 hour oral glucose tolerance test (OGTT) is offered to test for gestational diabetes at 24–28 weeks. For women who have had gestational diabetes in a previous pregnancy, a 75 g, 2 hour OGTT is offered as soon as possible after booking (whether in the first or second trimester), and a further 75 g, 2 hour OGTT at 24–28 weeks if the results of the first OGTT are normal.

Gestational diabetes is diagnosed if the woman has either:
- A fasting plasma glucose level of 5.6 mmol/L (100 mg/dL) or above or
- Or a 2 hour plasma glucose level of 7.8 mmol/L (140 mg/dL) or above.

According to *National Guidelines for Diagnosis and Management of GDM*, in India, screening for GDM is recommended twice during pregnancy. The first testing should be done during first antenatal contact as early as possible in pregnancy. The second testing should be done during 24–28 weeks of pregnancy if the first test is negative. There should be at least 4 weeks gap between the two tests. The method used includes, a single step testing using 75 g oral glucose and measuring plasma glucose 2 hour after ingestion. The threshold plasma glucose level of ≥140 mg/dL (more than or equal to 140) is taken as cut off for diagnosis of GDM.

Prevention of Gestational Diabetes Mellitus

It has been proved that exercise and healthy diet, before and during early pregnancies, are associated with reduction in GDM risk

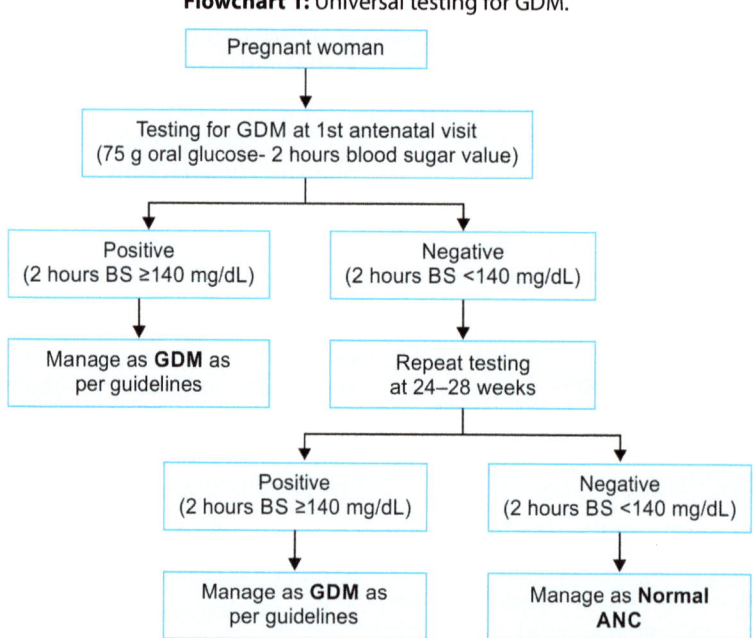

Flowchart 1: Universal testing for GDM.

(ANC: absolute neutrophil count; GDM: gestational diabetes mellitus)

(Flowchart 1). In particular, it has been shown a reduction of 51% in the development of GDM for women who practiced regular recreational physical activity in the year prior to pregnancy and a reduction of 48% in the development of GDM for women who had recreational physical activity during the first 20 weeks of pregnancy. If these two activities are combined together, a reduction of 60% of GDM risk has been documented.[8] Exercise and weight loss is able to improve insulin sensitivity, decreasing sympathetic activity, and/or increasing parasympathetic activity as well as lower resting heart rate and blood pressure. Nutritional therapy is essential in the treatment of GDM, as it helps to avoid an excessive increase in weight, minimizing the onset of macrosomic fetuses and neonatal complication.

Managing Diabetes during Pregnancy

Management of women diagnosed with gestational diabetes is a combination of lifestyle modification, with or without metformin/insulin **(Flowchart 2 and 3)**.

The 2005 Australian Carbohydrate Intolerance Study in Pregnant Women trial, the first large-scale (1,000 women), randomized treatment trial for GDM[10] found the treatment was associated with a significant reduction in the rate of the primary outcome, a composite of serious new-born complications (perinatal death, shoulder dystocia, and birth trauma, including fracture or nerve palsy). Treatment also reduced maternal complication like preeclampsia (from 18–12%) as well as reduced the frequency of infants who were large for gestational age (LGA) (from 22%–13%) and who had a birth weight >4,000 g (from 21%–10%). Another study from United States found that, although there were no differences in the frequency of the primary composite outcome (perinatal death, neonatal hypoglycemia, elevated umbilical cord C-peptide level, and birth trauma), several significant differences

CHAPTER 3: Glucose Intolerance in Pregnancy (DM + GDM)

Flowchart 2: Management of pregnant woman with GDM.

```
Pregnant woman with GDM
           │
           ▼
Medical nutrition therapy (MNT) and
        physical exercise
                    │ After 2 weeks
                    ▼
              2 hours PPBS
           ┌────────────┴─────────────┐
           ▼                          ▼
<120 mg/dL continue MNT and    ≥120 mg/dL start oral antidiabetic
   physical exercise            (metformin) or insulin therapy
           │                          │
           ▼                          ▼
Monitor 2 hours PPBS          • Monitor FBS and 2 hours PPBS every 3rd
• As per high risk pregnancy    days or more frequently for insulin and bi-
  protocol or as recommended    weekly for metformin dose adjustement to
  by physician (at least once   maintain normal blood sugar levels
  monthly)                    • As per high risk pregnancy protocol or as
                                recommended by physician (at least once
                                monthly)
```

(GDM: gestational diabetes mellitus; FBS: fasting blood sugar PPBS: post prandial blood sugar)

Flowchart 3: Management of postpartum screening results.

```
              Gestational diabetes
                       │
                       ▼
           FPG or 75g, 2 hours
           OGTT at 4–12 weeks postpartum
   ┌───────────────────┼───────────────────┐
   ▼                   ▼                   ▼
FPG >125 mg/dL or   FPG 100–125 mg/dL or  FPG <100 mg/dL or
2 hours glucose     2 hours glucose       2 hours glucose
>199 mg/dL          140–199 mg/dL         <140 mg/dL
   │                   │                   │
   ▼                   ▼                   ▼
Diabetes mellitus   Impaired fasting      Normal
                    glucose or IGT or both
   │                   │                   │
   ▼                   ▼                   ▼
Refer for diabetes  • Consider referral for    • Assess glycemic status
management            management                 every 1–3 years
                    • Weight loss and physical • Weight loss and physical
                      activity counseling as     activity counseling as
                      needed                     needed
                    • Consider metformin if
                      combined
                      impaired fasting glucose
                      and IGT
                    • Medical nutrition therapy
                      yearly assessment of
                      glycemic status
```

(FPG: fasting plasma glucose; OGTT: oral glucose tolerance test; IGT: impaired glucose tolerance)
Source: Reproduced from ACOG PRACTICE BULLETIN.

in secondary outcomes were observed with treatment, including a lower frequency of LGA infants, lower frequency of birth weight exceeding 4,000 g, and reduced neonatal fat mass.[11] Moreover, the rates of cesarean delivery, shoulder dystocia, and hypertensive disorders were significantly reduced in women who were treated for GDM.

From these studies, it can be inferred that women diagnosed with GDM should be managed with diet and exercise counseling and when this fails to achieve adequate glucose control medications should be added for maternal and fetal benefits.

Non-pharmacological methods for management of GDM: Diet, exercise, and glucose monitoring form the cornerstone of GDM management. The first step in management is medical nutrition therapy, which is offered for 2 weeks. The woman is also encouraged to walk for 30 minutes or do light exercises every day.

The goal of medical nutrition therapy in women with GDM is to achieve normal blood glucose levels, prevent ketosis, provide adequate weight gain, and contribute to appropriate fetal growth and development. The ADA recommends nutritional counseling by a registered dietitian and development of a personalized nutrition plan based on the individual's BMI for all patients with GDM. The following points are to be noted when patients are counseled regarding MNT:
- A diet composed of 50–60% carbohydrates often will result in excessive weight gain and postprandial hyperglycemia. Therefore, it has been suggested that carbohydrate intake be limited to 33–40% of calories, with the remaining calories divided between protein (20%) and fat (40%).
- Complex carbohydrates are recommended over simple carbohydrates because they are digested more slowly, are less likely to produce significant postprandial hyperglycemia, and potentially reduce insulin resistance.
- In practice, three meals and two to three snacks are recommended to distribute carbohydrate intake and to reduce postprandial glucose fluctuations.
- In terms of exercises, women with GDM should aim for 30 minutes of moderate-intensity aerobic exercise at least 5 days a week or a minimum of 150 minutes per week. Simple exercise such as walking for 10–15 minutes after each meal can lead to improved glycemic control and is commonly recommended.

Pharmacological methods for management of GDM: Pharmacological methods are used when sufficient control is not achieved after taking medical nutrition therapy and doing regular exercise for 2 weeks. There is no conclusive evidence for a specific threshold value at which medical therapy should be started but the Ministry of Health and Family Welfare recommends a threshold of 120 mg/dL, beyond which pharmacological interventions are to be initiated.

Role of insulin: Insulin, which does not cross the placenta, can achieve tight metabolic control and traditionally has been added to nutrition therapy if fasting blood glucose levels consistently are greater than or equal to 95 mg/dL, if 1 hour levels consistently are greater than or equal to 140 mg/dL, or if 2 hour levels consistently are greater than or equal to 120 mg/dL.

If insulin is used throughout the day in women in whom fasting and postprandial hyperglycemia are present after most meals, a typical starting total dosage is 0.7–1.0 units/kg daily. This dosage should be divided with a regimen of multiple injections using long-acting or intermediate acting insulin in combination with short-acting insulin.

If there are only isolated abnormal values at a specific time of day, focusing the insulin regimen to correct the specific hyperglycemia is preferred.

Oral antidiabetic medications: Oral antidiabetic medications (e.g., metformin and glyburide) are being popularly used in women with GDM, even though they have not been approved by the U.S. Food and Drug Administration for this indication[12] and in spite of the fact that insulin continues to be the ADA-recommended first-line therapy.

Metformin is a biguanide that inhibits hepatic gluconeogenesis and glucose absorption and stimulates glucose uptake in peripheral tissue. Metformin crosses the placenta with levels that can be as high as maternal concentrations

There have been multiple studies regarding metformin, and the fact that it may be a reasonable approach to treat gestational diabetes. It is important to note that there is a lack of superiority when compared with insulin, the placental transfer of the drug, and the absence of long-term data in exposed offspring and this needs to be counseled to patients accordingly.

The dosage for metformin usually starts at 500 mg nightly for 1 week at initiation, then increases to 500 mg twice daily. If higher doses are needed, the maximum dose is usually 2,500–3,000 mg per day in two to three divided doses. In women who decline insulin therapy or who the obstetricians or obstetric care providers believe will be unable to safely administer insulin, or for women who cannot afford insulin, metformin is a reasonable alternative choice.

Before initiation of metformin baseline creatinine is usually checked to rule out chronic kidney disease as it is contraindicated in it.

Glyburide is a sulfonylurea that binds to pancreatic beta-cell adenosine triphosphate potassium channel receptors to increase insulin secretion and insulin sensitivity of peripheral tissues. It is contraindicated in patients who report a sulpha allergy. The usual dosage of glyburide is 2.5-20 mg daily in divided doses, although higher doses may be necessary to achieve adequate control.

It was noted that 4–16% (or more) women required the addition of insulin to maintain good glycemic control when glyburide was used as initial treatment[13,14] and therefore it is not recommended as the initial treatment prior to insulin or metformin. There also have been studies reporting macrosomia and neonatal hypoglycemia with the use of glyburide.

There are also theoretical concerns with Metformin and Glyburide freely crossing the placenta.

To summarize, insulin remains the first line drug as the oral hypoglycemic agents freely cross the placenta, they lack good quality studies regarding neonatal safety and the fact that metformin is not US FDA approved for use in GDM. Having said that, there might be clinical situations that necessitate the use of oral hypoglycemic agents like in women who decline insulin or who the obstetricians or obstetric care providers believe will be unable to safely administer insulin, or for women who cannot afford insulin, metformin (and rarely glyburide) is a reasonable alternative choice in the context of discussing with the patient the limitations of the safety data and a high rate of treatment failure that requires insulin supplementation.

It is crucial to counsel women who are receiving insulin about the risks of hypoglycemia and impaired awareness of hypoglycemia in pregnancy, particularly in the first trimester and therefore to always have a fast-acting form of glucose for example, glucose containing drinks or glucose tablets.

Glucose monitoring: According to NICE guidelines, the frequency of glucose monitoring depends on the type of diabetes and what medications are used to control it.
- For women with type 1 diabetes, it is advised to test their fasting, pre-meal, 1 hour post-meal, and bedtime blood glucose levels daily.
- For women who are managing their diabetes with diet and exercise alone or are taking oral hypoglycemic agents are advised to check their fasting and 1 hour post-meal blood glucose levels daily.
- For women with type 2 DM or GDM, a multiple daily insulin injection regimen is advised to test their fasting, pre-meal, 1 hour post-meal, and bedtime blood glucose levels daily.

Target blood glucose levels to be maintained—pregnant women with any form of diabetes should maintain their capillary plasma glucose below the following target levels, if these are achievable without causing problematic hypoglycemia:
- Fasting: 5.3 mmol/L or 96 mg/dL
- 1 hour after meals: 7.8 mmol/L or 140 mg/dL
- 2 hours after meals: 6.4 mmol/L or 115 mg/dL

Role of hemoglobin A1c (HbA1c): HbA1c is used for monitoring glucose control in women with pre-existent diabetes. HbA1c can be repeated in each trimester in women with pre-existent diabetes to check control. The level of risk for the pregnancy for women with pre-existing diabetes increases with an HbA1c level >48 mmol/mol (6.5%). HbA1c can be used in women diagnosed with GDM, to differentiate it from pre-existing diabetes. Having said that, it should not be routinely used for monitoring control in second and third trimester.

ANTENATAL CARE IN WOMEN WITH DIABETES MELLITUS

As pregnancy with gestational diabetes is a high-risk condition, it needs to be managed by a consultant gynecologist in conjugation with a radiologist, nutritionist, physician, and a specialist nurse.

At each consultation offer pregnant women with diabetes ongoing opportunities for information and education.

If diagnosed before 20 weeks of gestation, it is essential to offer women with GDM a level 2 scan (anomaly scan), including examination of the fetal heart (four chambers, outflow tracts and three vessels to rule out any major structural abnormalities.

Pregnant women with diabetes should be offered ultrasound monitoring of fetal growth and amniotic fluid volume every 4 weeks from 28–36 weeks.

An individualized plan should be tailored for monitoring fetal growth and wellbeing for women with diabetes and a risk of fetal growth restriction (macrovascular disease or nephropathy).

Offer retinal assessment for women with pre-existing diabetes unless the woman has been assessed in the last 3 months. Repeat retinal assessment at 16–20 weeks for women who had diabetic retinopathy.

Offer a renal assessment for women with pre-existing diabetes, if they have not had 1 in the last 3 months.

At 36 weeks, offer information about:
- Timing, mode, and management of birth
- Analgesia and anesthesia

- Changes to blood glucose-lowering therapy during and after birth
- Care of the baby after birth
- Starting to breastfeed and the effect of breastfeeding on blood glucose control
- Contraception and follow-up.

Timing and mode of delivery: Women with GDM with good glycemic control and no other complications are commonly managed expectantly until term. As the fetal lung maturity is delayed in women with GDM there is no indication to offer delivery before 39 weeks of gestation.
- In women with diabetes controlled on diet and exercise, expectant management up to 40 6/7 weeks of gestation in the setting of indicated antepartum testing is generally appropriate.
- For women with GDM that is well controlled by medications, delivery is recommended from 39 0/7 weeks to 39 6/7 weeks of gestation.
- Consider elective birth before 37 weeks for women with type 1 or type 2 diabetes who have metabolic or other maternal or fetal complications
- Pre-existent or GDM is not an indication for caesarean section. It's a routine practice to offer caesarean section to LGA babies, to prevent shoulder dystocia or brachial plexus injury. But according to a study it has been estimated that up to 588 cesarean deliveries would be needed to prevent a single case of permanent brachial plexus palsy for an estimated fetal weight of 4,500 g, and up to 962 cesarean deliveries would be needed for an estimated fetal weight of 4,000 g.[15,16] Taking this into consideration it appears reasonable to counsel Indian women about the risks and benefits of performing a caesarean section at the birth weight of >4000 g.

Intrapartum Care of Women with Diabetes Mellitus

Pregnant women with GDM on medical management (metformin or insulin) require blood sugar monitoring during labor by a glucometer. The monitoring is to be performed hourly and the levels maintained between 4 mmol/L-7 mmol/L. The morning dose of insulin/metformin is withheld on the day of induction/labor. IV infusion with normal saline (NS) to be started and regular insulin to be added according to blood sugar levels in consultation with a physician or diabetic specialist.

■ NEONATAL CARE

- Initial assessment and need for admission to NICU: Babies of women with diabetes should stay with their mothers, unless there are complications or abnormal clinical signs that mean the baby needs to be admitted to intensive or special care unit. Carry out glucose testing 2-4 hours after birth and blood tests for babies with clinical signs of polycythemia, hyperbilirubinemia, hypocalcemia or hypomagnesemia.
- Monitor the baby for 24 hours, look for signs of hypoglycemia and make sure the baby is feeding well before transferring the baby to community care.
- Consider echocardiography for baby with signs of congenital heart disease or a heart murmur.
- Admit babies to the neonatal ICU if:
  - Hypoglycemia associated with abnormal clinical signs
  - Respiratory distress
  - Signs of cardiac decompensation from congenital heart disease or cardiomyopathy
  - Signs of neonatal encephalopathy

- Signs of polycythemia, and are likely to need partial exchange transfusion
- Need for intravenous fluids
- Need for tube feeding (unless adequate support is available on the postnatal ward)
- Jaundice requiring intense phototherapy and frequent monitoring of bilirubinemia
- Been born before 34 weeks (or between 34–36 weeks, if the initial assessment of the baby and their feeding suggests this is clinically appropriate).

Women with diabetes should feed their babies as soon as possible after birth (within 30 minutes) and then at frequent intervals (every 2–3 hours) until feeding maintains their pre-feed capillary plasma glucose levels at a minimum of 2.0 mmol/L.

Postnatal Care and Follow Up

Women with GDM can withhold their antidiabetic medications post-delivery as the carbohydrate intolerance resolves after delivery. Women with history of GDM are at 7-fold risk of developing type 2 diabetes later in life. Therefore, the Fifth International Workshop on Gestational Diabetes Mellitus recommends that women with GDM undergo a 75 g, 2 hour OGTT in the postpartum period.[17] This usually should include a fasting plasma glucose as well.

SUMMARY

Gestational diabetes mellitus can have serious implications on maternal and fetal outcome. Early diagnosis by adequate screening, effective treatment along with lifestyle modification can not only improve the pregnancy outcome but help prevent the long-term implications of GDM for the mother baby. A key factor in management is to involve a multidisciplinary team including consultant obstetrician, neonatologist, radiologist, dietician, physiotherapist, a specialist nurse and if need be, a psychologist. Counselling and patient education plays an important role in maintaining adherence to treatment. Its vital to keep patients informed of the likely complications, measures taken to prevent them and have a consultation with them to discuss the mode of delivery to allay anxiety. Patients should be supported during labour and the baby should receive adequate neonatal care.

■ REFERENCES

1. Kayal A, Anjana RM, Mohan V. Gestational diabetes-An update from India, 2013. Diabetes Voice. 2013;58.
2. Hadden DR. Maternal blood glucose and the baby. The origins of the hyperglycaemia and pregnancy outcome study. The Scott-Heron Lecture at the Royal Victoria Hospital—17 January 2001. Ulster Med J. 2001;70:119-35.
3. Duncan JM. On puerperal diabetes. Trans Obstet Soc Lond. 1882;24:256-85.
4. WHO Expert Committee on Diabetes Mellitus: Second report. World Health Organ Tech Rep Ser. 1980;646:1-80.
5. Diabetes mellitus. Report of a WHO Study Group. World Health Organ Tech Rep Ser. 1985;727:1-113.
6. American College of Obstetricians and Gynecologists (ACOG). (2021). ACOG Practice Bullet in Clinical Management Guidelines for Obstetrician–Gynaecologists. [online] Available from https://www.acog.org/clinical/clinical-guidance/practice-bulletin [Accessed November, 2022].
7. Hod M, Merlob P, Friedman S, Schoenfeld A, Ovadia J. Gestational diabetes mellitus: a survey of perinatal complications in the 1980s. Diabetes. 1991; 40:74-8.
8. Dempsey JC, Butler CL, Sorensen TK, Lee IM, Thompson ML, Miller RS, et al. A case control study of maternal recreational physical activity

and risk of gestational diabetes mellitus. Diabetes Res Clin Pract. 2004;66:203-15.
9. Moyer VA, U.S. Preventive Services Task Force. Screening for gestational diabetes mellitus: U.S. Preventive Services Task Force recommendation statement. U.S. Preventive Services Task Force. Ann Intern Med. 2014;160(6):414-20. (Level III)^
10. Crowther CA, Hiller JE, Moss JR, McPhee AJ, Jeffries WS, Robinson JS, et al. Effect of treatment of gestational diabetes mellitus on pregnancy outcomes. Australian Carbohydrate Intolerance Study in Pregnant Women (ACHOIS) Trial Group. N Engl J Med. 2005;352(24): 2477-86. (Level I)^
11. Landon MB, Spong CY, Thom E, Carpenter MW, Ramin SM, Casey B, et al. A multicenter, randomized trial of treatment for mild gestational diabetes. Eunice Kennedy Shriver National Institute of Child Health and Human Development Maternal-Fetal Medicine Units Network. N Engl J Med. 2009;361:1339-48. (Level I)^
12. Camelo Castillo W, Boggess K, Sturmer T, Brookhart MA, Benjamin DK Jr, Jonsson Funk M. Trends in glyburide compared with insulin use for gestational diabetes treatment in the United States, 2000-2011. Obstet Gynecol. 2014;123:1177-84. (Level II-3)^
13. Langer O, Conway DL, Berkus MD, Xenakis EM, Gonzales O. A comparison of glyburide and insulin in women with gestational diabetes mellitus. N Engl J Med. 2000;343(16):1134-8. (Level I)^
14. Jacobson GF, Ramos GA, Ching JY, Kirby RS, Ferrara A, Field DR. Comparison of glyburide and insulin for the management of gestational diabetes in a large managed care organization. Am J Obstet Gynecol. 2005;193:118-24. (Level II-3)^
15. Garabedian C, Deruelle P. Delivery (timing, route, peripartum glycemic control) in women with gestational diabetes mellitus. Diabetes Metab. 2010;36:515-21. (Level III)^
16. Fetal macrosomia. Practice Bulletin No. 173. American College of Obstetricians and Gynecologists. Obstet Gynecol. 2016;128:e195-209. (Level III)^
17. Metzger BE, Buchanan TA, Coustan DR, de Leiva A, Dunger DB, Hadden DR, et al. Summary and recommendations of the Fifth International Workshop-Conference on Gestational Diabetes Mellitus [published erratum appears in Diabetes Care. 2007;30: 3154]. Diabetes Care. 2007;30 (Suppl 2): S251-60. (Level III)^
18. Figure 1 National Guidelines for Diagnosis and Management of Gestational Diabetes Mellitus, Maternal Health Division Ministry of Health and Family Welfare Government of India December 2014: https://nhm.gov.in/images/pdf/programmes/maternal-health/guidelines/National_Guidelines_for_Diagnosis_&_Management_of_Gestational_Diabetes_Mellitus.pdf
19. Figure 2 National Guidelines for Diagnosis and Management of Gestational Diabetes Mellitus, Maternal Health Division Ministry of Health and Family Welfare Government of India December 2014: https://nhm.gov.in/images/pdf/programmes/maternal-health/guidelines/National_Guidelines_for_Diagnosis_&_Management_of_Gestational_Diabetes_Mellitus.pdf
20. Figure 3 ACOG Practice Bullet in Clinical Management Guidelines for Obstetrician-Gynecologists, Number 190, February 2018 (with the assistance of Aaron B. Caughey, MD, PhD, and Mark Turrentine, MD.)

CHAPTER 4

Thyroid Disorders

Aruna Verma

INTRODUCTION

Thyroid disorders are the second most common endocrinological problems during pregnancy after diabetes mellitus. Various physiological and endocrinological changes occur during pregnancy, which also alters the thyroid gland's functions.

FUNCTIONS OF THYROID HORMONE

- Growth and development
- Increased metabolic rate
- Regulation of cerebral conduction
- Sleep regulation
- Control of lipid metabolism.

Pregnant women with thyroid disease are generally evaluated and treated similarly to nonpregnant women, but they do experience certain particular issues.

THYROID ADAPTATION DURING PREGNANCY

- Increase in serum thyroid binding globulin (TBG)
- Stimulation of thyrotropin receptor by human chorionic gonadotropin (hCG).

Increase in serum thyroid binding globulin: Serum TBG production and sialylation rise almost twofold under increased progesterone during pregnancy. There is decreased clearance of TBG also.[1] TBG raises serum total but not free T4 and T3 concentrations. During the first half of pregnancy, T3 and T4 levels increase by 50% before remaining constant.

Human chorionic gonadotropin and thyroid function: Given that the beta subunits of hCG and thyroid stimulating hormone (TSH) are homologous[2], there is an increase in total serum T4 and T3 concentration with the rise in hCG levels, which peak at around 12 weeks. TSH usually remains within normal range but in 10–20% of normal pregnant females, it becomes transiently low or undetectable.[3] This temporary hyperthyroidism, which is typically asymptomatic, should be regarded as normal.

Assessment of Thyroid Function

- Serum TSH
- Serum FT4
- Serum FT3
- Antithyroid antibodies
- Nuclear scintigraphy (usually avoided during pregnancy)
- Fine-needle aspiration cytology (FNAC) of thyroid nodule.

IODINE REQUIREMENT

World Health Organization (WHO) recommends 250 µg of iodine daily during pregnancy and lactation.

THYROID FUNCTION IN THE FETUS (TABLE 1)

Fetal thyroid gland starts to form at 5 weeks → thyroid function starts at 10–12 weeks (concentrate iodine and synthesize iodothyronines) → formation of thyroid hormones at 18–20 weeks → gradual increase in fetal thyroid secretion.[4]

At term, fetal thyroid levels differ from mothers. Serum FT4 and serum FT3 levels are just half of the mother's levels, whereas, serum TSH levels are higher. At birth serum TSH concentration rapidly rises to 50–80 mIU/L and then falls to 10–15 mIU/L within 48 hours. Serum T3 and serum T4 are slightly higher than normal adults.

What Test to Order during Pregnancy

- *Routine:* TSH and FT4
- *Suspected hypothyroidism:* TSH alone
- *Suspected thyrotoxicosis:* FT3
- *Follow-up of T4 hypothyroidism:* TSH.

Evaluation of thyroid is depicted in **Figure 1**.

TABLE 1: Recommended reference ranges of thyroid function tests.

Guidelines	Country	Trimester wise serum TSH reference range
ITS (2012)	India	• First trimester: 2.5 mIU/L • Second trimester: 3.0 mIU/L • Third trimester: 3.0 mIU/L
ETA (2014)	European	• First trimester: 2.5 mIU/L • Second trimester: 3.0 mIU/L • Third trimester: 3.0 mIU/L
ATA (2017)	America	• Reference intervals derived locally from a particular community of expectant women • If the highest limit of serum TSH is not available, 4 mIU/L is used

(ATA: American Thyroid Association; ETA: European Thyroid Association; ITS: Indian Thyroid Society; TSH: thyroid stimulating hormone)

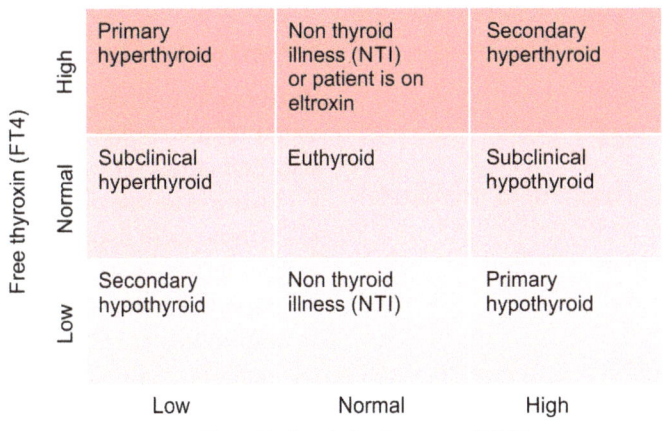

Fig. 1: The nine square thyroid evaluation.

HYPOTHYROIDISM

When the thyroid hormone levels are low, it may be primary or secondary.

Primary Hypothyroidism

It occurs after destruction of the thyroid gland because of autoimmunity (the most common cause), or medical intervention such as surgery, radioiodine, and radiation.

- *Overt hypothyroidism:* When serum TSH levels are high as a result of decreased thyroxin and negative feedback.
- *Subclinical hypothyroidism:* When thyroxin levels are within the normal range and serum TSH levels are between 4 and 10 mIU/L.
- *Maternal hypothyroxinemia (isolated low maternal FT4):* When there are isolated low levels of serum FT4 with normal TSH levels.

Secondary Hypothyroidism

It is because of low levels of TSH due to some defect in either pituitary or hypothalamus.

Incidence

- *Overt hypothyroidism:* 0.2–2.5%
- *Subclinical hypothyroidism:* 2–7%.[5,6]

Although rare, thyroid antibodies are found in nearly 60% of women of reproductive age.

Causes

- Autoimmunity (Hashimoto thyroiditis): most common
- Post-thyroidectomy
- Iodine deficiency.

Clinical Features

- Fatigue, cold intolerance, myalgia, and reflex delay
- Constipation
- Weight gain from fluid retention
- Memory loss, depression, and ataxia
- Dry skin, yellow skin, coarse hair, hair loss, and hypothermia
- Hoarseness of voice
- Goiter
- Hyperlipidemia
- Bradycardia.

Effect of Hypothyroidism on Pregnancy

Maternal

- Anemia and congestive heart failure (CHF)
- Preeclampsia
- Placental abnormalities (placental abruption)
- Low birth weight/preterm birth
- Postpartum hemorrhage.

Fetal

- Cognitive impairment
- Neurological abnormality
- Developmental abnormalities
- Congenital hypothyroidism.

Neonatal

- Hyperbilirubinemia
- Respiratory distress.

Whom to Screen during Pregnancy

Universal screening for thyroid function in asymptomatic pregnant women is controversial.[7] Screening to be done in the following:

- Living in iodine deficiency endemic area
- Symptoms of hypothyroidism
- Family history of thyroid disease
- Personal history of thyroid peroxidase antibodies (TPO ab) or type 1 diabetes mellitus
- Goiter
- Age >30 years
- Infertility

- Head and neck irradiation
- Recurrent miscarriages and preterm deliveries
- Class 3 obesity [body mass index (BMI) >40 kg/m^2]
- Prior thyroid surgery
- Use of amiodarone, lithium, or iodinated radiologic contrast medium.

Management Guidelines (Flowchart 1)

The 2017 ATA guidelines recommend treatment for hypothyroidism on TPO ab status.[8] TPO ab measurement should be done in all cases with levels >2.5 mIU/L.
- *Positive TPO ab:* L. thyroxin is prescribed if TSH is above 2.5 mIU/L.
- *Negative TPO ab:* L. thyroxin is prescribed if TSH is above 10 mIU/L.
- *Isolated hypothyroxinemia:* No treatment is required.

Monitoring and Dose Adjustment

- After initiation of therapy, the patient should be reevaluated and serum TSH is to be repeated after 4 weeks.
- If the levels are above the normal reference range, the dose should be increased by 12–25 μg/day. (Aim is to keep the values below the reference ranges, if available, or <2.5 mIU/L.)
- In the first half of pregnancy, TSH should be repeated every 4 weeks because of normal physiological changes during pregnancy.
- In the later half of pregnancy, TSH levels should be done once in every trimester.
- Overtreatment should be avoided.[9,10]

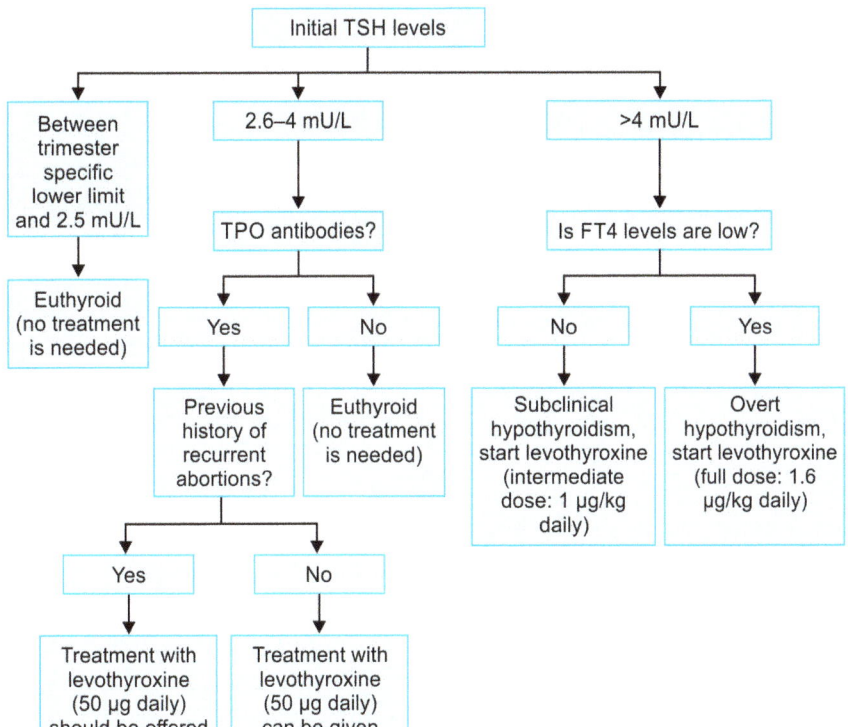

Flowchart 1: Management of hypothyroidism.

(TSH: thyroid stimulating hormone; TPO: thyroid peroxidase antibodies; FT4: Free T4/ thyroxine)

Postpregnancy Adjustment

- Patients who already have hypothyroidism should return to prepregnancy dosages, and TSH levels should be evaluated again after 6 weeks.
- In case who started thyroxin during pregnancy, may sometimes not require any treatment if dosages were ≤50 µg/day.
- If L. thyroxin is discontinued serum TSH should be repeated after 6 weeks.
- TSH levels should be checked annually on women with thyroid autoimmune disease.

HYPERTHYROIDISM

- Hyperthyroidism is relatively uncommon during pregnancy.
- Although there are certain specific issues, the diagnosis of hyperthyroidism in pregnant women is comparable to that in nonpregnant women.

Incidence

0.1–0.4 percent of all pregnancies.[11]

Clinical Manifestations

Numerous generalized symptoms of pregnancy, such as tachycardia, heat sensitivity, and increased sweating, are comparable to those linked to hyperthyroidism. Hand tremors, nervousness, and weight loss despite a regular or increased appetite are other symptoms.

Types

- *Overt hyperthyroidism:* Low TSH, free T4 and/or T3 levels above trimester-specific normal reference limits, or total T4 and T3 levels above 1.5 times the range seen in women who are not pregnant.
- *Subclinical hyperthyroidism:* Low TSH, normal free T4 and T3 using trimester-specific normal reference levels or total T4 and T3 are <1.5 times the nonpregnant range.
- *Free T4 in the upper-normal quintile:* A free T4 that is normal and in the higher quintile with a TSH that is normal.

Pregnancy Complications

Overt Hyperthyroidism

Premature labor, infection, preeclampsia, or cesarean delivery, as well as spontaneous abortion, low birth weight babies, stillbirths, preeclampsia, and heart failure (thyroid storm).

Subclinical Hyperthyroidism

- Lower incidence of spontaneous abortion
- Higher risk of preeclampsia.

Free T4 in the Upper-normal

- Lower birth weight
- Maternal hypertension.

Diagnosis

The diagnosis is made primarily on the basis of elevated thyroid hormone levels [serum free thyroxin (T4) and/or free triiodothyronine (T3) or total T4 and/or total T3] that are higher than the normal reference range during pregnancy and a suppressed (0.1 mIU/L) or undetectable (0.01 mIU/L) serum TSH value.

Establishing the Cause (Flowchart 2)

- Graves' (0.1–1% of all pregnancies)
- hCG-mediated hyperthyroidism (1–3% of pregnancies): hyperemesis gravidarum, gestational transient thyrotoxicosis (GTT), and trophoblastic hyperthyroidism.
- Silent or subacute thyroiditis

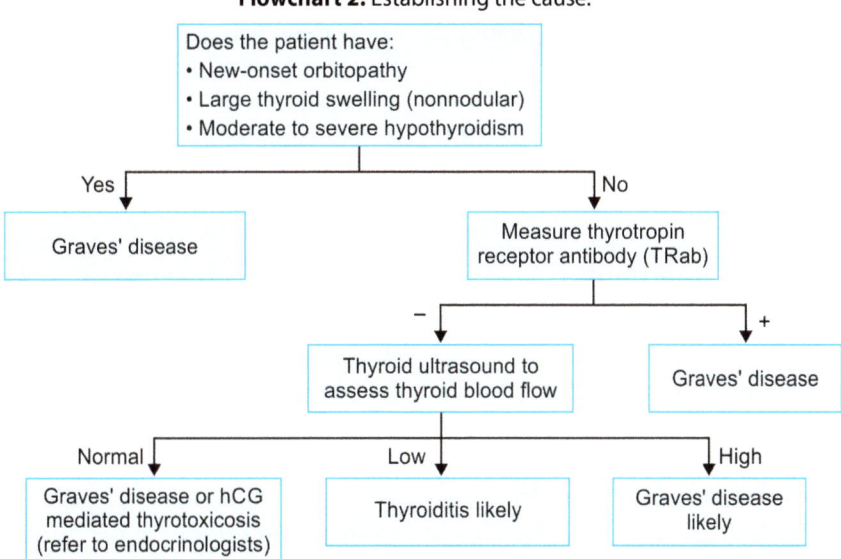

Flowchart 2: Establishing the cause.

(hCG: human chorionic gonadotropin)

- Toxic adenoma
- Toxic multinodular goiter
- Factitious thyrotoxicosis.

Gestational transient thyrotoxicosis: Total serum T4 and T3 levels rise while serum TSH levels decrease during the hCG peak (10-12 weeks). It could cause mild overt or subclinical hyperthyroidism. It happens near the end of the first trimester, and when hCG production decreases (usually between 14 and 18 weeks of gestation), symptoms (if any) and thyroid hyperfunction go away.

Hyperemesis gravidarum: These patients' serum hCG and estradiol levels are higher than those of typical pregnant women,[12] and their hCG also has a higher level of thyroid-stimulating activity.[13] Because it is moderate and self-limiting, thyroid hyperfunction in women with hyperemesis gravidarum typically does not require treatment. Any overt hyperthyroidism that persists through the first trimester should be investigated for other causes.

Trophoblastic hyperthyroidism: Hydatidiform moles are benign, however they can develop into choriocarcinomas. Both have aberrant hCG isoforms and elevated serum hCG concentrations.[14] While ophthalmopathy is absent in other cases, they have more typical clinical hyperthyroidism and diffuse goiter findings, e.g., with hyperemesis gravidarum, nausea and vomiting may be more prevalent.

Familial gestational hyperthyroidism: A mutant thyrotropin receptor that is hypersensitive to physiological amounts of hCG may be the cause of recurrent gestational hyperthyroidism in the families.[15]

Management
- In an effort to prevent fetal hypothyroidism, the goal is to maintain continuous, moderate hyperthyroidism. Since the fetal thyroid is very sensitive to the action of antithyroid drugs.[15]
- To achieve this goal, FT4 levels should be kept at or slightly above the normal range for each trimester of pregnancy,

or the combined T4 and T3 levels should be kept at 1.5 times more than the nonpregnant reference range.
- The serum TSH should be lower than the reference range for pregnancy (0.1-0.3 mIU/L), using the lowest possible dose of the drug.[16]

Indications for Treatment

In moderate to severe, overt hyperthyroidism due to:
- Graves' disease
- Toxic adenoma
- Toxic multinodular goiter
- Gestational trophoblastic disease.

Treatment is recommended in the following cases:
- Transient, subclinical hyperthyroidism
- hCG-mediated, overt hyperthyroidism (also called gestational transient thyrotoxicosis)
- Hyperemesis gravidarum-associated hyperthyroidism, because it is mild and usually subsides as hCG production decreases.

Subclinical and mild, asymptomatic, overt hyperthyroidism due to Graves' disease, toxic adenoma, or toxic multinodular goiter.

Therapeutic Options

- *Thionamides:* These are the primary modality for the treatment of hyperthyroidism due to Graves' disease, toxic adenoma, or toxic multinodular goiter during pregnancy.
- *Beta blockers:* Metoprolol or propranolol (but not atenolol), can be given to manage tremors and tachycardia. Long treatment with beta blockers (>2-6 weeks) should be avoided in pregnant females because of the risk of FGR and hypoglycemia, especially with atenolol.[17]
- *Thyroidectomy:* It is rarely necessary but is done where women are intolerable to thionamides due to agranulocytosis or allergy.
- *Plasmapheresis:* It has been used to quickly manage severe hyperthyroidism in women with trophoblastic illness.[18]

Approach to Treatment

According to the Endocrine Society and American Thyroid Association (ATA), the recommended approach is as follows:
- *Control of symptoms:* Metoprolol 25-50 mg daily or propranolol 20 mg every 6-8 hours, is given to ameliorate the symptoms of hyperthyroidism. Due to the sporadic occurrences of infant growth restriction, hypoglycemia, respiratory depression, and bradycardia, these should be discontinued as soon as the hyperthyroidism is under thionamide management.[19]
- *Decrease thyroid hormone synthesis by thionamide:* The choice of thionamide depends upon which trimester the drug is being initiated. Methimazole is preferred to propylthiouracil (PTU) except during the first trimester of pregnancy.
- *Pretreatment evaluation:* Complete blood counts and liver function tests should be done before starting antithyroid medication. Do not use thionamides when a baseline absolute neutrophil count <1,000 cells/μL or elevated liver transaminases (more than five-fold) except in selected patients.

Diagnosed Prior to Pregnancy

- Definitive therapy with either surgery or radioiodine to be done before conception.
- Switch to PTU before trying to conceive. This option is most reasonable in younger

women with normal periods who are expected to conceive within 1-3 months.
- Switch to PTU as soon as the pregnancy test is confirmed. This option is more reasonable for older women and women having difficulty conceiving.
- Stop methimazole while closely observing thyroid function tests (weekly throughout the first trimester, then monthly). PTU (if recurrence in the first trimester) or methimazole should be administered to the patient if hyperthyroidism returns after discontinuance (if relapse after the first trimester).

Diagnosed during the First Trimester

The best option is PTU. At 16 weeks of pregnancy, patients have the option of returning on methimazole or continuing PTU.

Diagnosed after the First Trimester

After the first trimester, women with symptoms of moderate to severe hyperthyroidism should start taking methimazole.

Compared to PTU, methimazole and carbimazole have more severe teratogenic effects. Aplasia cutis, a scalp abnormality, has been documented in multiple case series in babies exposed to methimazole in utero.[20]

Maternal usage of methimazole and carbimazole but not PTU has also been linked to more severe congenital malformations such as tracheoesophageal fistulas, patent vitellointestinal duct, choanal atresia, omphalocele, and omphalomesenteric duct abnormality.[21] So, throughout the first trimester, PTU is preferable.

Initial Dosing

Start with the minimum dose of thionamide needed to control thyroid function:
- PTU 50 mg BD or TDS
- Methimazole 5-10 mg OD, or
- Carbimazole 5-15 mg OD.

For women with severe hyperthyroidism, full starting doses of PTU (100 mg TDS) or methimazole (10-30 mg OD) may be required to control the disease.

Thyroid Function Tests

- Thyroid function tests should be obtained every 4 weeks throughout pregnancy.
- If thionamides are stopped in early pregnancy, tests should be done weekly throughout the first trimester, then monthly.
- Thyroid tests should be performed 2 weeks after switching.

Thyrotropin Receptor Antibody

- For women diagnosed with hyperthyroidism during pregnancy who will be taking thionamides, serum thyrotropin receptor antibody (TRAb) should be measured at diagnosis and, if elevated, again at 18-22 weeks and at 30-34 weeks of gestation.
- Disappearance of TRAb indicates potential remission of Graves' disease, and the dose of thionamides can be reduced and potentially discontinued.

Thionamide Intolerance

- Thyroidectomy during pregnancy can be required for Graves' disease sufferers who are allergic to or have agranulocytosis and cannot take thionamides.
- Prior to thyroidectomy, pregnant women with intolerance to thionamides should be pretreated with beta blockers (metoprolol or propranolol) and a short course (i.e., 7-10 days) of potassium iodine solution (35-50 mg iodine per drop, 1-3 drops daily).

POSTPARTUM ISSUES

- Given the worries about possible hepatotoxicity linked to PTU, we advise methimazole over PTU for lactating women.
- Women with Graves' disease who have received treatment before or during pregnancy require close observation after delivery because they are at-risk of aggravation.

Postpartum Thyroiditis

- Incidence are 5–10% of all pregnancies.
- Occurs after 3–4 months of delivery.
- Autoimmune disorder and three times more common in patients with type 1 diabetes.[22]

Mechanism: Destruction induced hormone release (hyperthyroidism) followed by thyroid insufficiency (hypothyroidism). Almost two-third of the patients has full recovery.

Management: β-blockers are given for hyperthyroid symptoms and then thyroxin therapy is given for next 6–12 months. These patients are at increased risk for postnatal depression.

THYROID NODULE

- These individuals should be assessed as if they were not pregnant.
- TSH and ultrasonography testing should be done.
- Radionuclide screening of the thyroid is not advised while pregnant.
- The reasons for performing a fine-needle aspiration (FNA) biopsy of the nodule are the same as for patients who are not pregnant.[23]

THYROID CANCER DURING PREGNANCY

- To reduce problems for both the mother and the fetus, women with newly diagnosed differentiated thyroid cancer can postpone thyroidectomy until after delivery.[24]
- In rare cases, when a patient has a cancer that is larger, more aggressive, or growing quickly, or when there are significant nodal or distant metastases, surgery during pregnancy may be indicated.
- The second trimester of pregnancy is the safest time for any sort of operation.[25]
- The patient should be observed during pregnancy with thyroid ultrasounds performed during each trimester[26] when surgery for thyroid cancer is postponed. We advise thyroid hormone suppressive medication in these situations where thyroid surgery is postponed. The TSH should be kept within a range of 0.3–2.0 mIU/L.

CONCLUSION

Hypothyroidism

- Thyroxin is very essential for early fetal development.
- After first trimester only small amount of thyroxin crosses the placenta.
- There is good outcome after appropriate treatment.

Hyperthyroidism

- Careful evaluation of cause is necessary as if left untreated, poor outcome is the rule.
- As antithyroid drugs crosses the placenta, lowest optimal dosage should be started.
- Cord blood thyroid function should be done after delivery to check the fetal thyroid functions.

Postpartum Thyroiditis

- Autoimmune disorder and occurs usually after 3–4 months postpartum.

- Phases of hyperthyroidism followed by hypothyroidism and recovery in almost two-thirds of patients.
- Annual thyroid function tests should be done in these patients.

Thyroid Nodule and Cancer

- These should be managed as same as in nonpregnant patients.
- Radioactive iodine for diagnosis and treatment is contraindicated.
- Surgery should be deferred, if indicated, should be done in second trimester.

REFERENCES

1. Ain KB, Mori Y, Refetoff S. Reduced clearance rate of thyroxine-binding globulin (TBG) with increased sialylation: a mechanism for estrogen-induced elevation of serum TBG concentration. J Clin Endocrinol Metab 1987;65(4):689-96.
2. Ballabio M, Poshychinda M, Ekins RP. Pregnancy-induced changes in thyroid function: role of human chorionic gonadotropin as putative regulator of maternal thyroid. J Clin Endocrinol Metab. 1991;73(4):824-31.
3. Yeo CP, Khoo DH, Eng PH, Tan HK, Yo SL, Jacob E. Prevalence of gestational thyrotoxicosis in Asian women evaluated in the 8th to 14th weeks of pregnancy: correlations with total and free beta human chorionic gonadotrophin. Clin Endocrinol (Oxf). 2001;55(3):391-8.
4. Burrow GN, Fisher DA, Larsen PR. Maternal and fetal thyroid function. N Engl J Med. 1994;331(16):1072-8.
5. Allan WC, Haddow JE, Palomaki GE, Williams JR, Mitchell ML, Hermos RJ, et al. Maternal thyroid deficiency and pregnancy complications: implications for population screening. J Med Screen. 2000;7(3):127-30.
6. Klein RZ, Haddow JE, Faix JD, Brown RS, Hermos RJ, Pulkkinen A, et al. Prevalence of thyroid deficiency in pregnant women. Clin Endocrinol (Oxf). 1991;35(1):41-6.
7. Thyroid Disease in Pregnancy: ACOG Practice Bulletin Summary, Number 223. Obstet Gynecol. 2020;135(6):e261-74.
8. Alexander EK, Pearce EN, Brent GA, Brown RS, Chen H, Dosiou C, et al. 2017 Guidelines of the American Thyroid Association for the Diagnosis and Management of Thyroid Disease During Pregnancy and the Postpartum. Thyroid. 2017; 27(3):315-89.
9. Lemieux P, Yamamoto JM, Nerenberg KA, Metcalfe A, Chin A, Khurana R, et al. Thyroid Laboratory Testing and Management in Women on Thyroid Replacement Before Pregnancy and Associated Pregnancy Outcomes. Thyroid. 2021;31(5):841-49.
10. Hales C, Taylor PN, Channon S, Paradice R, McEwan K, Zhang L, et al. Controlled Antenatal Thyroid Screening II: Effect of Treating Maternal Suboptimal Thyroid Function on Child Behavior. J Clin Endocrinol Metab. 2018;103(4):1583-91.
11. Lo JC, Rivkees SA, Chandra M, Gonzalez JR, Korelitz JJ, Kuzniewicz MW, et al. Gestational thyrotoxicosis, antithyroid drug use and neonatal outcomes within an integrated healthcare delivery system. Thyroid. 2015; 25(6):698-705.
12. Goodwin TM, Montoro M, Mestman JH, Pekary AE, Hershman JM. The role of chorionic gonadotropin in transient hyperthyroidism of hyperemesis gravidarum. J Clin Endocrinol Metab. 1992;75(5):1333-7.
13. Hershman JM. Human chorionic gonadotropin and the thyroid: hyperemesis gravidarum and trophoblastic tumors. Thyroid. 1999;9(7):653-7.
14. Yoshimura M, Pekary AE, Pang XP, Berg L, Goodwin TM, Hershman JM. Thyrotropic activity of basic isoelectric forms of human chorionic gonadotropin extracted from hydatidiform mole tissues. J Clin Endocrinol Metab. 1994;78(4):862-6.
15. Smits G, Govaerts C, Nubourgh I, Pardo L, Vassart G, Costagliola S. Lysine 183 and glutamic acid 157 of the TSH receptor: two interacting residues with a key role in determining specificity toward

TSH and human CG. Mol Endocrinol. 2002;16(4):722-35.
16. Ross DS, Burch HB, Cooper DS, Greenlee MC, Laurberg P, Maia AL, et al. 2016 American Thyroid Association Guidelines for Diagnosis and Management of Hyperthyroidism and Other Causes of Thyrotoxicosis. Thyroid. 2016;26(10):1343-1421.
17. Lydakis C, Lip GY, Beevers M, Beevers DG. Atenolol and fetal growth in pregnancies complicated by hypertension. Am J Hypertens. 1999;12(6):541-7.
18. Adali E, Yildizhan R, Kolusari A, Kurdoglu M, Turan N. The use of plasmapheresis for rapid hormonal control in severe hyperthyroidism caused by a partial molar pregnancy. Arch Gynecol Obstet. 2009;279(4):569-71.
19. Rubin PC. Current concepts: beta-blockers in pregnancy. N Engl J Med. 1981;305(22):1323-6.
20. Bowman P, Osborne NJ, Sturley R, Vaidya B. Carbimazole embryopathy: implications for the choice of antithyroid drugs in pregnancy. QJM. 2012;105(2):189-93.
21. Andersen SL, Olsen J, Wu CS, Laurberg P. Birth defects after early pregnancy use of antithyroid drugs: a Danish nationwide study. J Clin Endocrinol Metab. 2013;98(11):4373-81.
22. Nicholson WK, Robinson KA, Smallridge RC, Ladenson PW, Powe NR. Prevalence of postpartum thyroid dysfunction: a quantitative review. Thyroid. 2006;16(6): 573-82.
23. Haugen BR, Alexander EK, Bible KC, Doherty GM, Mandel SJ, Nikiforov YE, et al. 2015 American Thyroid Association Management Guidelines for Adult Patients with Thyroid Nodules and Differentiated Thyroid Cancer: The American Thyroid Association Guidelines Task Force on Thyroid Nodules and Differentiated Thyroid Cancer. Thyroid. 2016;26(1):1-133.
24. Nam KH, Yoon JH, Chang HS, Park CS. Optimal timing of surgery in well-differentiated thyroid carcinoma detected during pregnancy. J Surg Oncol. 2005;91(3): 199-203.
25. Chong KM, Tsai YL, Chuang J, Chen KT, Hwang JL. Thyroid cancer in pregnancy: a report of 3 cases. J Reprod Med. 2007; 52(5):416-8.
26. Kuy S, Roman SA, Desai R, Sosa JA. Outcomes following thyroid and parathyroid surgery in pregnant women. Arch Surg. 2009;144(5):399-406.

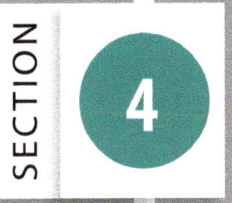

SECTION 4: Systemic Diseases

- **Cardiac Diseases (Commonly found Disorders be Discussed)**
  Sheeba Marwah, Anshika Rakesh

- **Hepatic Diseases in Pregnancy**
  Riddhi Desai

- **Respiratory and Pulmonary Diseases**
  Monisha Singh, Amit Singh, Juhi Deshpande

- **Renal Disorders**
  Ankita Jain

- **Haemtological and Coagulation Disorders (VTE)**
  Nidhi Bansal

- **Neurological Disorders in Pregnancy**
  Prabhat Agrawal

- **Hypertensive Disorders in Pregnancy**
  Parul Sinha, Garima Gupta

CHAPTER 5

Cardiac Diseases (Commonly found Disorders be Discussed)

Sheeba Marwah, Anshika Rakesh

INTRODUCTION

It is observed that 1–3% of pregnancies are complicated by cardiac diseases. In developing countries like India rheumatic heart disease (RHD), continues to be a major contributor to cardiac illness (69%). The majority of cases include mitral stenosis (38.5%) and atrial septal defects (25%). Maternal mortality increases up to 7% during pregnancy associated with cardiac disease and morbidity increases up to 30%.[1]

Women should be stratified according to the risk factors in prepregnancy period and managed by a multidisciplinary team including cardiologists, obstetricians, fetal medicine specialists, obstetric anesthetists, and pediatricians.[2] This chapter briefly explores the common cardiac diseases in pregnancy with their management.

PHYSIOLOGICAL CHANGES IN PREGNANCY

Many physiological changes embark in pregnancy which predisposes women to various complications.

Plasma volume increases up to 40% and red cell mass increases only 30% resulting in "physiological anemia of pregnancy", which is most apparent at 30–34 weeks of pregnancy. Up to 40% increase in cardiac output in early pregnancy is due to increased stroke volume, however, later on, increased heart rate is a major contributory factor. Due to decreased systemic vascular resistance the systemic blood pressure falls early in pregnancy; however, diastolic blood pressure starts to rise in the third trimester of pregnancy. The changes are summarized in **Table 1**.

TABLE 1: Physiological changes during pregnancy.

Hemodynamic parameter	Pregnancy
Blood flow	↑
Blood volume [plasma and red blood cells (RBC)]	↑
Systemic vascular resistance	↓
Stroke volume	↑
Cardiac output	↑
Heart rate	↑
Blood pressure	↓
Pulmonary capillary wedge pressure	↔
Colloid oncotic pressure	↓
Central venous pressure	↔
Maternal oxygen consumption	↑

SIGNS AND SYMPTOMS OF HEART DISEASE

The symptoms of heart disease in pregnancy are of concern to an obstetrician because they can be masked by physiological changes of pregnancy.

TABLE 2: Normal signs and symptoms of pregnancy.

Symptoms	Signs	ECG changes
Tiredness	Increased heart rate	Left axis deviation
Dyspnea	Peripheral edema	ST segment changes
Orthopnea	Bounding pulses	Small Q
Syncope	Loud S1	Inverted P wave in lead III abolished by inspiration
	Grade 1 and 2 systolic murmur	T wave inversion in lead III

Normal signs and symptoms of pregnancy are enumerated in **Table 2**.

SIGNS AND SYMPTOMS OF SUSPECTED HEART DISEASE

Symptoms

- Progressive severe dyspnea/orthopnea
- Nocturnal cough
- Hemoptysis
- Exertional syncope
- Exertional chest pain
- Progressive edema/anasarca
- Tachycardia 120 beats per minute (BPM)
- History of heart failure in previous pregnancy also increases the risk.

Physical Signs

- Cyanosis
- Clubbing
- Persistent neck vein distension
- Persistent systolic murmurs (grades 3 and 4)
- Any diastolic murmurs
- Unequivocal enlargement of heart on chest X-ray (CXR)
- Heave
- Persistent arrhythmias (atrial fibrillation/flutter)
- Persistent split in S2
- Pulmonary hypertension
- Murmurs associated with stenotic lesions accentuated [(due to increased blood volume and carbon monoxide (CO)], murmurs of aortic stenosis (AR), mitral regurgitation (MR), and ventricular septal defect (VSD) may become attenuated [due to decrease in systemic vascular resistance (SVR)].

INVESTIGATIONS

- Electrocardiography (ECG) and CXR if indicated.
- A 24-hour Holter monitoring may be required to diagnose arrhythmias.
- Echocardiography is noninvasive and safe.
- Transesophageal echocardiography (TOE) is useful in selected cases, e.g., assessment of infective endocarditis (IE), aortic dissection, or a technically difficult transthoracic study.
- Magnetic resonance cardiac imaging is useful when other modalities fail. However, safety in pregnancy and its effects on the fetus have not been established.
- Radionuclide cardiac imaging and left heart catheterization are not recommended in pregnancy.

MANAGEMENT

Preconceptional Counseling[3]

- Baseline cardiac function status and calculation of risk prediction according to cardiac disease in pregnancy (CARPREG) risk scoring.

- Counseling the patient regarding pregnancy risk to female and fetus.
- Opinion of cardiologists for optimization of their conditions.
- Review current medications to determine appropriateness of drugs.
- Co-ordination between cardiologist, obstetrician, physician, and anesthesiologist is necessary for a successful outcome of pregnancy.
- Absolute contraindications for conception are as follows:
  - Primary pulmonary hypertension
  - Eisenmenger's syndrome
  - Coarctation of aorta with valvular involvement
  - Marfan syndrome with aortic involvement
  - Peripartum cardiomyopathy with persistent left ventricular dysfunction.

NEW YORK HEART ASSOCIATION FUNCTIONAL CLASSIFICATION OF HEART FAILURE (TABLE 3)[4]

TABLE 3: New York heart association functional classification of heart failure.

Class 1	Patients with cardiac disease but without resulting limitations of physical activity
Class 2	Patients with cardiac disease result in slight limitations of physical activity. They are comfortable at rest
Class 3	Patients with cardiac disease resulting in marked limitation of physical activity. They are comfortable at rest
Class 4	Patients with cardiac disease resulting in an inability to carry on any physical activity without discomfort. Symptoms of cardiac insufficiency may even be present at rest

WORLD HEALTH ORGANIZATION CLASSIFICATION FOR CARDIOVASCULAR RISK IN PREGNANCY[5]

World Health Organization classification for cardiovascular risk in pregnancy is depicted in **Table 4**.

RISK PREDICTION ACCORDING TO THE CARPREG RISK SCORE[6]

Risk prediction according to the CARPREG risk score is depicted in **Table 5**.

ANTEPARTUM CARE

- Regular evaluation of patients for any deterioration of symptoms.
- Twice weekly follow-up till 28 weeks and weekly afterward.
- Antenatal care (ANC) checkup should be done by the same clinician so that significant changes can be detected early, allowing timely intervention.
- ECG and echocardiogram (ECHO) to evaluate any clinical deterioration.
- Anomaly scan and fetal ECHO (in cases of congenital heart disease) between 18 and 22 weeks.
- Antepartum fetal surveillance at 30–34 weeks in case of fetal growth restriction.
- Admission according to the functional status of patient.
- Multidisciplinary team approach involving obstetricians, cardiologists, pediatricians, and anesthetists.

LABOR AND DELIVERY

- Strict input output charting.
- Avoid the supine position.
- Propped up position and O_2 supplementation.

TABLE 4: WHO classification for cardiovascular risk in pregnancy.

WHO pregnancy risk classification (risk of pregnancy by medical condition)	Cardiovascular conditions by WHO risk class
WHO risk class I: No detectable increased risk of maternal mortality and no or mild increase in morbidity	• Uncomplicated, small, or mild: – Pulmonary stenosis – Patient ductus arteriosus – Mitral valve prolapse • Successfully repaired simple lesions (atrial or ventricular septal defect, patent ductus arteriosus, and anomalous pulmonary venous drainage) • Atrial or ventricular ectopic beats and isolated
WHO risk class II (if otherwise well and uncomplicated): Small increased risk of maternal mortality or moderate increase in morbidity	• Unoperated atrial or ventricular septal defect • Repaired tetralogy of Fallot • Most arrhythmias
WHO risk class II (if otherwise well and uncomplicated): Small increased risk of maternal mortality or moderate increase in morbidity	• Mild left ventricular impairment • Hypertrophic cardiomyopathy • Native or tissue valvular heart disease not considered WHO I or IV • Marfan syndrome without aortic dilatation • Aorta
WHO risk class III: Significantly increased risk of maternal mortality or severe morbidity. Expert counseling is required. If pregnancy is decided upon, intensive specialist cardiac and obstetric monitoring are needed throughout pregnancy, childbirth, and the puerperium	• Mechanical valve • Systemic right ventricle • Fontan circulation • Cyanotic heart disease (unrepaired) • Other complex congenital heart disease • Aortic dilatation 40–45 mm in Marfan syndrome • Aortic dilatation 45–50 mm in aortic disease associated with bicuspid aortic valve
WHO risk class IV (pregnancy contraindicated): Extremely high risk of maternal mortality or severe morbidity; pregnancy is contraindicated. If pregnancy occurs, then the termination should be discussed. If the pregnancy continues, care as for class III	• Pulmonary arterial hypertension of any cause • Severe systemic ventricular dysfunction (LVEF 45 mm) • Aortic dilation >50 mm in aortic disease associated with bicuspid aortic valve • Native severe coarctation

(IV: intravenous; LVEF: left ventricular ejection fraction; WHO: World Health Organization)

- Frequent chest auscultation.
- Consultant delivery with high dependency care.
- Vaginal delivery preferable, lower segment cesarean section (LSCS) only for obstetric indication.
- Endocarditis prophylaxis: (a) In the Indian scenario, prophylaxis was given to patients with a history of infective endocarditis, congenital cyanotic heart disease, prosthetic valve, and cardiac transplantation with valvulopathy. Drugs used are ampicillin, amoxicillin, and gentamicin. Vancomycin is given in resistant cases (b) injection penicillin 1.2 MU 3 weekly—in rheumatic heart disease.

POSTPARTUM CARE[7]

- Not to be discharged before 1 week.

- In the first 72 hours pulmonary oedema can develop so strict monitoring is done.
- Antibiotics to continue for 7 days after delivery
- Breastfeeding to continue, except in Class III and IV.

CONTRACEPTION[8]

- Oral contraceptives (OC) pills, barrier contraceptives—not recommended
- Intrauterine contraceptive devices (IUCDs) can be used in uncomplicated heart disease
- Progestin-only pills (desogestrel) or long-acting injectable progesterone are better [medroxyprogesterone 150 mg intramuscular (IM) for every 3 months]
- Permanent sterilization (by MiniLap/partner's vasectomy) is best and considered if a family is complete.

FOLLOW-UP

- At 6 weeks.
- To the cardiologist as indicated according to the functional status of the patient.

Approach to a patient of heart disease in pregnancy is described in **Figure 1**.

Elucidation on valvular heart disease is enumerated in **Box 1**.

Elucidation on regurgitant lesion is enumerated in **Box 2**.

Elucidation on anticoagulation in valvular heart disease is enumerated in **Box 3**.

Elucidation for peripartum cardiomyopathy is enumerated in **Box 4**.

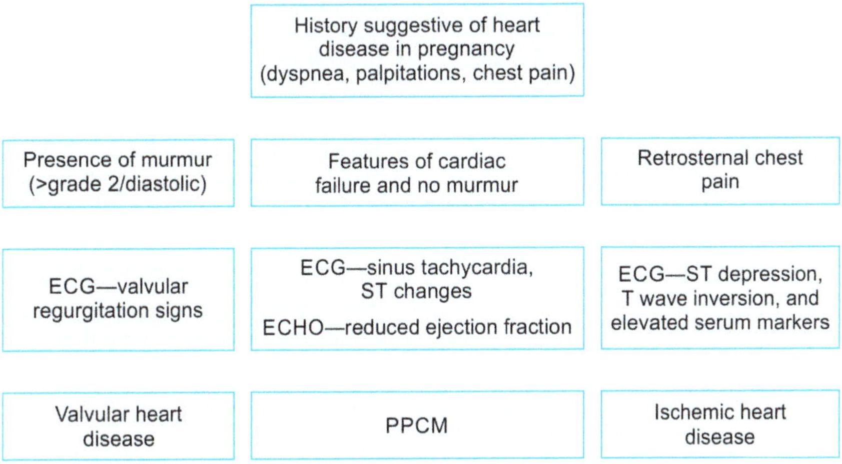

TABLE 5: Risk prediction according to the CARPREG risk score.

Predictors of maternal cardiovascular events
- NYHA Class >II
- Cyanosis
- Prior cardiovascular event
- Systemic ventricular ejection fraction

For each CARPREG predictor a point is assigned

No of predictors	Risk of cardiac events in pregnancy (%)
0	5
1	25
>1	75

(CARPREG: cardiac disease in pregnancy; NYHA: New York Heart Association)

Fig. 1: General approach for a patient with heart disease. (ECG: electrocardiography; ECHO: echocardiogram; PPCM: peripartum cardiomyopathy)

BOX 1: Valvular heart disease.

Valvular heart disease
- Mitral stenosis (MS):[9]
  - In patients with symptoms of pulmonary hypertension, restricted activities, and β-1-selective blockers (metoprolol or bisoprolol) are recommended
  - Diuretics are recommended when congestive symptoms persist despite β-blockers
  - Patients with severe MS should undergo intervention before pregnancy. If at all it is planned percutaneous mitral commissurotomy is preferably performed after a 20-week gestation and only in NYHA class III/IV and/or estimated systolic PAP >50 mm Hg at echocardiography despite optimal medical treatment, in the absence of contraindications and if patient characteristics are suitable
  - Therapeutic anticoagulation is recommended in the case of atrial fibrillation, left atrial thrombosis, or prior embolism
- Aortic stenosis:
  - Echocardiography is mandatory for diagnosis
  - Patients with severe AS should undergo intervention prepregnancy if they are symptomatic or have LV dysfunction (LVEF <50%)
  - Asymptomatic patients with severe AS should undergo intervention prepregnancy when they develop symptoms during exercise testing
  - A β-blocker or a nondihydropyridine calcium channel antagonist should be considered for rate control in AF. If both are contraindicated, digoxin may be considered
  - During pregnancy in severely symptomatic patients not responding to medical therapy, percutaneous valvuloplasty can be undertaken. If not possible and patients have life-threatening symptoms, valve replacement should be considered after early delivery by caesarean section

(AF: atrial fibrillation; AS: aortic stenosis; LV: left ventricle; LVEF: left ventricular ejection fraction; PAP: pulmonary artery pressure; NYHA: New York Heart Association)

BOX 2: Regurgitant lesions.

Regurgitant lesions:[10]
- In asymptomatic women with preserved left ventricle (LV) function the most frequent complications are arrhythmias
- Patients with severe aortic or mitral regurgitation and symptoms or impaired ventricular function or ventricular dilatation should be treated surgically prepregnancy
- Medical therapy is recommended in pregnant women with regurgitant lesions when symptoms occur

BOX 3: Anticoagulation for valvular disease.

Anticoagulation for valvular disease:[11]
- High-dose LMWH therapy throughout gestation. Start enoxaparin 1 mg/kg every 12 hours. Goal anti-Xa level 4 hours postinjection is 1 U/mL (0.7–1.2 U/mL).
- High-dose UFH throughout gestation. UFH subcutaneously every 12 hours. Goal anti-Xa level midinterval is 0.35–0.7 U/mL or goal midinterval activated partial thromboplastin time ≥2 times control.
- Either of the first two regimens through completed week 12, then change to warfarin until 36 weeks or close to delivery. Goal INR w3 (2.5–3.5). UFH or LMWH can then be resumed until delivery.

(INR: international normalized ratio; LMWH: low-molecular-weight heparins; UFH: unfractionated heparin)

BOX 4: Peripartum cardiomyopathy (PPCM).

Peripartum cardiomyopathy:
It is defined as heart failure in the last month of pregnancy or within 5 months postpartum in absence of prior heart disease. There is no determinable cause and ECHO findings suggest left ventricular dysfunction. The latter includes an ejection fraction (EF) of 2.7 cm/m^2. The incidence is 1:1,500 to 1:4,000 with 90% occurring in the first 2 months postpartum. Fifty percent of deaths occur in the first 6 weeks postpartum. Mortality ranges from 18 to 56%.

- *Management:*
  - *ECG:* Normal sinus rhythm or sinus tachycardia, T wave inversion, Q wave, and nonspecific ST segment
  - X-ray chest: Cardiomegaly
  - Blood samples – C- Reactive protein is ↑, Brain natriuretic peptide (BNP) ↑↑, LDL ↑, Interferon gamma ↑
  - Drugs:
    - Salt restriction
    - Reduce preload: Diuretics—furosemide 20–40 mg PO everyday
    - Reduce afterload: Vasodilators—
      - Hydralazine 25–100 mg PO everyday
      - Amlodipine 5–10 mg PO everyday
      - Postpartum—enalapril 5 mg BD reduces myocardial oxygen requirement, and maintains HR between 80 and 100 BPM 1. Metoprolol 25–100 mg PO every day or 2. Carvedilol 3.25–25 mg PO every day
      - Reduce inflammation pentoxifylline 400 mg PO TDS, inhibits prolactin secretion
    - Anticoagulation—(if cardiomegaly and reduced EF): Heparin/LMWH/oral anticoagulants

(BPM: beats per minute; HR: heart rate; ECG: electrocardiography; ECHO: echocardiogram; LDL: low-density lipoprotein; LMWH: low-molecular-weight heparins)

REFERENCES

1. Simpson LL. Maternal cardiac disease: update for the clinician. Obstet Gynecol. 2012;119(2 Pt. 1):345-59.
2. European Society of Gynecology (ESG); Association for European Paediatric Cardiology (AEPC); German Society for Gender Medicine (DGesGM); Regitz-Zagrosek V, Blomstrom Lundqvist C, Borghi C, et al. ESC Guidelines on the management of cardiovascular diseases during pregnancy: the task force on the management of cardiovascular diseases during pregnancy of the European Society of Cardiology (ESC). Eur Heart J. 2011;32(24):3147-97.
3. Ray P, Murphy GJ, Shutt LE. Recognition and management of maternal cardiac disease in pregnancy. Br J Anaesth. 2004;93(3):428-39.
4. Dolgin M; New York Heart Association. Nomenclature and Criteria for Diagnosis of diseases of the heart and great vessels, 6th edition. Boston: Little, Brown; 1964.
5. Jastrow N, Meyer P, Khairy P, Mercier LA, Dore A, Marcotte F, et al. Prediction of complications in pregnant women with cardiac diseases referred to a tertiary Center. Int J Cardiol. 2010;151(2):209-13.
6. Siu SC, Sermer M, Colman JM, Alvarez AN, Mercier LA, Morton BC, et al. Prospective multicenter study of pregnancy outcomes in women with heart disease. Circulation. 2001;104(5):515-21.
7. Keizer JL, Zwart JJ, Meerman RH, Harinck BI, Feuth HD, Van RJ. Obstetric intensive care admissions: a 12-year review in a tertiary care centre. Eur J Obstet Gynecol Reprod Biol. 2006;128(1-2):152-6.
8. World Health Organization. (2015). Medical eligibility criteria for contraceptive use. [online] Available from https://www.who.int/

publications/i/item/9789241549158 [Last accessed November, 2022].
9. Vahanian A, Baumgartner H, Bax J, Butchart E, Dion R, Filippatos G, et al. Guidelines on the management of valvular heart disease: the Task Force on the Management of Valvular Heart Disease of the European Society of Cardiology. Eur Heart J. 2007; 28(2):230-68.
10. Lesniak-Sobelga A, Tracz W, KostKiewicz M, Podolec P, Pasowicz M. Clinical and echocardiographic assessment of pregnant women with valvular heart diseases—maternal and fetal outcome. Int J Cardiol. 2004;94(1):15-23.
11. Guyatt GH, Akl EA, Crowther M, Gutterman DD, Schuünemann HJ; American College of Chest Physicians Antithrombotic Therapy and Prevention of Thrombosis Panel. Executive summary: Antithrombotic Therapy and Prevention of Thrombosis, 9th ed: American College of Chest Physicians Evidence-Based Clinical Practice Guidelines. Chest. 2012;141(2 Suppl):7S-47S.

CHAPTER 6

Hepatic Diseases in Pregnancy

Riddhi Desai

■ INTRODUCTION

Hepatic diseases can complicate pregnancy in approximately 3% of pregnant women. When severe they can cause significant maternal as well as fetal morbidity and mortality. A mortality rate as high as up to 25% has been reported in women with pregnancy-related liver diseases.[1] While managing women with suspected liver disease, it should be kept in mind that normal physiological changes in pregnancy can mimic liver disease. It is imperative that clinicians are familiar with these disorders and can differentiate them so as to facilitate prompt and appropriate management in all of these situations.

Types of Liver Disease Associated with Pregnancy[2]

- Liver disease specific to pregnancy, which can occur at a specific time during pregnancy.
- Liver disease not related to pregnancy, which can occur at any time, such as viral- or drug-induced hepatitis.
- Pregnancy in women with pre-existing liver disease.

■ NORMAL PHYSIOLOGICAL CHANGES OF PREGNANCY[3]

Physical changes occur in pregnancy, which impact the normal ranges for liver function tests (LFTs) **(Table 1)**. Therefore, the interpretation of LFTs during pregnancy must take these changes into account.

TABLE 1: Physiological changes in pregnancy.

• Albumin	Decreases
• Hemoglobin	
• Bilirubin	Unchanged
• Transaminases	
• PT INR	
• Bile acids	
• Gamma GT	
• Alkaline phosphatase (ALP)	Increases
• Alfa-fetoprotein (AFP)	

(INR: international normalized ratio; PT: prothrombin time)

Physiological changes in pregnancy are enumerated in **Table 1**.

Classification of Hepatic Diseases in Pregnancy[4]

The various Liver diseases need to be differentiated so as to allow proper management of the patient. This chapter will cover liver diseases specific to pregnancy and cirrhosis. Classification of Hepatic diseases in pregnancy is given in **Table 2**.

■ HYPEREMESIS GRAVIDARUM[5]

- It is defined as nausea and intractable vomiting that results in dehydration, ketosis, and weight loss >5% of body weight.

TABLE 2: Classification of hepatic diseases in pregnancy.

Liver diseases specific to pregnancy	Trimester
Hyperemesis gravidarum	First, but can persists in second/third
Preeclampsia and eclampsia	Second/third/immediately postpartum
HELLP syndrome	Third/immediately postpartum
Intrahepatic cholestasis	Second/third
Acute fatty liver	Third
Liver disease not related to pregnancy	**Trimester**
Viral hepatitis	Any time during pregnancy
Drug-induced hepatotoxicity	Any time during pregnancy
Gall stones	Second/third, can occur in first
Budd–Chiari syndrome	Anytime during pregnancy/postpartum
Sepsis	Anytime during pregnancy
Pregnancy in pre-existing liver diseases	**Trimester**
Autoimmune hepatitis	Present all throughout pregnancy with a variable course
Primary biliary cirrhosis	
Cirrhosis from any cause	
Wilson's disease	
Primary sclerosing cholangitis	

- 0.3–2.0% of pregnancies during the first trimester can be complicated by it.
- Symptoms begin before the 9th week of gestation and disappear after the 20th week.
- It is not a true liver disease in itself but >50% of cases are associated with abnormal liver tests.
- Risk factors are hyperemesis gravidarum in a previous pregnancy, multiple gestations, increased body mass index (BMI), pre-existing diabetes, and psychiatric illness.
- Patients present with dehydration, electrolyte abnormalities, metabolic alkalosis, increased renal values, and erythrocytosis.
- There is an elevation in serum aminotransferases (usually >200 U/L), serum amylase, and lipase values.
- Abdominal ultrasound shows normal liver parenchyma without biliary obstruction. Obstetric ultrasound is to be done to exclude hydatidiform mole and multiple gestations.
- Supportive management includes intravenous fluid, antiemetics, parenteral nutrition, correction of electrolyte abnormalities, and vitamin supplementation.

INTRAHEPATIC CHOLESTASIS OF PREGNANCY[6]

- It is the most common pregnancy-related liver disease and results from idiosyncratic exaggeration of normal bile stasis due to hormonal changes.
- It is a reversible condition with an onset in the late second and third trimesters. There have been rare reports of cases as early as 7 weeks of gestation.
- It resolves rapidly postpartum within 6 weeks of delivery.
- Risk factors are multiple gestations, history of use of oral contraceptive pills, maternal age >35 years, multiparity, history of assisted reproductive

techniques, and history of intrahepatic cholestasis in a previous pregnancy.
- Etiology is multifactorial with genetic, hormonal, and environmental factors playing a role. It is associated with abnormal biliary transport across the canalicular membrane.
- It presents as pruritus, which typically predominates on the palms and soles of the feet and worsens at night. It develops after 25 weeks of gestation, with 80% of cases occurring after the 30th week.
- 14–25% present with jaundice that may develop 1–4 weeks after the onset of pruritus. Other symptoms include dark urine, pale stools, steatorrhea, malabsorption of fat-soluble vitamins, and weight loss.
- Total bile acids are the most important biochemical test for diagnosis and prognosis. Usually, it can be the first, and sometimes only, laboratory abnormality. The levels should be checked weekly since the values fluctuate and increase with advancing pregnancy.
- Nonfasting serum bile acid levels ≥40 μmol/L increase the risk of perinatal complications and can be associated with poor perinatal outcome and increased risk of preterm labor, fetal distress, and sudden intrauterine fetal death.
- Aminotransferases are increased 2–20 times. Serum gamma-glutamyl transferase (GGT) levels are normal or moderately elevated. Bilirubin levels rarely increase more than 100 μmol/L. Alkaline phosphatase (ALP) is elevated. There are no abnormal findings for the liver parenchyma and no dilatation of biliary ducts on ultrasound.
- The treatment goals are to manage maternal symptoms and keep total bile acids in the normal range, thereby improving both maternal and fetal outcomes.
- The first-line therapy is ursodeoxycholic acid (UDCA), 15 mg/kg/day in divided doses. UDCA is safe in the third trimester and no maternal or fetal side effects have been reported.

ACUTE FATTY LIVER OF PREGNANCY[7]

- It is a rare medical and obstetric emergency, which in the absence of early recognition and appropriate management can be fatal for both mother and fetus. It can complicate pregnancies in up to 1:7,000 to 1:16,000 pregnancies, usually occurring in the third trimester.
- Risk factors are multiparity, multiple gestations, preeclampsia, male fetus, and underweight women.
- The pathogenesis is poorly understood. Investigations suggest that it may result from mitochondrial dysfunction with a defect in mitochondrial fatty acid oxidation in both the mother and fetus.
- Clinical presentation is variable and patients present with nonspecific symptoms such as malaise, nausea, vomiting, headache, and abdominal pain. Complications of acute liver failure are encephalopathy, jaundice, and coagulopathy.
- Laboratory tests show elevated aminotransferase levels, hyperbilirubinemia, leukocytosis, elevated uric acid, thrombocytopenia, normochromic anemia, hypoalbuminemia, hyperammonemia, renal dysfunction, metabolic

acidosis, and biochemical pancreatitis. Hypoglycemia is a predictor of poor prognosis. Disseminated intravascular coagulation can occur in 10% of cases.
- Coagulopathies can lead to Infections and bleeding from the vagina or from a cesarean section wound.
- Current imaging methods have limited utility in the diagnosis, abdominal ultrasonography, or computed tomography (CT) can show signs of fat infiltration.
- Swansea criteria, for diagnosis **(Box 1)**, has a sensitivity of 100% and specificity of 57%, with positive and negative predictive values of 85 and 100%, respectively, for the diagnosis.
- Early recognition and delivery of the fetus regardless of gestational age are the keys to good outcomes, followed by supportive maternal care.

BOX 1: Swansea criteria, for the diagnosis of acute fatty liver in pregnancy.

(The presence of any 6 of the 14 is diagnostic)
- Symptoms:
  - Vomiting
  - Abdominal pain
  - Polydipsia/polyuria
  - Encephalopathy
- Laboratory tests:
  - Elevated bilirubin (>0.82 mg/dL)
  - Hypoglycemia (5.7 mg/dL)
  - Leukocytosis (>11 × 109 /L)
  - High AST or ALT (>42 IU/L)
  - High ammonia (>66 μmol)
  - Renal impairment (Cr >1.7 mg/dL)
  - Coagulopathy [PT >14s or activated partial thromboplastin clotting time (aPTT) >34s]
- Imaging:
  - Ascites or bright liver on ultrasound
- Histology:
  - Microvesicular steatosis on liver biopsy

PREECLAMPSIA, ECLAMPSIA, AND HEMOLYSIS, ELEVATED LIVER ENZYMES, LOW PLATELET COUNT SYNDROME[8]

- Preeclampsia is a multisystem disorder. It is defined by de novo hypertension after the 20th week of pregnancy with blood pressure (BP) ≥140/90 mm Hg and proteinuria of >300 mg/day in association with other organ dysfunction of the mother such as renal and liver involvement, neurological or hematological complications, and uteroplacental dysfunction, as well as, fetal growth restriction. Eclampsia is preeclampsia complicated with seizures.
- Onset is between 27 and 30 weeks in 70% of women or postpartum within the first 48 hours.
- HELLP syndrome is characterized by the presence of hemolysis, elevated liver aminotransferases, and low platelet counts. It is seen in up to 12% of cases with preeclampsia, but can also occur in normotensive patients.
- The diagnosis of HELLP syndrome is by on clinical features and abnormal laboratory values. Patients present with colic-like pain in the epigastric or in the right upper quadrant along with hypertension and proteinuria.
- Laboratory parameters and the various classification systems are mentioned in **Table 3**.
- Liver complications, such as liver infarction, intraparenchymal hemorrhage, subcapsular hematoma, and hepatic rupture can be diagnosed on ultrasonography, computed tomography (CT), and magnetic resonance imaging (MRI).
- HELLP syndrome must be distinguished from other rare life-threatening, diseases

TABLE 3: Classification of HELLP.

HELLP class	Mississippi classification	Tennessee classification
Class 1 (severe)	• AST or ALT ≥70 IU/L • LDH ≥600 IU/L • Platelet count ≤50 × 10⁹L	• AST ≥70 IU/L • LDH ≥600 IU/L or billirubin ≥1.2 mg/dL
Class 2 (moderate)	• AST or ALT ≥70 IU/L • LDH ≥600 IU/L • Platelet count 50–100 × 10⁹L	N/A
Class 3 (mild)	• AST or ALT ≥40 IU/L • LDH ≥600 IU/L • Platelet count 100–150 × 10⁹L	N/A
Partial HELLP syndrome	Presence of severe preeclampsia plus one of the following: ELLP, EL, HEL, LP	

(ALT: alanine transaminase; AST: aspartate transaminase; EL: elevated liver enzymes; ELLP: absence of hemolysis; HEL: absence of low platelets; HELLP: hemolysis, elevated liver enzymes, low platelet count; LDH: lactate dehydrogenase; LP: low platelets)

TABLE 4: Differential diagnosis.

Disorder	Hyperemesis gravidarum	HELLP	Acute fatty liver	Intrahepatic cholestasis
Incidence	0.3–2%	0.2–0 6%	0.005–0.01%	0.1–0.01%
Onset (Trimester)	First	Third/postpartum	Third	Third and rarely second
Presence of preeclampsia	No	Yes	>50%	No
Clinical features	Intense nausea and vomiting, dehydration, and electrolyte imbalance	Hemolysis and thrombocytopenia	Liver failure with coagulopathy, encephalopathy, hypoglycemia, and DIC	Generalized pruritus and elevated bile acids
Aminotransferases	<300 units/L	>500 units/L	300–500 units/L	Mild to 20-fold increase
Bilirubin	<4 mg/dL	<5 mg/dL	<5 mg/dL	<5 mg/dL
Imaging	Normal	May show hepatic rupture or infarction	May show fatty infiltrate	Normal
Histology	Normal or bland cholestasis	Patchy/extensive necrosis	Microvesicular steatosis	Cholestasis
Perinatal and fetal outcomes	Preterm and low birth	Perinatal mortality and premature delivery	Fetal mortality 9–23%	Preterm and low birth weight and fetal distress

such as thrombotic thrombocytopenic purpura (TTP) and hemolytic uremic syndrome.

- The differential diagnosis of various liver disorders are enumerated in **Table 4**.

TABLE 5: Management of pregnancy-specific liver disease.

Disorder	Management
Hyperemesis gravidarum	Supportive management
Preeclampsia and eclampsia	Delivery
HELLP	Delivery—consider platelet transfusion before delivery especially if C section.
Intra hepatic cholestasis	Ursodeoxycholic acid 10–15 mg/kg in divided doses, early delivery at 37 weeks
Acute fatty liver in pregnancy	Prompt delivery—newborn to be monitored for manifestations of deficiency of long-chain 3-hydroxyacyl coenzyme A dehydrogenase

SUMMARY OF MANAGEMENT OF PREGNANCY SPECIFIC LIVER DISEASE[9]

Management of pregnancy-specific liver disease is depicted in **Table 5**.

PRE-EXISTING LIVER DISEASES AND PREGNANCY

Cirrhosis and Portal Hypertension[10]

- Pregnancy occurs rarely in women with liver cirrhosis, although pregnancy is not contraindicated in these women. If pregnancy occurs, it is associated with the risk of spontaneous abortion, prematurity, and perinatal death.
- Variceal bleeding is the most dreaded complication in pregnant women with cirrhosis. It occurs mainly during the second trimester and the in the second stage of labor. This is due to impaired venous return caused by increased circulating blood volume and direct pressure of the gravid uterus on the inferior vena cava and worsening of portal hypertension (PH).
- Treatment for an episode of acute variceal bleeding during pregnancy is focused on the resuscitation and hemodynamic stabilization of the mother, antibiotic prophylaxis, and endoscopic variceal band ligation.

CONCLUSION

Hepatic diseases in pregnancy is a complex and poorly understood condition that deserves a multidisciplinary approach. The diagnosis and management can pose a great challenge to the clinician. Liver diseases can complicate approximately 3% of pregnancies with poor maternal and fetal outcomes. It is imperative that clinicians are familiar with these disorders and can differentiate them so as to facilitate prompt and appropriate management.

REFERENCES

1. Westbrook RH, Dusheiko G, Williamson C. Pregnancy and liver disease. J Hepatol. 2016;64(4):933-45.
2. Mikolasevic I, Filipec-Kanizaj T, Jakopcic I, Majurec I, Brncic-Fischer A, Sobocan N, et al. Liver disease during pregnancy: a challenging clinical issue. Med Sci Monit. 2018;24:4080-90.
3. Tran, Tram T, Ahn, Joseph, Reau, Nancy S. ACG clinical guideline: liver disease and pregnancy. Am J Gastroenterol. 2016;111(2): 176-94.
4. Verma D, Saab AM, Saab S, El-Kabany M. A systematic approach to pregnancy-specific liver disorders. Gastroenterol Hepatol (NY). 2021;17(7):322-9.
5. Lim E, Mouyis M, MacKillop L. Liver diseases in pregnancy. Clin Med (Lond). 2021;21(5):e441-5.

6. Palmer KR, Xiaohua L, Mol BW. Management of intrahepatic cholestasis in pregnancy. Lancet. 20192;393(10174):853-4.
7. Naoum EE, Leffert LR, Chitilian HV, Gray KJ, Bateman BT. Acute fatty liver of pregnancy: pathophysiology, anesthetic implications, and obstetrical management. Anesthesiology. 2019;130(3):446-1.
8. Guntupalli SR, Steingrub J. Hepatic disease and pregnancy: an overview of diagnosis and management. Crit Care Med. 2005; 33(10 Suppl):S332-9.
9. Morrison MA, Chung Y, Heneghan MA. Managing hepatic complications of pregnancy: practical strategies for clinicians. BMJ Open Gastroenterol. 2022;9(1):e000624.
10. Arora A, Kumar A, Anand AC, Puri P, Dhiman RK, Acharya SK, et al. Indian National Association for the Study of the Liver-Federation of Obstetric and Gynaecological Societies of India Position Statement on Management of Liver Diseases in Pregnancy. J Clin Exp Hepatol. 2019;9(3):383-406.

CHAPTER 7

Respiratory and Pulmonary Diseases

Monisha Singh, Amit Singh, Juhi Deshpande

■ INTRODUCTION

Pregnancy causes altered anatomical and physiological changes in cardiovascular and respiratory system causing any pathology difficult to treat and manage. Firstly, all of pathologies and treatment can directly or indirectly affect various other systems, impacting her quality of life and fetus. Secondly, with regards to fetal well-being, various restrictions are put on in terms of diagnosing and treating the pregnant woman. In many life threatening conditions, a careful risk benefit analysis (in terms of investigations and management) has to be done in order to come to a wise decision.[1]

When it comes to respiratory diseases, an understanding related to its pathophysiology should be taken into consideration. Because of prior statement, there has been poor control when it comes to respiratory illness in pregnancy. It has been seen that asthma still is leaking preexisting medical disorder encountered in pregnancy. Despite the changes in immunity, the incidence of respiratory infections is not higher in pregnancy.

Physiology of respiratory system in pregnancy has been described with flow diagrams as shown in **Figure 1**.

Dyspnea in Pregnancy (Table 1)

Differential diagnosis of dyspnea in pregnancy:
- Physiological dyspnea of pregnancy
- Pulmonary edema
- Pulmonary embolism
- Pneumothorax
- Pneumonia
- Worsening Asthma
- Severe Asthma
- Cardiovascular issues.

Causes of Acute Respiratory Failure in the Obstetric Patient

The causes of acute respiratory failure in the obstetric patient are given in **Table 2**.

■ PNEUMONIA

Cause

Pregnant women may be more susceptible to organisms that are controlled by cell-mediated immune processes. The incidence of pneumonia is 1.5 cases per 1,000 pregnancies. Pneumonia may produce pregnancy complications, including preterm labor, small-for-gestational-age, and intrauterine and neonatal death and acute respiratory distress syndrome (ARDS) in women.

Bacterial pneumonia presents with fever, chills, and productive cough. The two most common bacterial pathogens are *Streptococcus pneumoniae* (*Pneumococcus*) and *Haemophilus influenzae*. When bacterial pneumonia complicates viral pneumonia, *Staphylococcus aureus* or Gram negative

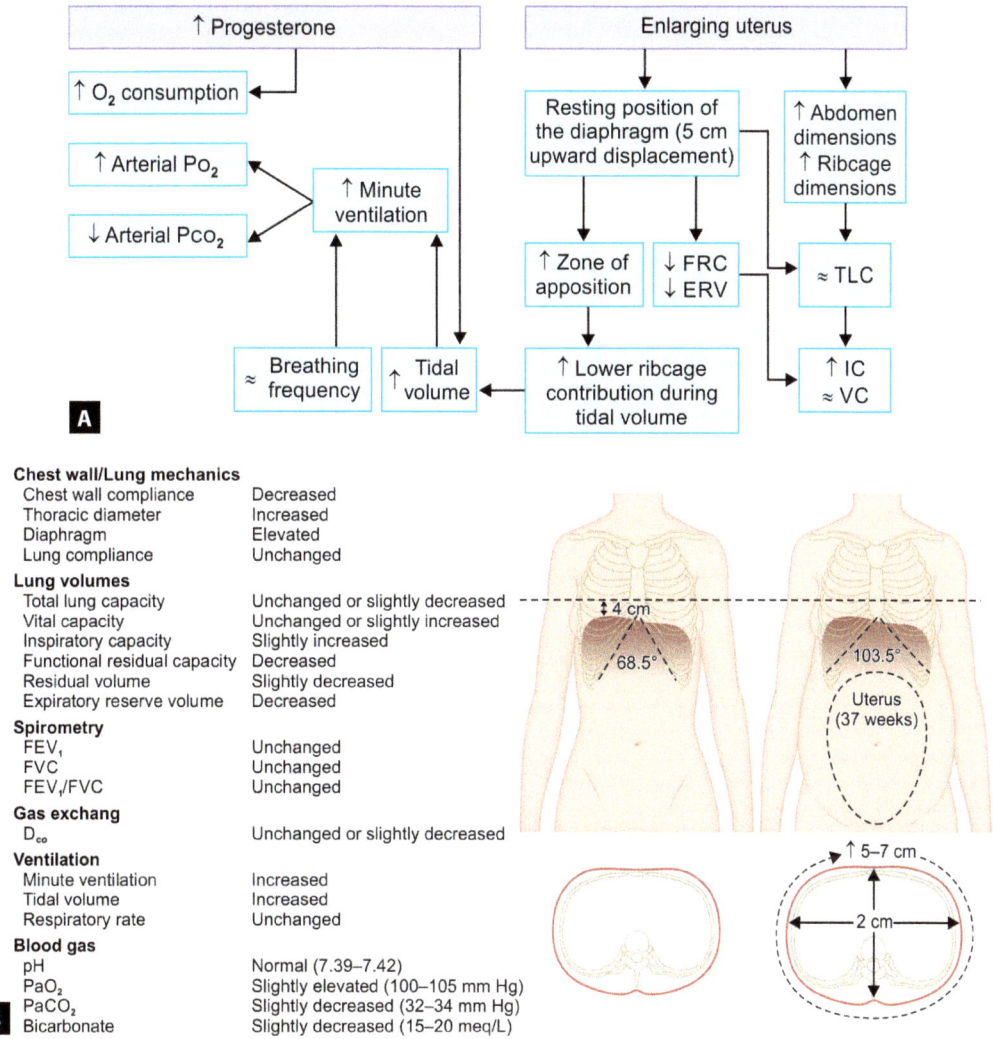

Figs. 1A and B: Flow diagram summarizing the most important effects of (A) biochemical (left) and (B) Mechanical (right) pregnancy-induced factors on pulmonary function, ventilatory pattern and gas exchange. (PO_2: oxygen tension; PCO_2: carbon dioxide tension; FRC: functional residual capacity; ERV: expiratory reserve volume; TLC: total lung capacity; IC: inspiratory capacity; VC: vital capacity; ↑: increased; ↓: decreased; ≈: no change).

organisms should be considered as potential pathogens. β-Lactam and macrolide antibiotics are safe in pregnancy and are effective in treating community acquired infections.

Viral pneumonia presents with high fever, bodyache, postnasal drip, and cough, lasting for around a week depending on the immunity. If symptoms persist, it should be investigated and consulted with pulmonologist. Pneumonia can occur from a viral inflammation of lung parenchyma or from a secondary bacterial infection.

Although routine vaccination of pregnant females against influenza with inactivated trivalent influenza vaccine is recommended,

TABLE 1: Important causes of dyspnea in pregnancy.[2]

Cause of dyspnea	Clinical characteristics	Helpful investigations	Interventions
Dyspnea of pregnancy	Need to take a deep breath intermittently, or inability to get a deep enough breath	None	Reassurance
Asthma/airways disease	Dyspnea with chest tightness or wheezing	Spirometry, pre and post bronchodilator	Inhaled β-agonists +/− inhaled steroids
Cardiac disease	Myocardial/valvular dysfunction: Progressive orthopnea or orthopnea with paroxysmal nocturnal dyspnea. Often present at end of second trimester or in early postpartum period when fluid shifts occur	Echocardiogram	Diuretics, β-blockers as indicated. ACE inhibitors contraindicated in pregnancy
Arrhythmia	Sudden onset and cessation, associated sensation of palpitations or chest discomfort	Electrocardiogram, holter or event monitor	β-blockers, calcium channel blockers
Venous thromboembolism	Sudden onset, any trimester. May have associated DVT features	Computerized tomography pulmonary angiogram, V/Q scan, lower extremity dopplers	Anticoagulation with injectable heparins in pregnancy, warfarin in the postpartum period

TABLE 2: Causes of acute respiratory failure in the obstetric patient.

Specific to pregnancy	Pulmonary edema (from preeclampsia and Tocolytic-associated), ARDS (from chorioamnionitis, placental abruption), peripartum cardiomyopathy, pulmonary embolism (amniotic fluid, trophoblastic embolism)
Risk increased by pregnancy	VTE, gastric acid aspiration, TRALI related acute lung injury, asthma ARDS due to sepsis, , pneumonia, stenotic valvular heart disease, and pulmonary hypertension
Nonspecific conditions	Trauma/drugs/toxins/acute organ inflammation

(ARDS: Acute respiratory distress syndrome; TRALI: Transfusion-related acute lung injury; VTE: venous thromboembolism)

it has been only recently endorsed by the Federation of Obstetricians and Gynecologists of India (FOGSI). Amantadine has been used in pregnancy as treatment and as prophylaxis, and oseltamivir was used quite extensively in pregnancy in the 2009 epidemic. Varicella pneumonia is also associated with significant morbidity and mortality during pregnancy. Treatment with acyclovir is necessary and reduces mortality in gravid patients.

Fungal pneumonia: Coccidioidomycosis is one of the most common fungal infection in pregnancy followed by cryptococcosis, blastomycosis, and sporotrichosis. Mortality can be avoided by early diagnosis and treatment of disseminated disease with antifungal agents, such as amphotericin B.[1,3]

TUBERCULOSIS

Incidence of tuberculosis among pregnant women would be as high as in the general population, with possibly higher incidence in developing countries. For India alone, their estimated burden of active tuberculosis (TB) among pregnant women was 44,500 (95% uncertainty range 36,000–62,000), which contributes 20.6% of global burden of all active TB among pregnant woman.[4] Factors affecting outcomes of TB in Pregnancy are given in **Figure 2** and modes of transmission of tuberculosis from mother to newborn infant are shown in **Figure 3**.

Symptoms

Cough with sputum (morning rise in frequency), fever, generalized weakness,

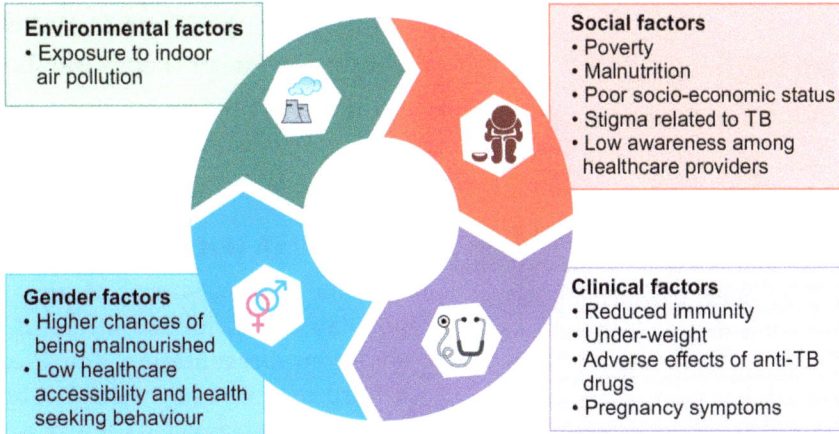

Fig. 2: Factors affecting outcomes in pregnancy.

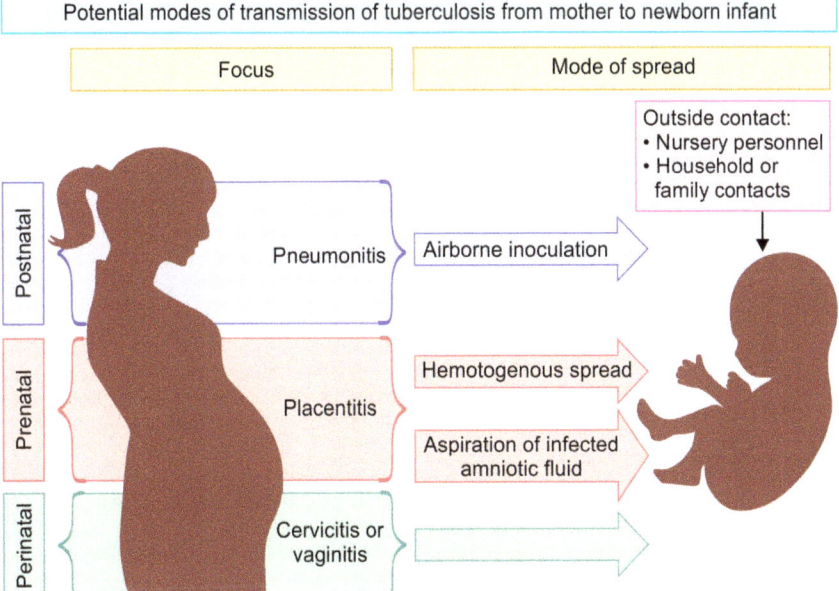

Fig. 3: Modes of transmission of tuberculosis from mother to newborn infant.

loss of weight, loss of appetite, night sweats, hemoptysis, lymphadenopathy, joint pain and swelling, and disorientation.[4]

Diagnosis

The diagnosis is confirmed with sputum examination for acid-fast bacilli (Ziehl–Neelsen stain). Although pregnancy and TB have little effect on each other, treatment should not be delayed in pregnancy.

Treatment Regimen

Drug Sensitive Tuberculosis

- Standard regimen for 6 months of which four drugs (rifampicin, isoniazid, ethambutol, pyrazinamide) to be given for first 2 months and three drugs for next 4 months (excluding pyrazinamide).
- Although the drugs used in the initial treatment regimen for TB cross the placenta, they do not have harmful effects on the fetus.

- In breast feeding women full course of anti-TB treatment is recommended. The dosage and the duration of anti-TB therapy is not modified due to pregnancy.
- Pyridoxine, 10 mg/day should be given with isoniazid during pregnancy because of increased requirement in pregnant women and to prevent potential neurotoxicity in the fetus.

Management of Pregnant Women Diagnosed with Tuberculosis

Management of pregnant women diagnosed with tuberculosis is depicted in **Flowchart 1** and **Table 3**.

■ ASTHMA (FIGS. 4 AND 5)

Asthma affects 4–8% of the general population and follows a rule of third as symptom presentation (approximately a third of asthmatics remain unchanged during pregnancy, while a similar proportion

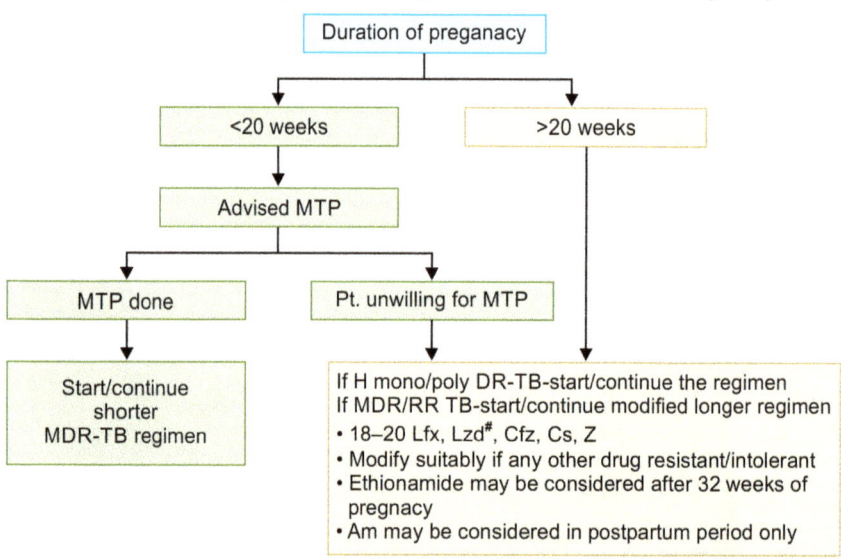

Flowchart 1: Management of drug-resistant tuberculosis in pregnancy.

(DR-TB: drug-resistant tuberculosis; MTP: medical termination of pregnancy; MDR-TB: multidrug-resistant tuberculosis)

TABLE 3: Postdelivery management of tuberculosis.

Drug sensitive tuberculosis (TB)	Drug resistant tuberculosis
• Both microbiological and histopathological examination of the placenta (using RKS funds) • Rule out neonatal TB (refer to updated pediatric TB guidelines) • Ensure initiation of INH chemoprophylaxis to the newborn of active TB affected pregnant mother if neonatal TB has been ruled out • Continue treatment of mother during the breastfeeding period and breastfeeding should not be stopped • Lactating women (0–6 months) require an additional 600 kcal and 19 g protein making their RDA 2,500 kcal of energy and 74 g of protein. For a sedentary lactating woman suffering from TB, an addition of 10% calories increases the requirement to 2,750 kcal, protein 74 g, 300 µg folic acid, 1200 mg calcium, 21 mg iron and 950 µg of vitamin A • Under Nikshay Poshan Yojana, nutritional support through direct benefit transfer of 500 INR per month for all patients on TB treatment throughout duration of treatment.	• Both microbiological and histopathological examination of the placenta (use RKS funds to conduct these investigations if not available in the hospital) • Rule out neonatal TB chemoprophylaxis to the newborn of active TB affected pregnant mother if neonatal TB has been ruled out • Continue treatment of mother during the breastfeeding period and breastfeeding should not be stopped • Lactating women (0–6 months) require an additional 600 kcal and 19 g protein making their RDA 2,500 kcal of energy and 74 g of protein. For a sedentary lactating woman suffering from TB, an addition of 10% calories increases the requirement to 2750 kcal, protein 74 g, 300 µg folic acid, 1200 mg calcium, 21 mg iron and 950 µg of vitamin A • Under Nikshay Poshan Yojana, nutritional support through direct benefit transfer of 500 INR per month for all patients on TB treatment throughout duration of treatment.[4]

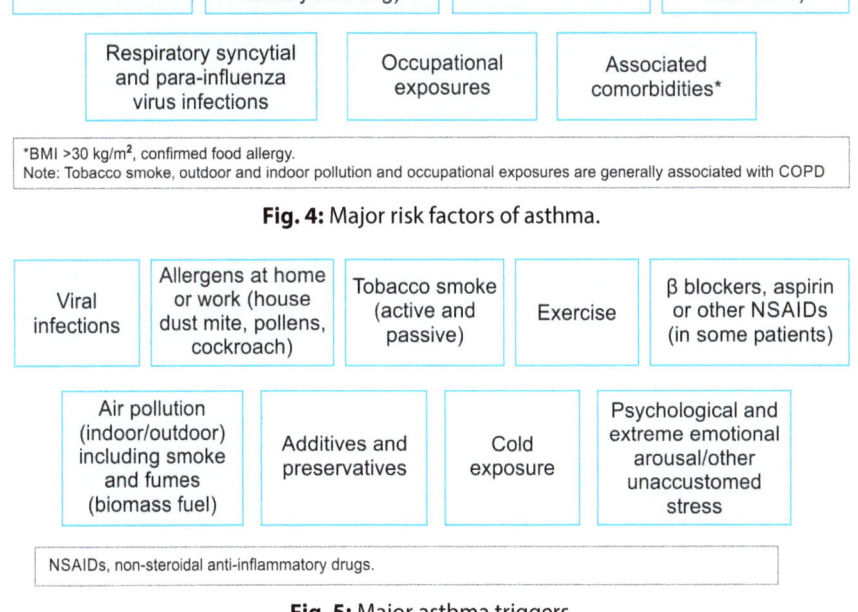

*BMI >30 kg/m², confirmed food allergy.
Note: Tobacco smoke, outdoor and indoor pollution and occupational exposures are generally associated with COPD

Fig. 4: Major risk factors of asthma.

NSAIDs, non-steroidal anti-inflammatory drugs.

Fig. 5: Major asthma triggers.

deteriorate or improve). Asthma during pregnancy can lead to increase in incidence of preterm labor, low neonatal birth weight, increased perinatal mortality, and can sometimes be associated with raised blood pressure. Most exacerbations of asthma symptoms occur during the last trimester. 90% has no symptoms during labor and delivery and within 3 months of delivery nearly 7.5% of women go back to their prepregnancy status. ACAAI – ACOG Recommendations: step therapy during pregnancy is given in **Table 4**.

Drugs to Avoid in Pregnancy for Asthma

Leukotriene receptor antagonists (LTRAs), systemic glucocorticoids (first and second trimester), prostaglandin F2α, theophylline (during pregnancy and lactation).

Management of the Acute Asthmatic Attack During Pregnancy

Selective short-acting β2-agonists have demonstrated an acceptable safety profile for the fetus. Halogenated corticosteroids (such as prednisolone and prednisone) do not cross the placenta to a significant degree, so fetal and neonatal adrenal suppression is not a major concern with these drugs. *Labor and delivery* carry some risks for asthmatic patients, partly due to the drugs commonly administered. Narcotics other than fentanyl may release histamine, which can worsen bronchospasm. Oxytocin is the optimal agent for labor induction and for postpartum hemorrhage, but 15-methyl prostaglandin F_2-alpha, methylergonovine, and ergonovine may cause bronchospasm and should be avoided in asthmatics.

TABLE 4: Step therapy during pregnancy.

Medication	Category	Category	Step therapy
Bronchodialators		Mid intermittent	Inhaled β2-agonists as needed (for all categories)
• Albuterol	C		
• Levalbuterol	C	Mid persistent	• Inhaled cromolyn
• Salmeterol	C		• Continue inhaled nedocromil in patients who have shown a goodresponse before pregnancy
• Fromoterol	C		
• Ipratropium	B		
Cromolyn sodium	B		• Substitute inhaled corticosteroids if above not adequate
Nedocromil	B		
Inhaled corticosteroids		Moderate persistent	• Inhaled corticosteroids
• Budesonide	B		• Continue inhaled salmeterol in patients who have sown a very good response before pregnancy
• Beclomethasone	C		
• Fluticasone	C		
• Triamcinolone	C		• Add oral theophylline and/or inhaled salmeterol for patients inaequately controlled by medium-dose inhaled corticosteroids
Leukotriene agents			
• Zafirlukast	B		
• Montelukast	B		
• Zileuton	C	Severe persistent	Above + oral corticosteroids (burst for active symptoms, alternate-day, or daily if necessary)
Oral corticosteroid	C		
Theophylline	C		

PULMONARY EDEMA

Pregnant women with pre-existing heart disease are at risk of cardiac decompensation especially in later stages of trimester, labor, and postpartum. Features are ↑ cardiac output, ↑ heart rate, ↓ systemic vascular resistance, and ↓ colloid osmotic pressure.

The most common cause of acute pulmonary edema in pregnancy is in association with severe preeclampsia followed by peripartum cardiomyopathy, multiple pregnancy, infections, and fluid overload. The treatment has to be done with oxygen support with respiratory support along with diuretics.

PULMONARY THROMBOEMBOLISM

Venous thromboembolism (VTE) in pregnancy is leading cause of direct maternal mortality in developed world and is 10 times more common in pregnancy (especially in postnatal period). The initial diagnostic test for venous thrombosis should be duplex ultrasonography if symptoms or signs of deep vein thrombosis (DVT) are present. Ventilation perfusion scanning is usually the preferred initial test to detect pulmonary embolism during pregnancy.[4] Treatment should be commenced on clinical suspicion and not be withheld until an objective diagnosis is obtained. The mainstay of treatment for pulmonary thromboembolism in pregnancy is low molecular weight heparin for a minimum of 3 months in total duration and until at least 6 weeks postnatal.

AMNIOTIC FLUID EMBOLISM

Risk factors for amniotic fluid embolism include older maternal age, high parity, cesarean section, low uterine segment laceration, and meconium staining of amniotic fluid. It may occur following early or late abortion, invasive procedures such as transabdominal amniocentesis, blunt abdominal trauma, or any surgical procedure. Radiographically, the patients usually develop bilateral pulmonary infiltrates. The cardinal criteria of amniotic fluid embolism are acute hypoxia diagnosed by dyspnea, cyanosis, and respiratory distress, followed by pulmonary edema, left sided heart failure, hemorrhagic shock, confusion, convulsion, coma, severe coagulopathy, and disseminated intravascular coagulation (DIC). If patient survives, injury to brain, lungs, and renal systems establish, which may last many weeks. Patient may die as a result of severe brain and lung injury, infection and multi organ failure. In acute phase, pulmonary hypertension may develop due to vascular occlusion (debris or vasoconstriction). If resolved, this may lead to left ventricular dysfunction or failure.

Plan: Immediate termination of pregnancy, multiple blood, plasma, and platelet transfusions. Cardiopulmonary resuscitative measures, inotropes, oxygen by using tracheal tube or mechanical ventilation.[5]

ACUTE RESPIRATORY DISTRESS SYNDROME

Symptoms

Dyspnea, tachypnea, cyanosis, tachycardia, and changes in mental status that occur 12–72 hours after the inciting event. Martin and associates developed the mnemonic GESTOSIS: Gestational complications; Embolic events; Sepsis; Transfusion (rapid and massive); Other (diabetic ketoacidosis, sickle cell crisis); Substance abuse; Irritants (aspiration, burns); and Severe pregnancy-induced hypertension.

Diagnosis

The ARDS include (1) Radiologic evidence of pulmonary edema; (2) Elimination of cardiac causes for pulmonary edema (i.e., a pulmonary capillary wedge pressure of <12 mmHg); (3) Severe hypoxemia requiring >50% inspired oxygen; and (4) Reduced lung compliance. The overall mortality rate for ARDS in the general population ranges from 30 to 70%, the highest mortality rate being among patients suffering from multisystem organ failure.

Treatment

Consists of elimination of the cause and supportive care consisting of hemodynamic and nutritional support and mechanical ventilation. The most important treatment is delivery of the baby if the patient can tolerate it and the baby is at a safe gestational age.[2]

Preeclampsia: The most common obstetric disorder, with multisystem ramifications, ↑ minute ventilation because of ↑ concentration of blood leptin (a ventilation-stimulating hormone), ↓ vital capacity secondary to lower transverse section area of the upper airways, pharyngeal edema, and excessive weight gain with higher adipose deposition around the neck.

Cardiopulmonary transplantation: It is crucial not to conceive within 2 years of transplantation as it can lead to potential pregnancy-related complications—prematurity, low weight at birth, and postpartum graft loss. There is an absolute need for maintenance of immunosuppression with close monitoring of cyclosporine blood levels during gestation.

Hereditary neuromuscular disorders: There is an ↑ respiratory muscle load by higher airway resistance and impaired bulbar load, leading to overwhelmed respiratory muscle capacity. It is important that monitoring of respiratory and cough function is done. They also have high aspiration risk in the third trimester because of ↑ abdominal pressure and ↓ gastroesophageal sphincter tone.

Others: Mendelson/*gastric acid aspiration* is related to the increased intra-abdominal pressure caused by the enlarged uterus, the effect of progesterone lowering the tone of the esophageal sphincter, as well as use of the supine position for delivery. Aspiration of gastric contents with pH 2.5 or lower causes chemical pneumonitis with permeability edema. *Transfusion related acute lung injury (TRALI)* is a complication of blood component therapy, which may occur in pregnancy. The clinical presentation is of sudden onset of dyspnea during, or within 6 hours, of transfusion of plasma-containing blood products.

■ CYSTIC FIBROSIS

Cystic fibrosis is a single gene mutation on chromosome 7. It is characterized by exocrine gland dysfunction, with the lungs and pancreas being primarily affected.

Symptoms

Chronic, recurrent infections, bronchiectasis, and airway obstruction. Those with mild disease, early diagnosis and good nutritional status tend to tolerate pregnancy well.[6,7]

■ RESTRICTIVE LUNG DISEASES

Interstitial lung diseases (ILD) are not very common in woman in their childbearing years. There are conditions which may occur in this age-group and some, including lymphangioleiomyomatosis and systemic lupus erythematosus, may worsen as a result of pregnancy. ILD in pregnancy may present as hypoxemia and difficulty in meeting the increased oxygen requirements of pregnancy.

Women with chest wall restrictive disease (e.g., kyphoscoliosis) or neuromuscular weakness may not be able to meet the increased ventilation demands of pregnancy, putting them at-risk of respiratory failure. Due to the lack of pulmonary parenchymal disease, oxygenation problems are less of a concern. Minimal complication includes preterm delivery with newborn needing high-dependency support. Lung function and oxygen saturation should be monitored with need of oxygen therapy and noninvasive ventilation.[8]

VENTILATORY MANAGEMENT OF PREGNANT WOMEN

Intubation: Nasal intubation has to be avoided and a smaller size endotracheal tube should be kept in emergency trolley. Preoxygenation is essential, although arterial blood gas (ABG) has to be maintained avoiding respiratory alkalosis. Mendelson aspiration should always be considered.

Noninvasive ventilation can be performed on pregnant woman who is alert and conscious and need of ventilator is brief.

Invasive mechanical ventilation: Hyperventilation and alkalosis should be avoided to prevent uterine vasoconstriction. Slightly higher airway pressures may be needed to achieve appropriate tidal volumes in pregnant women near term. A maternal oxygenation goal of pO_2 greater than 70 mm Hg has been advised.

DELIVERY OF THE FETUS

If the fetus is at a viable gestation and is at-risk due to intractable maternal hypoxia, then it is better to deliver the fetus. The mode of delivery should be determined by standard obstetrical principles. Although cesarean section may allow more rapid delivery in the critically-ill patient, there is significantly increased physiological stress, and operative delivery has been associated with higher mortality in these patients. Delivery should not be performed solely in an attempt to improve maternal oxygenation or ventilation. It is essential that the intensive care unit (ICU) have prearranged plans for urgent delivery and neonatal resuscitation in the event of spontaneous labor or sudden maternal or fetal deterioration. This should include immediate availability of all necessary equipment, drugs, and staff contact details.

CONCLUSION

Dyspnea and hyperventilation are common symptoms of pregnancy, they are usually benign and not indicative of serious underlying pathology. Commonly encountered acute respiratory conditions include thromboembolic disease, amniotic fluid embolism, aspiration, pneumonia, and pulmonary edema. Chronic pulmonary diseases especially asthma and tuberculosis can poorly affect both mother and fetus.[3,4] Women with a chronic respiratory disease should receive prepregnancy counseling and education regarding the risks of pregnancy and the importance of continuing their medications and pregnancy. Women should be managed in a multidisciplinary setup with regular review by chest physicians and access to chest physiotherapy if necessary.[9]

REFERENCES

1. Leighton B, Fish J. Pulmonary Disease in Pregnancy. GLOWM. 2008;1756-2228.
2. Mehta N. Respiratory Disease in Pregnancy. Reproductive Immunol Open Acc. 2016; 1:14.

3. Stone S, Nelson-Piercy C. Respiratory disease in pregnancy. Obstet Gynaecol Reprod Med. 2007;17(5):140-6.
4. Ministry of Health and Family welfare. Central Tuberculosis Division, Government of India, National Tuberculosis Elimination Programme. [online] Available from tbcindia.gov.in [Last accessed November, 2022].
5. British Thoracic Society Standards of Care Committee. BTS Guidelines for the Management of Community Acquired Pneumonia in Adults. *Thorax.* 2001;56 (suppl IV):IV1-64.
6. De Swiet M. Respiratory disease. In: de Swiet M (Ed). *Medical disorders in obstetric practice,* 4th edition. London: Blackwell Science; 2002. pp. 1-28.
7. Kothari A, Mahadevan N, Girling J. Tuberculosis and pregnancy—Results of a study in a high prevalence area in London. Eur J Obstet Gynecol Reprod Biol. 2006;126(1):48-55.
8. Murphy VE, Clifton VL, Gibson PG. Asthma exacerbations during pregnancy: incidence and association with adverse pregnancy outcomes. Thorax. 2006;61(2):169-76.
9. Nelson-Piercy C. Respiratory disease. In: Nelson-Piercy C (Ed). Handbook of obstetric medicine, 3rd edition. London: Informa Healthcare; 2006. pp. 65-90.

CHAPTER 8

Renal Disorders

Ankita Jain

INTRODUCTION

The maternal and perinatal outcomes in pregnancies with kidney disorders have drastically improved in the past four to five decades.[1] This can be accounted for a better understanding of renal physiology in pregnancy as well as early recognition and prompt treatment. Renal disorders in pregnancy include asymptomatic bacteriuria, acute kidney insufficiency, chronic kidney disease, a renal disease requiring dialysis, acute cortical and tubular necrosis, end-stage renal disease, pregnancy after renal transplant, glomerulonephritis, and nephropathy due to collagen vascular diseases. Some of the important disorders commonly encountered in the Indian scenario have been discussed in this chapter.

RENAL PHYSIOLOGY DURING PREGNANCY

The physiological changes in the renal system have been depicted in **Table 1**.[2-4]

ASYMPTOMATIC BACTERIURIA AND URINARY TRACT INFECTION

- Asymptomatic bacteriuria (ASB)
- Lower urinary tract infection (UTI) (acute cystitis)
- Upper UTI (acute pyelonephritis).

These account for frequent complications in pregnancy, if left untreated. These have been discussed in further detail in **Table 2**.[5-14]

TABLE 1: Renal physiology during pregnancy.[2-4]

	Renal	Renal hemodynamics	Cardiovascular	Volume hemostasis	Acid-base balance
↑	• Size and volume of kidney and collecting system • Glomerular membrane porosity • Ureteral smooth muscle hypertrophy	• RPF (50–85%) • GFR (40–65%) • Creatinine clearance • Filtration of sugar and protein	• Stroke volume • Cardiac output	• Total body water (6.5 L at term) • Plasma volume (40–50%)	• pH (7.42–7.46) • Bicarbonate reabsorption
↓		Renal vascular resistance	Systemic vascular resistance	Plasma osmolality (by 10 mOsm/kg) S. albumin	pCO_2 (18–22 mmol/L)

(GFR: glomerular filtration rate; RPF: renal plasma flow; S. albumin: serum albumin)

TABLE 2: ASB and UTI in pregnancy.[5-14]

	Asymptomatic bacteriuria (ASB)	*Acute cystitis (lower UTI)*	*Acute pyelonephritis (upper UTI)*
Definition	Positive urine culture in an asymptomatic person	Positive urine culture with lower urinary tract symptoms (refer below)	Positive urine culture with upper urinary tract symptoms (refer below)
Incidence	2–7%		
Complications	Maternal: Ascending infection: • ASB → Lower UTI → Upper UTI → Urosepsis • Preterm labour • PPROM • Fever/hyperpyrexia Fetal: • IUD • Preterm birth • LBW • NICU admission • Neonatal sepsis		
Signs and symptoms	None	• Frequency • Dysuria • Lower abdominal pain • Low grade fever	• Features of acute cystitis • Fever ± chills • Renal angle tenderness • Features of sepsis
Screening	• At booking visits in all pregnant women • Once in every trimester		
Diagnosis	• "Clean catch sample" of midstream urine • Urine routine and microscopy and urine culture • USG–KUB—acute pyelonephritis • Significant bacteriuria: >10^5 CFU/mL		
Treatment	• Increased water intake • Antibiotic (as per culture sensitivity) for 7 days		
	• Fosfomycin 3 g stat dose • Nitrofurantoin 100 mg BD PO for 7 days • Amoxicillin 500 mg TDS PO × 7 days	• Fosfomycin 3 g stat dose • Nitrofurantoin 100 mg BD PO for 7 days • Amoxicillin 500 mg TDS PO × 7 days	• Ceftriaxone 1 g daily until afebrile for 48 h → oral cephalexin 500 mg 6 h for 10 days • Clindamycin IV 900 mg TDS and gentamicin IV 1.5 mg/kg TDS

(CFU: colony-forming units; IUD: intrauterine death; NICU: neonatal intensive care unit; TDS: three times daily; UTI: urinary tract infection; USG–KUB: ultrasonography–kidneys, ureters, and urinary bladder)

PREGNANCY-RELATED ACUTE KIDNEY INJURY

Pregnancy-related acute kidney injury (PRAKI), although a rare event in developed countries, still remains a significant cause for maternal morbidity and mortality in developing countries. In India, its incidence has decreased from 22% in 1960 to 3–7% in the 2000s.[15,16] Hence, it

TABLE 3: AKI definition, classification and staging systems.[15]

AKI definition, classification, and staging systems

	RIFLE criteria			AKIN criteria			KDIGO criteria	
Stage	Increase in S. Cr.	Urine output	Stage	Increase in S. Cr.	Urine output	Stage	Increase in S. Cr.	Urine output
R	X1.5	<0.5 mL/kg/h for 6–12 h	1	≥1.5–2.0 × or ≥0.3 mg/dL	<0.5 mL/kg/h for 6–12 h	1	≥1.5–1.9 × or ≥ 0.3 mg/dL	<0.5 mL/kg/h for 6–12 h
I	X2.0	<0.5 mL/kg/h for 12 h	2	≥2.0–3.0	<0.5 mL/kg/h for 12 h	2	≥2.0–2.9 × or ≥ 3 mg/dL	<0.5 mL/kg/h for 12 h
F	X3.0 Or S. Cr. >4 mg/dL	<0.3 mL/kg/h for 24 h or anuria for 12 h	3	≥3.0 × or ≥4 mg/dL or received RRT	<0.3 mL/kg/h for 24 h or anuria for 12 h	3	≥3.0 × or ≥4 mg/dL or received RRT	<0.3 mL/kg/h for 24 h or anuria for 12 h
L	Persistent ARF>4 weeks							
E	ESKD >4 months							

(AKIN: acute kidney injury network; ESKD: end-stage kidney disease; GFR: glomerular filtration rate; KDIGO: kidney disease improving global outcomes; RIFLE: risk of renal failure, injury to the kidney, failure of kidney function, loss of kidney function, end-stage renal failure;; RRT: renal replacement therapy; S. Cr.: serum creatinine; X: times)

is important to be aware of the causes of acute kidney injury (AKI) in pregnancy and the measures that can be taken to prevent it.

Till date, there has been no consensus on a standard definition of PRAKI. **Table 3** depicts the commonly used classification systems in non-pregnant adults.

Etiology of AKI is multifactorial. Causes of PRAKI based on pathophysiological mechanism and location of pathology have been tabulated in **Table 4**.[16]

Management of PRAKI

Table 5 summarizes the management of patients of PRAKI.[16]

PREGNANCY WITH CHRONIC KIDNEY DISEASE

Chronic kidney disease (CKD) is defined as abnormal kidney structure or function documented or inferred for >3 months with implications for health and one of the following two criteria:

1. GFR <60 mL/min/1.73 m^2
2. Markers of kidney damage including albuminuria.[17]

Although the incidence of such pregnancies in low (2–12/10,000 women) it poses a challenging scenario for obstetricians.[18] The outcome of pregnancy depends on the degree of renal impairment, the presence of chronic hypertension, the presence of proteinuria, and the underlying renal pathology.

Table 6 enumerates the complications of CKD in pregnancy.

The various renal diseases and their effects on pregnancy are depicted in **Table 7** and **Table 8** discusses the guidelines on the management of these renal diseases.[18]

TABLE 4: Causes of PRAKI.[16]

Causes of PRAKI

Prerenal causes

Pregnancy-related conditions:
- Hypovolemia due to water loss:
  – Hyperemesis gravidarum
  – Vomiting due to preeclampsia, HELLP, and AFLP
- Hypovolemia due to hemorrhage:
  – Early pregnancy bleeding (abortion, ectopic, and molar pregnancy)
  – APH and placental abruption
  – APH and placenta previa
  – PPH (uterine atony, bleeding during surgery, and uterine laceration)
  – Uterine rupture/perforation
- Hypotension due to decreased effective circulating volume
  – Septic abortion
  – Puerperal sepsis

Pregnancy-unrelated conditions:
- Acute gastroenteritis (AGE)
- Pyelonephritis/urosepsis

Renal causes

Pregnancy-related conditions:
- Preeclampsia, eclampsia, and HELLP syndrome
- FLP
- Hepatorenal syndrome (HRS)
- Hemolytic uremic syndrome (HUS)
- Thrombotic thrombocytopenic purpura (TTP)
- DIC
- Glomerulonephritis
- Autoimmune disorders

Postrenal causes

Pregnancy-related conditions:
- Multifetal gestation
- Trauma to the ureters and bladder during cesarean section

Pregnancy-unrelated conditions:
- Renal/ureteral stones
- Large uterine fibroid

(AFLP: acute fatty liver of pregnancy; APH: antepartum hemorrhage; DIC: disseminated intravascular coagulation; HELLP: hemolysis, elevated liver enzymes, and low platelet count; PPH: postpartum hemorrhage)

TABLE 5: Management of PRAKI.[16]

General principles	Specific management
• Stabilize the patient • HDU/ICU care • Involve nephrologists • Treat the pathology • Avoid nephrotoxic drugs • Prevent further kidney damage • Supportive care for mother (priority) • Monitor fetal well-being	• Patient vitals and intake-output • Assessment of respiratory, circulatory, and hemodynamic systems • CBC, blood group, KFT with SE, ABG (where necessary), USG–KUB • Volume resuscitation—oral fluids (where possible), IV crystalloids and colloids, and blood products • Treat underlying cause—antihypertensive and delivery • Loop diuretics • Low-dose dopamine infusion • RRT (where necessary) • Correction of acid-base imbalance • Correct dyselectrolytemia

(ABG: arterial blood gas; CBC: complete blood count; HDU: high dependency unit; ICU: intensive care unit; KFT: kidney function tests; RRT: renal replacement therapy; USG–KUB: ultrasonography–kidneys, ureters, and urinary bladder)

TABLE 6: Complications of CKD in pregnancy.[17-18]

Complications	Degree of renal impairment (%)		
	Mild	Moderate	Severe
Chronic hypertension	25	30–70	50
Gestational hypertension	20–50	30–50	75
Further impairment of renal function	8–15	20–43	35
Preterm delivery	7	30–60	73
Fetal growth restriction	8–14	30–38	57
Perinatal mortality	5–14	4–7	0

(CKD: Chronic kidney disease)

TABLE 7: Renal diseases and their effects on pregnancy.[18]

Chronic glomerulonephritis and focal glomerular sclerosis	• Urinary tract infection is more common • No adverse effect unless hypertensive
IgA nephropathy	• Risk of uncontrolled hypertension worsening renal function
Pyelonephritis	• Urosepsis • Multiorgan failure • Acute respiratory distress syndrome
Urolithiasis	• More prone to infection • Can be managed with stents and ureterostomy
Diabetic nephropathy	• No change in renal lesion • Increased risk of infection and preeclampsia
Systemic lupus erythematosus	Higher doses of steroids may be needed postpartum
After nephrectomy or solitary kidney	• Association with other malformations • Pregnancy rarely affected
Renal artery stenosis	Chronic hypertension or as recurrent isolated preeclampsia

TABLE 8: Guidelines for management of renal disease in pregnancy.[18]

General	Multidisciplinary team: • Obstetrician • Renal/obstetric physician • Specialist midwife
Prepregnancy	• Couple counseling • Modify risk factors • Optimize medications • If considering IVF—single embryo transfer is preferred
Antenatal	• Low-dose aspirin in first trimester—prophylaxis against preeclampsia • Quantification of proteinuria—24 hours urine protein and protein/creatinine ratio (PCR) • Persistent proteinuria (>500 mg/day) before 20 weeks—nephrology referral • Nephrotic syndrome—thromboprophylaxis with heparin in the antenatal and postpartum period • Lesser degree of proteinuria—may need thromboprophylaxis • Treat asymptomatic bacteriuria and UTI • Recurrent UTI and kidney disease—antibiotic prophylaxis target blood pressure <140/90 mm Hg *Drugs:* • Should not be discontinued—prednisolone, azathioprine, cyclosporine, or tacrolimus (teratogenicity unknown) • Uncertain safety—mycophenolate mofetil/enteric-coated mycophenolic acid, sirolimus, everolimus, and rituximab
Postpartum	• Planned early postpartum renal review • Offer early contraceptive advice • Evaluate for underlying kidney disease in early-onset preeclampsia (<32 weeks)

CONCLUSION

Screening of asymptomatic bacteriuria and early recognition of urinary tract infections can present many of the complications in pregnancy, especially preterm premature rupture of membranes and preterm delivery. Pregnancy with renal disorders poses a challenging situation for obstetricians and requires management through a multidisciplinary team approach. Pregnant mothers with only mildly deranged renal function usually have few complications in pregnancy. Moderate to severe impairment of renal function leads to increased pregnancy complications and raises the risk of long-term renal impairment. Appropriate counseling and management by an expert team is necessary when handling these women.

REFERENCES

1. Wiles K, Chappell L, Clark K, Elman L, Hall M, Lightstone L, et al. Clinical practice guideline on pregnancy and renal disease. BMC Nephrol. 2019;20(1):401.
2. Gonzalez Suarez ML, Kattah A, Grande JP, Garovic V. Renal Disorders in Pregnancy: Core Curriculum 2019. Am J Kidney Dis. 2019;73(1):119-30.
3. Erratum in: Am J Kidney Dis. 2019;73(6):897.
4. Belzile M, Pouliot A, Cumyn A, Côté AM. Renal physiology and fluid and electrolyte disorders in pregnancy. Best Pract Res Clin Obstet Gynaecol. 2019;57:1-14.
5. Davison JM. Renal disorders in pregnancy. Curr Opin Obstet Gynecol. 2001;13(2):109-14.
6. Mussap M, Noto A. Renal disorders in pregnancy. J Lab Precis Med. 2020.
7. Hnat M, Sibai B. Renal disease and pregnancy. Glob Libr Women's Med. 2008.
8. Bayrak O, Cimentepe E, Inegol I, Atmaca AF, Duvan CI, Koc A, et al. Is single-dose fosfomycin trometamol a good alternative for asymptomatic bacteriuria in the second trimester of pregnancy?" Int Urogynecol J Pelvic Floor Dysfunct. 2007;18(5):525-9.
9. Brost BC, Campbell B, Stramm S, Eller D, Newman RB. Randomized clinical trial of antibiotic therapy for antenatal pyelonephritis. Infect Dis Obstet Gynecol. 1996;4:294-7.
10. Cunningham FG, Lucas MJ. Urinary tract infections complicating pregnancy. Baillieres Clin Obstet Gynaecol. 1994;8(2):353-73.
11. Guinto VT, De Guia B, Festin MR, Dowswell T. Different antibiotic regimens for treating asymptomatic bacteriuria in pregnancy. Cochrane Database Syst Rev. 2010;8(9):CD007855.
12. Kenyon SL, Taylor DJ, Tarnow-Mordi W. Broad-spectrum antibiotics for preterm, prelabour rupture of fetal membranes: the ORACLE I randomised trial. Lancet. 2001;357:979-88.
13. Krcmery S, Hromec J, Demesova D. Treatment of lower urinary tract infection in pregnancy. Int J Antimicrob Agents. 2001;17(4):279-82.
14. Smaill F, Vazquez JC. Antibiotics for asymptomatic bacteriuria in pregnancy. Cochrane Database Syst Rev. 2019; 2019:CD000490.
15. Palevsky PM, Liu KD, Brophy PD, Chawla LS, Parikh CR, Thakar CV, et al. KDOQI US commentary on the 2012 KDIGO clinical practice guideline for acute kidney injury. Am J Kidney Dis. 2013;61(5):649-72.
16. Davison J, Nelson-Piercy C, Kehoe S, Baker P. Renal disease in pregnancy. United Kingdom: Cambridge University Press; 2008.
17. Kapoor N, Makanjuola D, Shehata H. Management of women with chronic renal disease in pregnancy. Obstet Gynecol. 2009; 11(3):185-91.
18. Bramham K, Hall M, Nelson-Piercy C. Renal disease in pregnancy. United Kingdom: Cambridge University Press; 2018.

Hematological and Coagulation Disorders (VTE)

Nidhi Bansal

BACKGROUND

- Women with hematological disorders, including inherited and acquired blood disorders, can face many problems during pregnancy.[1]
- Among all the disorders during pregnancy major is anemia in developing world. More than 70% women in developing countries suffer from nutritional anemia but global prevalence is 42%. It may be mild, moderate, and severe type but when it is severe, it may cause significant risks to mother and fetus both.[2]
- Normally pregnancy is a state of physiological anemia so if patient is already anemic then it may worsen the situations. In developing countries, anemia is associated with up to 13% of maternal deaths.[3]
- All the three types of cell lines may be associated with hematological disorders including red blood cells (RBCs), white blood cells (WBCs), and platelet disorders, coagulation disorders, and hematological malignancies.
- So, it is very important to understand types of all disorders to make a correct diagnosis and to insure a proper treatment according to the guidelines.

PHYSIOLOGICAL CHANGES DURING PREGNANCY

The most dramatic changes occur in hematological system during pregnancy. The RBCs increase by 30% while plasma volume increases by 40-50%, resulting in hemodilutional state by 5-15% normally in pregnancy. This is known as physiological anemia of pregnancy. In pregnancy a total of 1 g iron is required of which 500 mg goes to fetus and placenta and 250 mg is lost during delivery. So, exact daily need of iron is 4-6 mg/day in second trimester but it increases to 6-8 mg/day in third trimester.[4,5]

ICMR Classification of Anemia in Pregnancy

Indian Council of Medical Research (ICMR) classifies anemia as:
- Mild: 10-10.9 g/dL
- Moderate: 7-9.9 g/dL
- Severe: <7 g/dL
- Very severe: <4 g/dL.

Classification of Anemia

- *Nutritional:*
    - Iron deficiency } Microcytic anemia
    - Folic acid deficiency } Megaloblastic anemia
    - Vitamin B_{12} deficiency
    - Dimorphic/mixed
- *Hemoglobinopathies:*
    - Thalassemia
    - Sickle cell anemia
- *Miscellaneous:*
    - Protein malnutrition
    - Acquired/heredity hemolytic anemia
    - Anemia due to:

- Chronic infection (malaria, hookworm)
- Chronic diseases
- Malignancy.

HEMATOLOGICAL CHANGES DURING PREGNANCY

Table 1 depicts the hematological changes during pregnancy.

Effect of Anemia on Mother and Fetus[6,7]

Maternal anemia may lead to complications in pregnancy **(Table 2)**.

Diagnosis of Anemia in Pregnancy

Symptoms and signs: Generally nonspecific clinical features are seen in anemia and they are like normal pregnancy symptoms. Fatigue, weakness, palpitations, dizziness dyspnea, and headache are few of them.

Most important way to diagnose and differentiate anemia is by laboratory diagnosis.

Laboratory tests **(Table 1)**:[8]
- Hb%
- Red cell indices [mean corpuscular volume (MCV), mean corpuscular hemoglobin (MCH), and mean corpuscular hemoglobin concentration (MCHC)]
- Peripheral blood picture (microcytic, macrocytic, dimorphic, or hemolytic anemia)
- Complete urine examination
- Stool examination on three consecutive days by concentration method
- Serum ferritin—the most useful parameter for assessing iron deficiency; levels <15 pg/L are diagnostic of established iron deficiency while levels <30 pg/L in pregnancy should prompt treatment.
- Reticulocyte count (to observe response to treatment).

Management of Iron Deficiency Anemia in Pregnancy (Flowchart 1)

The principles of management are as follows:
- Ideally, the woman should approach labor with a hemoglobin level 100%.

TABLE 1: Hematological changes during pregnancy.

Parameter	Nonpregnant	Pregnant
Hemoglobin	12–16	11.5–13.5
Hematocrit (vol)	37–44	34–31
MCV (fl)	86–96	84–95
MCH (pg)	28–32	27–32
MCHC (g/dL)	32–34	32–35

(MCV: mean corpuscular volume; MCH: mean corpuscular hemoglobin; MCHC: mean corpuscular hemoglobin concentration)

TABLE 2: Effect of anemia on mother and fetus.

Effect on mother and pregnancy	Effect on fetus and infant
• Increased susceptibility to infection (immunity) • Disturbances of postpartum cognition and emotions • Preterm delivery • Intrauterine growth restriction (IUGR) • Preeclampsia • Abruptio placentae • Uterine atony and postpartum hemorrhage (PPH)	• Fetus relatively protected from the effects of iron deficiency by upregulation of placental iron transport proteins • Prematurity • Increased risk of iron deficiency in the first 3 months of life • Impaired psychomotor and mental development

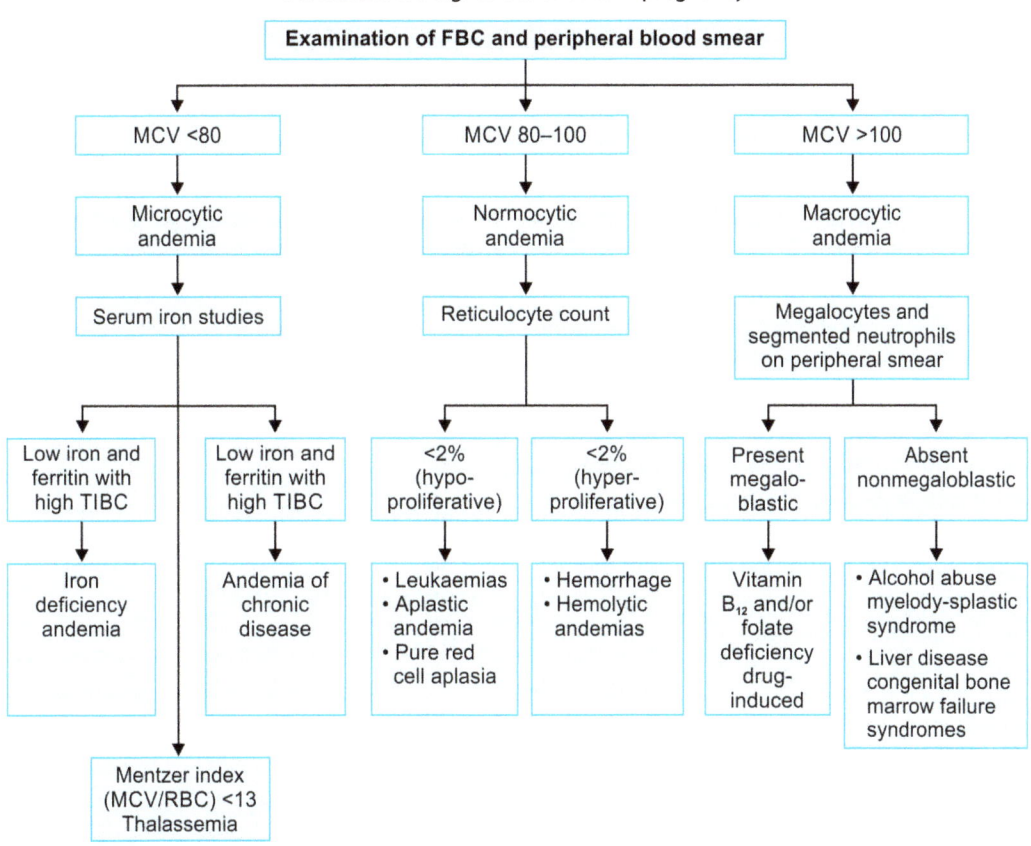

Flowchart 1: Diagnosis of anemia in pregnancy.

(FBC: full blood count; MCV: mean corpuscular volume; RBC: red blood cell; TIBC: total iron-binding capacity)

- Oral iron is the preferred choice of treatment.
- Dietary modifications may be advised to promote oral iron absorption.
- Parenteral iron therapy and blood transfusion are indicated only in specific circumstances.

Diet is the main cause of iron deficiency in India. Most dietary iron is unutilized or unabsorbed due to the predominance of phytates in our diet, which chelate iron away from the gut. Also, 95% of dietary iron intake is from nonheme sources, whose absorption may decrease due to a diet poor in Vitamin C. The following modifications should be suggested to pregnant women to increase the absorption of dietary iron:

- Germination and fermentation of cereals and legumes to increase bioavailability.
- Reduction in the phytate content of food by using mixed cereals.
- Inclusion of a source of Vitamin C (citrus) in the daily diet.
- Avoidance of tea and coffee shortly after meals.

The therapeutic dose of iron in the deficiency state is 180 mg/day three divided doses; this is continued at the same dosage till the blood indices return to normal. Thereafter, therapy is maintained using supplemental

TABLE 3: Percentage and amount of iron in common iron preparations.

Preparation	Molecular iron (mg/tablet)	Percentage of iron (%)	Elemental iron (mg/tab)
Ferrous sulfate	200	30	60
Ferrous fumarate	200	33	66
Ferrous gluconate	300	12	36

doses as it takes a considerable time (preferably continued in the postpartum period till such time as the woman breastfeeds her baby) to replenish the iron stores. The supplementation dose in pregnancy is provided by 60 mg daily of elemental iron **(Table 3)**.

Oral iron should be taken on empty stomach, 1 hour before meals, with a vitamin C source such as dilute lemon/orange juice or amla. Antacids should not be taken at the same time. The Hb rise with oral iron therapy is nearly 1.0 g/dL/day from the second week of treatment, though the reticulocyte counts starts rising within 5-10 days of initiating treatment **(Box 1)**.[9,10]

Routine daily supplementation of 100 mg of elemental iron and 500 μg of folic acid is recommended for all pregnant women in India for at least 100 days.

The reasons for failure to respond to oral iron therapy (refractory anemia) may be:
- Inaccurate diagnosis (thalassemia, pyridoxine deficiency, lead poisoning)
- Noncompliance
- Continued blood loss (hookworm infestation, bleeding piles)
- Coexisting infection (malaria, pyogenic infection)
- Concomitant folate deficiency.

Parenteral iron can be given by intramuscular (IM) and intravenous (IV) routes. The dose calculation is as follows:

[(Normal Hb − Patient's Hb) × Weight* (kg) + 1000**] mg of elemental iron

___
*Prepregnancy weight
**To replenish iron stores

BOX 1: Indication for parenteral iron treatment (can be started from the second trimester till the postpartum period).

- Intolerance to oral iron
- Noncompliance
- Malabsorption syndromes
- Development of serious side effects with oral iron which cannot be treated by simple measures

The rise in Hb is the same as with oral iron (1 g/dL/week from the second week)

Parenteral Iron Treatment

Intramuscular injections:
- Iron dextran complex (Imferon)
- Iron sorbitol citrate (Jectofer)
- Given by deep IM injection using Z technique
- Not more than 100 mg of elemental iron injected daily
- Adverse effects include pain and skin discoloration at the site of injection, abscess formation, nausea, vomiting, headache, fever, lymphadenopathy, allergic reactions, arthritis, and rarely anaphylaxis.

Intravenous infusion:
- Iron dextran complex
- Total dose calculated dissolved in 0.9% saline or 5% dextrose solution and infused slowly
- Test dose administered and the patient observed for adverse reactions before infusing the total dose
- If the calculated dose is >2,500 mg, it is divided and infused in 2 consecutive days hemolysis and anaphylactic reaction.

Iron sucrose complex:
- Ferric hydroxide saccharide complex
- Ferric carboxymaltose
- Available as 2.5 mL and 5 mL vials containing 20 mg elemental iron per mL
- Given by IV infusion, diluted in 100 mL 0.9% saline (100 mg at one sitting)
- Given on alternate days or twice weekly; cannot be given as total dose infusion
- Does not require a test dose
- Anaphylaxis is rare.

Indications for blood transfusion in pregnancy with anemia:
- Severe anemia detected in the last 4 weeks or pregnancy
- Associated infection resulting in refractory anemia
- Blood loss due to antepartum or postpartum hemorrhage
- Anemia not responding to oral or parenteral iron therapy.

Management of Delivery[11,12]
- Hospital delivery in cases of moderate and severe anemia
- Antibiotic prophylaxis (amoxicillin 500 mg IV, eight hourly till delivery of the baby)
- Digitalization in cardiac failure due to very severe anemia
- Prolongation of second stage of labor to be avoided
- Active management of third stage of labor (10 IU oxytocin IM, immediately after the delivery of the baby + controlled cord traction)
- Intravenous infusion of 40 IU oxytocin continued for 2-4 hours in cases of prolonged labor or instrumental delivery
- Misoprostol 600–800 μg per rectally, a good alternative for management of third stage of labor.

Management of Puerperium
- Oral iron and folate supplementation continued for at least 3 months postpartum, if not for the whole lactation period.
- Careful watch for the development of puerperal sepsis, thromboembolism, subinvolution of uterus, and failure of lactation.

■ MEGALOBLASTIC ANEMIA

This is due to deficiency of either folic acid or vitamin B_{12} or both. Vitamin B_{12} deficiency is rare. In India, iron deficiency anemia and folic acid deficiency coexist because of cooking methods, where the folate is destroyed at high temperatures. This is an addition to the increased demand for folic acid in pregnancy. Folate deficiency in pregnancy is commonly associated with twin pregnancy, chronic malaria, and antifolate medication (antiepileptic drugs, trimethoprim, and pyrimethamine).[13]

Folate deficiency in pregnancy is responsible for the increased incidence of miscarriage, intrauterine growth restriction (IUGR), placental abruption, and preeclampsia (PEC). It is an established cause of neural tube defects, prematurity, and growth restriction in the fetus. It is also responsible for folate deficiency in the newborn.

Clinical Features
Tables 4 and 5 list the clinical features of megaloblastic anemia.

Diagnosis
- Peripheral blood picture
- Serum folate <3 ng/mL
- Red cell folate <150 ng/mL.

Treatment
- Prophylaxis in pregnancy—300–500 μg/day

- Treatment in pregnancy—5 mg/day, to be continued for at least 4 weeks in puerperium.

HEMOGLOBINOPATHIES

Hemoglobinopathies are a diverse group of inherited disorders that can vary from asymptomatic laboratory abnormalities to life-threatening manifestations.[1] Hemoglobinopathies can be classified broadly as disorders that result from structurally altered hemoglobin molecules (e.g., sickle cell anemia) or disorders that arise from imbalance of otherwise normal globin chain synthesis (e.g., β-thalassemia).[2] There are five major classes of hemoglobinopathies as shown in **Box 2**.

Of all these, the most common type encountered in India is thalassemias.

Structural Hemoglobinopathy: Sickle Cell Disease[14]

Due to abnormal structure of hemoglobin chain, polymerization of the abnormal hemoglobin occurs in low oxygen conditions, which leads to the formation of rigid and fragile sickle-shaped red cells. These cells are generally hemolyzed causing the hemolytic anemia, and vaso-occlusion in the small blood vessels leading to multiple problems.

Genetics

It is a group of inherited single-gene autosomal recessive disorders caused by[6] a mutation in beta globin gene in which sixth amino acid of beta chain glutamic acid is replaced by valine. Sickle cell disease (SCD) includes sickle cell anemia (HbSS) and the heterozygous conditions of hemoglobin S and other variants (genotypes). All of these genotypes give similar clinical presentations of varying severity.[7] Hemoglobin S combined with normal hemoglobin (A) is also known as sickle trait (AS).

Clinical Features

Most common clinical feature is acute painful crises. Other complications of SCD include stroke, pulmonary hypertension, renal dysfunction, retinal disease, leg ulcers, cholelithiasis, and avascular necrosis of femoral head depending upon "where is vaso-occlusion occurring?" Carriers of one HbS gene (sickle trait) lead normal healthy life but in pregnancy they can have pyelonephritis and bacteriuria.

Maternal and Fetal Outcome

Generally in sickle cell anemia patient not reach up to pregnancy levels due to more mortality but in trait patients may be associated with an increased incidence of perinatal mortality, premature labor, fetal

TABLE 4: Sign and symptoms of megaloblastic anemia.

Symptoms	Signs
• Asymptomatic	• Pallor
• Loss of appetite	• Bleeding spots in skin
• Vomiting	• Hepatosplenomegaly
• Diarrhea	• Polyneuropathy
• Unexplained fever	

TABLE 5: Folate deficiency—peripheral blood picture.

Red cells	White cells	Hematological values
• Macrocytic and normochromic	• Hypersegmented neutrophils	• ↑ Hemoglobin
• Anisocytosis	• Leukopenia	• ↓ MCV or normal
• Poikilocytosis		• ↑ MCH
• Sometimes nuclear material		• ↑ Serum iron
		• ↓ Red cell folate or B_{12}

(MCV: mean corpuscular volume; MCH: mean corpuscular hemoglobin)

> **BOX 2:** Classification of hemoglobinopathies.[3]
> - Structural hemoglobinopathies as sickle cell disease
> - Thalassemias
> - Thalassemic hemoglobin variants as HbE, Hb Constant Spring, Hb Lepore
> - Hereditary persistence of fetal hemoglobin
> - Acquired hemoglobinopathies as methemoglobin, sulfhemoglobin, carboxyhemoglobin, HbH in erythroleukemia
>
> (HbH: hemoglobin H)

growth restriction, and acute painful crises during pregnancy and thromboembolism and pregnancy-induced hypertension (PIH).

Management in Sickle Cell Disease

Women with SCD should be seen preconceptionally by a specialist to receive all information about SCD along with routine antenatal care. Information regarding planning to conceive including effects of dehydration, overexertion, warning signs, and possible effects on fetus should be given.[8-24] Genetic screening for hemoglobinopathy status of the partner is also tested. If a partner is a carrier or affected by a major hemoglobinopathy, the couple should receive appropriate counseling regarding the risk of having affected fetus.[13] Folic acid 5 mg daily should be definitely prescribed during pregnancy to reduce the risk of neural tube defect and to compensate for the increased demand of folate during pregnancy due to increased destruction of RBC.

Some drugs like hydroxycarbamide and angiotensin-converting enzyme (ACE) inhibitors which are used in SCD should be stopped in pregnancy. Low-dose aspirin 75 mg once daily from 12 weeks of gestation can be started to reduce the risk of developing PEC along with prophylactic low-molecular-weight heparin (LMWH). Blood pressure and urine analysis with regular ultrasounds for fetal growth should be done to detect early detection of fetal growth restriction and help in deciding appropriate time of delivery to reduce perinatal mortality and morbidity. Most common problem is painful crisis during pregnancy which can occur. The management of these episodes is analgesia, hydration, treatment of infection, thromboprophylaxis, oxygen therapy, blood transfusion/exchange transfusion, and supportive treatment as needed.[25] Mode of delivery should be spontaneous labor but cesarean section is reserved for obstetric indications.[26]

Quantitative Disorders of Hemoglobin: Thalassemia and Thalassemic Hemoglobin Variants

These are a group of genetic disorders that result in quantitative defects in the biosynthesis of the globin chains and also result from diminished production of a structurally abnormal chain, such as in Hb Lepore disease or Hb E-β-thalassemias. The decreased hemoglobin production leads to a microcytic, hypochromic anemia. Accumulation of unpaired globin subunits leads to ineffective erythropoiesis and hemolytic anemia.

Beta Thalassemia

Beta thalassemias are characterized by diminished production of β-globin chains, which causes accumulation of α-globin chains leading to microcytic hypochromic anemia, an abnormal peripheral blood smear with nucleated RBCs, and reduced amounts of HbA on hemoglobin analysis. The deficiency of β-globin synthesis may be compensated partially by an increase in δ and γ chain synthesis. This leads to variable increase in levels of HbA2 ($\alpha 2 \delta 2$) and HbF ($\alpha 2 \gamma 2$) on hemoglobin electrophoresis.

Maternal and fetal outcome: Beta thalassemia minor (β-thalassemia trait) affected individuals have mild or no anemia and is well tolerated in pregnancy. Thalassemia intermedia and major are associated with very poor maternal and fetal outcomes due to iron overload causing multiple complications including cardiomyopathy leading to congestive heart failure, increased susceptibility to both maternal and fetal infections and damage to the fetus.[27] These women may have impaired liver function due to iron overload and also risk of cholelithiasis due to hemolytic anemia and diabetes mellitus.

Diagnosis: Generally the peripheral smear shows hypochromia and microcytosis with basophilic stippling. Splenomegaly is found occasionally. β-thalassemia major (Cooley's anemia) and β-thalassemia intermedia have more severe anemia presenting earlier during life.

Hemoglobin electrophoresis is done for confirmation and ascertaining the variant depending on ratios of HbA, HbA2, and HbF. The spectrum of thalassemia is broad and ranges from asymptomatic to profound transfusion-dependent anemia.[16]

Management during pregnancy: Preconceptional evaluation of thalassemic women who are considering pregnancy includes assessment of the patient's transfusion needs, compliance with chelation therapy, iron load status, assessment for end organ damage from iron overload, endocrine and hormonal function, and indirect Coombs status and exposure or chronic infection with hepatitis B, hepatitis C, and HIV. Genetic evaluation of her partner should also be done.[28] Patients who have significant iron overload should refrain from becoming pregnant. Also hormonal dysfunction due to iron overload in transfusion-dependent patients can lead to a variety of hormonal insufficiencies, including hypopituitarism leading to infertility. Folic acid supplementation during the periconceptional period is must. A full evaluation of the patient's medical status should be performed. Ideally, asplenic patient should be vaccinated. Ferritin levels and blood counts should be done to assess iron overload and fetal well-being should be closely monitored because of the increased risk of growth restriction by serial ultrasounds.

Due to high rate of infertility and morbidity in patients who have β-thalassemia major, pregnancy experience is very little. Most cases of pregnancy are seen in patients who had β-thalassemia intermedia. Thalassemia minor carries normal pregnancy till term with only few blood transfusion requirements. The mode of delivery should be individualized in β-thalassemia patients. Patients who do not have myocardial dysfunction can be delivered vaginally and cesarean section can be reserved for obstetric indications.[17]

Alpha Thalassemia

Alpha thalassemias include a group of syndromes that is characterized by deficient production of the α-globin chain usually due to gene deletion in chromosome 16. Four classic α-thalassemia syndromes are recognized based on the number and configuration of α-globin deletions, which are silent carrier state, α-thalassemia trait, hemoglobin H (HbH), and hemoglobin Bart's (Hb Bart's).[2] Clinical features, laboratory evaluation, maternal and fetal outcomes, and management during pregnancy are not different than β variant. It is also having variants from nearly normal to a vigorous risk patient.[18]

WBC Disorders

Hodgkin's Lymphoma

Hodgkin's lymphoma is the most common lymphoma in women of childbearing age but can be found approximately 1 in 6,000 pregnancies.

Clinical findings: Patients may be asymptomatic or have fever, weight loss, and pruritus. The most common finding is peripheral lymphadenopathy. Careful staging is essential prior to the initiation of treatment with radiotherapy or chemotherapy. Modifications of standard staging modalities, such as the use of magnetic resonance imaging (MRI), can allow for adequate staging during pregnancy.[19]

Complications associated with Hodgkin's lymphoma during pregnancy are related to treatment of the disease, not the disease itself. Chemotherapy during the first trimester is associated with an increased risk of fetal structural malformation. During the second and third trimesters, chemotherapy is associated with intrauterine growth restriction, preterm birth, stillbirth, and adverse fetal neurodevelopmental outcomes such as mental retardation and learning disabilities.

Treatment: Treatment is individual based on the extent of disease and the gestational age. Radiotherapy is an effective treatment option if the risk to fetus can be minimized. Chemotherapy is relatively safe later in gestation but best avoided in the first trimester. Pregnancy termination is an alternative if Hodgkin's lymphoma is diagnosed early in gestation. If the diagnosis is made later in gestation and the patient is asymptomatic, delaying therapy until fetal lung maturity is established may be reasonable.

Women with Hodgkin's lymphoma are extremely susceptible to infection and sepsis. Sequelae of treatment include radiation pneumonitis causing restrictive lung disease, pericarditis leading to congestive heart failure, hypothyroidism, and ovarian failure.

Non-Hodgkin's Lymphoma

Until recently, non-Hodgkin's lymphomas were encountered infrequently in pregnancy. However, because 5–10% of individuals infected with the human immunodeficiency virus (HIV) will develop a lymphoma, the incidence of non-Hodgkin's lymphomas is rising. Similar to Hodgkin's lymphoma, extensive staging is essential. Treatment with radiotherapy is indicated for localized disease, whereas chemotherapy is used for more extensive disease. Care of the pregnant patient with lymphoma requires a multidisciplinary approach by obstetrician-gynecologists, hematologic oncologists, perinatologists, and neonatologists. With careful treatment, the fetuses of affected women appear to tolerate treatment of lymphoma quite well.[20]

Leukemia

Leukemias are malignant proliferations of cells of the hematopoietic system. Acute leukemias are derived from primitive progenitor cells of either the myeloid lineage [acute myelogenous leukemia (AML)] or the lymphocytic lineage [acute lymphocytic leukemia (ALL)]. Chronic leukemias are also derived from either myeloid cells [chronic myelogenous leukemia (CML)] or lymphocytic cells [chronic lymphocytic leukemia (CLL)]. All leukemias are rare before the age of 40 years with the exception of ALL, a childhood disease with a median age at diagnosis of 10 years.[21]

Clinical findings: Affected individuals often present with the symptoms of anemia (fatigue, weakness), thrombocytopenia (bleeding, bruising), or neutropenia (infection) caused by the replacement of normal hematopoietic cells with leukemia cells in the bone marrow. WBC count in the serum can be low, normal, or extremely elevated. Diagnosis is made by cytochemical, genetic, and immunochemical evaluations of the cells of a bone marrow biopsy or aspirate.

Treatment: Treatment of acute leukemia is based on immediate initiation of chemotherapy. For example, the median survival time of untreated patients with AML is 3 months or less. Exposure to chemotherapy during organogenesis frequently results in fetal death. However, many consider chemotherapy safe in the second and third trimesters. A period of pancytopenia following chemotherapy can be complicated by infection and hemorrhage. Patients often require erythrocyte and platelet transfusions, as well as antibiotic medications.

Acute leukemia during pregnancy is associated with premature delivery, fetal growth restriction, and fetal loss, but these findings are more likely due to chemotherapy and its complications rather than the leukemia itself.

■ PLATELET DISORDERS

Thrombocytopenia

Thrombocytopenia is defined as platelet counts below 150×10^9/L. During pregnancy it may result from several causes, which can be either immune-mediated platelet destruction or platelet consumption. Some of these disorders require early termination of pregnancy while others respond to conservative therapy.[22] Thrombocytopenia develops in 5-10% of women during pregnancy or in the immediate postpartum period. Some commonly encountered causes of thrombocytopenia during pregnancy are gestational thrombocytopenia (GT), immune thrombocytopenia (ITP), hereditary thrombocytopenia (HT), thrombotic thrombocytopenic purpura (TTP), hemolytic-uremic syndrome (HUS), PEC, hemolysis elevated liver enzyme and low platelet (HELLP) syndrome, and acute fatty liver of pregnancy (AFLP).

Gestational Thrombocytopenia

Gestational thrombocytopenia occurs in 4.4-11.6% of pregnancies, accounting for about 75% of all cases of thrombocytopenia in pregnancy more often seen in twin and triplet gestations. Platelet counts in some women show a gradual downward trend in the second trimester due to hemodilution during pregnancy and possibly increased platelet clearance. A subset of women with GT develop a more significant decline in platelet count suggesting that pathogenesis may be like HELLP syndrome and AFLP, and it may be associated with a higher risk of recurrence in subsequent pregnancies.

Maternal and fetal outcome: Gestational thrombocytopenia does not affect the health of the mother and fetal thrombocytopenia is uncommon and mild.[9]

Diagnosis: There are no biomarkers to provide a confirmed diagnosis, which can differentiate GT from mild ITP or onset of PEC/HELLP (or other diagnosis of exclusion). If thrombocytopenia does not resolve within 1-2 months after delivery, the diagnosis of ITP or HT should be considered.[2]

Management: No treatment is required as GT is a benign condition but it does not respond to IV immune globulin (IVIG) or corticosteroids.[23]

Immune Thrombocytopenia

Immune thrombocytopenia occurs in 1 in 1,000–10,000 pregnancies and it is the most common cause of a platelet count below $50 \times 10^9/L$ usually detected in the first and second trimesters. Platelet counts may fall during gestation, and at least 15–35% of mothers require treatment even prior to delivery.

Maternal and fetal outcome: Maternal and neonatal outcomes are generally favorable. So, ITP is not a contraindication to pregnancy. However, in unusually severe or refractory cases or for women reliant on potentially teratogenic medications, avoiding pregnancy is advised.[24]

Diagnosis: There is no specific laboratory test to distinguish ITP from GT or other causes of thrombocytopenia. The peripheral blood smear may show large platelets, with otherwise normal morphology. Therefore, the diagnosis of ITP is based on history of bleeding, low platelet count prior to pregnancy, and/or a family history that excludes HT; the diagnosis of ITP is made by excluding other disorders when possible or may be made only after monitoring response to therapy given for ITP. For excluding secondary causes of ITP, testing for HIV infection and hepatitis C infection is indicated. Serologic testing for systemic lupus erythematosus (SLE), serum protein electrophoresis, immunoglobulin (Ig) levels, direct Coombs test, and a bone marrow examination may also be done in cases of diagnostic dilemma.

Management: Treatment of ITP aims to decrease antibody production or increase platelet production or decrease platelet destruction or a combination of these. Treatment is initiated for bleeding when the platelet count falls below $20 \times 10^9/L$, for procedures and delivery. There is an increased risk of bleeding if platelet count is below $20 \times 10^9/L$ to $30 \times 10^9/L$ for a vaginal delivery or below $50 \times 10^9/L$ for a cesarean section.[11,12] Epsilon aminocaproic acid is a safe and effective option as an additional therapy that can be considered before and after delivery in women with severe ITP. Initial short-term treatment with daily oral prednisone (1 mg/kg) may be started. In case of inadequate response or intolerance to corticosteroids IVIG (1–2 g/kg total, given over 1–5 days) is used. Splenectomy can be performed safely in the second trimester, but is rarely required. Persistent exposure to high-dose corticosteroids in the first trimester is associated with an increased risk of cleft palate and exposure throughout gestation may increase the risk of preterm birth and gestational diabetes. Therefore, often a repeated administration of IVIG is done which is not usually done in the nonpregnant counterparts. A combination therapy using both corticosteroids and IVIG can be considered in severe nonresponding cases. ITP does not provide protection from thrombosis so anticoagulation is recommended as per standard protocols taking into account the presence of thrombocytopenia and the associated risks.[29]

Inherited Thrombocytopenia

Inherited platelet function disorders are rare, presence of thrombocytopenia since childhood and a family history is highly suggestive. These can be either autosomal dominant or recessive. Rare disorders include the autosomal recessive disorders—Glanzmann's thrombasthenia (absence of the platelet Gp llb/llla receptor) and Bernard-Soulier syndrome [absence of the platelet glycoprotein (GP) Ib-IX-V receptor]—present with bleeding symptoms in childhood.

Platelet storage pool disorder (SPD) is the classic autosomal dominant qualitative platelet disorder. The milder variants can go undetected. In case of known disorders of platelet function, genetic counseling must be done.[30]

Thrombotic Microangiopathies (TMA): Pregnancy-Associated Microangiopathies

Preeclampsia and HELLP

Preeclampsia is the most common cause of thrombocytopenia presenting in the late second or in the third trimester of pregnancy but sometimes with associated thrombocytopenia may develop during postpartum period also. HELLP can be a variant of PEC characterized by more severe thrombocytopenia, more fulminant microangiopathic hemolytic anemia, and more profoundly elevated liver function tests. Disseminated intravascular coagulation is uncommon, but if present it is a marker of disease progression.[31]

Diagnosis: PEC is defined as the onset of hypertension beginning after 20 weeks of gestation that may or may not be accompanied by 1 or more of the "severe features" which are thrombocytopenia (100×10^9/L), impaired liver function or injury (liver transaminases elevated to twice the normal concentration), new-onset renal insufficiency (serum creatinine 1.1 mg/dL) or doubling of the baseline creatinine in the absence of known renal disease, pulmonary edema, new-onset cerebral or visual disturbances, and persistent systolic blood pressure ≥160 mm Hg or diastolic blood pressure ≥110mm Hg.

Maternal and fetal outcome: Risk for sudden and severe progression of disease, including deterioration of mental status and development of disseminated intravascular coagulation (DIC) with associated hemorrhage. Neonatal thrombocytopenia is uncommon. If present the neonate is usually premature or small for gestational age.[32]

Management: The diagnosis of PEC and HELLP, and their distinction from TTP and HUS, is vital because the only treatment of PEC and HELLP is delivery. Use of corticosteroids to reduce maternal complications is not effective.[24] Regular monitoring throughout gestation, especially after 34 weeks, for clinical as well as laboratory indicators of worsening can be useful in guiding timing and mode of delivery. Most women improve clinically soon after delivery. The diagnosis of TTP or HUS should be considered in any woman who does not show clinical and laboratory improvement within 48–72 hours postdelivery or in woman whose clinical situation deteriorates after delivery. In high-risk mothers low-dose aspirin may be helpful in reducing the risk of developing PEC, the incidence of preterm birth, and fetal growth restriction and should be initiated early in gestation.[33]

Acute Fatty Liver of Pregnancy

It occurs in 1 in 5,000–10,000 pregnancies and is more common with multiple gestations than in single ones. Maximum women present with nausea or vomiting and few have abdominal pain or signs and symptoms overlapping with PEC.

Maternal and fetal outcome: Both maternal and fetal outcomes are adverse unless the condition is diagnosed and managed aggressively.

Diagnosis: It is based on impaired renal and hepatic function, including impaired synthesis of clotting factors, accompanied by abdominal pain, nausea, and vomiting. Reduction in plasma antithrombin III may be an early marker of AFLP and sometimes coagulopathy is disproportionately severe as compared to severity of liver dysfunction. Hypoglycemia is present in severe cases and is a key diagnostic feature, which is not seen in related conditions such as PEC, HELLP, TTP, and HUS. Although it is often difficult to differentiate HELLP from AFLP, evidence of hepatic insufficiency including hypoglycemia, DIC, or encephalopathy is seen more often in AFLP. Imaging modalities are not of much help. Maternal thrombocytopenia is seen, but severe thrombocytopenia is unusual.[34]

Management: Treatment consists of supportive management and resuscitation of the mother with aggressive replacement with packed red cells and fresh-frozen plasma to maintain adequate perfusion to vital organs. Antithrombin III concentrate and platelets may be useful in severely affected mothers.[21] Stabilization of the mother and prompt delivery of the fetus is indicated, irrespective of gestational age. The risks of recurrent AFLP remain to be high during subsequent pregnancies.

Thrombotic Microangiopathies: Not Specific to Pregnancy

Thrombotic Thrombocytopenic Purpura

Acquired, antibody-induced TTP (aTTP) is estimated to occur in 1 in 200,000 pregnancies.[31,32] Approximately 10% of women with aTTP and a quarter to half of those with congenital TTP (cTTP) present for the first time during pregnancy, often during the first pregnancy or postpartum period. This predisposition may reflect the fall in ADAMTS13 and rise in Von Willebrand factor (VWF) that occurs normally during gestation.[35]

Maternal and fetal outcome: Fetal loss caused by widespread placental ischemia is frequent when TTP occurs in the first and second trimester, but the incidence of healthy live births approaches 75–90% when TTP develops closer to term and when maternal treatment has been successful.

Diagnosis: Prompt diagnosis is important because maternal mortality can be reduced by 80–90% with timely recognition and treatment. TTP presents more commonly during the latter part of gestation or postpartum period.[31-35] Diagnosis is straight forward when a previously healthy mother presents in the first trimester with severe MAHA (microangiopathic hemolytic anemia), thrombocytopenia, and neurologic dysfunction that may or may not be accompanied by renal insufficiency and fever. Diagnosis becomes more difficult as term approaches due to the overlap between key features of TTP with severe PEC. Full-term pregnancy (FTP) should be a prominent consideration when a woman with TMA does not meet criteria for severe PEC or HELLP or in the presence of neurologic findings such as weakness, numbness, aphasia, or an overt change in mental status or when the platelet count is below $20 \times 10^9/L$.[35-37] An abundance of schistocytes and nucleated RBCs on the peripheral blood smear and a marked elevation in serum LDH favor the diagnosis of TTP, but is not always found on presentation. TTP can be differentiated from atypical HUS (aHUS) by presence of neurologic complications and platelet count below $20 \times 10^9/L$ and by the absence of severe and progressive renal insufficiency (creatinine above 2.2 mg/dL). The diagnosis of TTP should become a prominent consideration when clinical signs and symptoms do not resolve and the platelet count does not increase above $100 \times 10^9/L$ by 48–72 hours postdelivery.[37] cTTP comprises up to 50% of all cases of gestational TTP.[32] It should be suspected when severe ADAMTS13 is detected even if family history is not present. Gene sequencing is required for definitive diagnosis and to guide management of subsequent pregnancies. ADAMTS13 activity and antibody should be measured early during the first trimester to identify women at highest risk who shall require close monitoring.[36]

Management: Quick clinical diagnosis is critical because the decision to start plasmapheresis for aTTP, plasma infusion for cTTP, or a complement inhibitor for aHUS as opposed to early delivery for PEC/HELLP often leaves the clinician in a difficult situation. Confirmation of the diagnosis of TTP is based on an ADAMTS13 level below 10% of normal. Pregnancy does not impair response to plasma infusion in cTTP or plasmapheresis and corticosteroid in aTTP. There is no data suggesting that termination of pregnancy improves maternal outcome.[38] Use of low-dose aspirin and LMWH has been suggested but their role is doubtful. The risk of recurrence of AFLP in a subsequent pregnancy is as high as 50%.

Atypical Hemolytic–Uremic Syndrome

Atypical HUS is estimated to occur in 1 in 25,000 pregnancies. 10–20% of all women present with aHUS for the first time during pregnancy. This may be related complement activation that develops normally during gestation. 80% of affected women develop aHUS postpartum although no trimester is exempt.

Maternal and fetal outcome: There is no evidence that delivery alters outcome of aHUS.[37] Risk of fetal loss is 10–20%.[39] There is some evidence that there is a 10–30% risk of recurrence in subsequent pregnancies depending on the underlying mutation.[37]

Diagnosis: Atypical HUS is suspected when a woman presents with progressive renal failure, thrombocytopenia with platelet counts above $50 \times 10^9/L$, MAHA, and occasionally, evidence of ischemic tissue injury in the absence of fulfillment for PEC/HELLP. Differentiation from TTP may be difficult before renal failure becomes the predominant feature. The diagnosis is supported in about two-thirds of patients by identifying a mutation that impairs expression or function of proteins that regulate the alternative pathway C3 convertase. However, because these tests are time consuming and results are often inconclusive they can only be used for long-term prognostic evaluation. Clinical decision and differentiation from closely related conditions is most important to start early management.

Management: Plasmapheresis should be initiated upon diagnosis and continued. The development of end-stage renal disease may be prevented by start of plasma exchange or plasmapheresis. Majority of patients require dialysis at some point.

Other TMAs: Conditions which may lead to potential worsening of clinical condition during pregnancy are active SLE, other forms of vasculitis, scleroderma, and antiphospholipid syndrome (APS). But these causes have to be treated as specific disease entities and whether pregnancy poses an increased risk for TMA in these settings is not clear.[25,26,38-40]

COAGULATION DISORDERS IN PREGNANCY

Normally during pregnancy fibrinogen, VWF, factors 2, 7, 8, 9, and 10 levels increase by 20–1000%. And also increase in levels of antifibrinolytic plasminogen inhibitors, thus pregnancy is a hypercoagulable state to prevent excessive blood loss during pregnancy and delivery.[27]

Thrombophilic Disorders

Acquired Thrombophilias

The most common acquired disorder is antiphospholipid antibody syndrome. It is an autoimmune condition which is associated with venous and arterial thrombosis leading to adverse pregnancy outcome in the form of pregnancy loss, PEC, and placental insufficiency and preterm births.

It is diagnosed by laboratory criteria of titers of anticardiolipin (aCL) antibodies, anti-β2 Glycoprotein I (ab2 GP I) IgG, and IgM antibodies.

Management Options during Pregnancy

Recurrent preembryonic and embryonic loss; no history of (H/o) thrombotic events:

- Low-dose aspirin alone or with LMWH (prophylactic dose)
- Prior fetal death or preterm labor (PTL) due to severe PIH; no H/o thrombotic events
- Low-dose aspirin plus LMWH (prophylactic dose)
- Anticoagulation regimen for women with a history of thrombotic events
- Low-dose aspirin plus LMWH (in therapeutic dose) which is enoxaparin 1 mg/kg every 12 hours.[28]

These patients should be regularly monitored during antenatal period by frequent color Doppler and regular BP check and clinical evaluation for stroke and thrombosis. Postnatally these patients should stop aspirin and heparin after 6 weeks. But those patients who were on Warfarin, they should start this again once baby is delivered.

Paroxysmal Nocturnal Hemoglobinuria

It is a rare disorder characterized by absence of complement regulatory proteins causing complement-mediated hemolysis leading to dark urine at night. These patients present with symptoms of anemia, abdominal pain, bone marrow suppression, and renal insufficiency. Especially thrombotic events occurring at specific sites may cause death in pregnant patients and risk of preterm labor is also very common. Diagnosis is made by flow cytometry only. Management is done by iron folic acid supplementation and blood and platelet products but we should avoid fresh frozen plasma (FFP) as it is rich in complements. Eculizumab is a drug which is commonly used in nonpregnant patients, and can be used in pregnancy also. However, safety data is not much available. Also prophylactic anticoagulation should also be continued during whole pregnancy and 6 weeks postpartum.[41,42]

Essential Thrombocythemia or Thrombocytosis

It is a rare chronic myeloproliferative disorder with unknown etiology but females are more affected by this disease. The effect in gene causes reduced apoptosis of platelets leading to thrombocythemia. Mostly patients are asymptomatic but may present with headaches, syncope transient ischemic attacks (TIAs). Diagnosis can be made by persistent platelet count >450/L. Risk to fetus include in the form of miscarriages and intrauterine fetal death and hemorrhage during pregnancy. These patients should be treated by low-dose aspirin during pregnancy and platelet lowering agents in patients with history of TIAs.

Inherited Thrombophilias

- Factor 5 Leiden deficiency
- Factor 2 gene mutation
- Protein C deficiency
- Protein S deficiency
- Antithrombin deficiency
- Methylene tetrahydrofolate reductase mutation and other thrombophilias.

All the abovementioned thrombophilias increase the risk of nonphysiologic thrombosis so deserve a careful attention during pregnancy and during postpartum periods. Fetal risks in the form of fetal demise and abruption of placenta and PIH.[43]

Management goals are to prevent VTE in patients with a known inherited thrombophilias. We should closely monitor the patients without anticoagulation therapy. Mostly used LMWH enoxaparin 40 mg subcutaneous (SC) daily or unfractionated heparin 7,500 IU twice daily. With these dose regimens no monitoring by blood tests is required and it should be hold for few days and delivery should be planned. If heparin is hold during delivery then it should be resumed 6–12 hours after delivery. Therapeutic dose anticoagulation is enoxaparin 1 mg/kg SC twice daily. But in this dose monitoring by anti X a levels should be done during pregnancy. If in any case urgent reversal is needed then protamine sulfate is used in the dose like 1 mg protamine sulfate neutralizes 100 IU of unfractionated heparin (UFH). But this is less effective with LMWH but can be used in dose of 1 mg for 1 mg dose of enoxaparin and a second dose of 0.5 mg if bleeding persists. Other oral anticoagulants warfarin is contraindicated in pregnancy but can be given in postpartum period. Patients with heparin-induced thrombocytopenia can be managed by fondaparinux in pregnancy.[44,45]

Thromboembolic Disease in Pregnancy (Acute Venous Thromboembolism)

Venous thromboembolism affects approximately 1 in 1,000 pregnancies. Indeed, all the elements of *Virchow's triad* (circulatory stasis, vascular damage, and hypercoagulability of blood) are present during pregnancy. Increased venous capacity during pregnancy coupled with compression of large veins by the gravid uterus causes venous stasis. Endothelial damage occurs at delivery and is more extensive after cesarean delivery, contributing to the increased risk of VTE after cesarean section. Coagulation is favored during pregnancy due to estrogen stimulation of coagulation factors and decreased activity of the fibrinolytic.

Inherited thrombophilias such as *activated protein C resistance* (most commonly due to the *factor V Leiden* mutation), prothrombin gene mutation *antithrombin III deficiency*, and *protein C and protein S deficiency*, along with acquired thrombophilias such as the *APS*, have emerged as important risk factors for VTE. Other risk factors include prior VTE, older age, smoking, and immobilization.

Superficial Thrombophlebitis

Patients with thrombosis of the superficial veins of the saphenous system present with tenderness, pain, or erythema along a vein. A palpable cord is sometimes present. Because of the possibility of concurrent deep vein thrombosis (DVT), compression ultrasound is reasonable to confirm the diagnosis and exclude DVT. Treatment consists of compression stockings, ambulation, leg elevation, local heat, and analgesic medications. Of note, the superficial femoral vein belongs to the deep venous system despite its name. A thrombus in this vein requires treatment for DVT.

Deep Vein Thrombosis

Approximately half of DVT in pregnancy occurs antepartum and half occurs postpartum. Previous clinical practices that contributed to thrombosis, such as prolonged postpartum bed rest, likely falsely elevated the risk of DVT in the puerperium. Most of DVT in pregnancy occurs in the left lower extremity rather than the right.[46]

Clinical Findings

The presentation of DVT is variable but frequently includes lower extremity tenderness, swelling, color changes, and a palpable cord. *Homan's sign*, pain elicited by passive dorsiflexion of the foot, may be present.

Diagnosis

The modality of choice for diagnosis of DVT is real-time ultrasound, used with duplex and color Doppler ultrasound. Venography remains the standard but has been largely replaced by the less invasive diagnostic tests.

Treatment

Anticoagulation, bed rest, and analgesia are the fundamental treatments of DVT. Ambulation with elastic stockings begins once all symptoms have abated, usually in 7-10 days. Patients are initially anticoagulated with unfractionated heparin or LMWH. Due to embryopathy and fetal hemorrhage, warfarin is contraindicated during pregnancy. Antepartum DVT is treated with anticoagulation for the rest of pregnancy and then for 6-12 weeks postpartum for at least a total of 3-6 months of therapy. DVT occurring postpartum should be treated with anticoagulation for 3-6 months.

Pulmonary Embolism

Pulmonary embolism accounts for approximately 20% of maternal deaths. Its antepartum and postpartum prevalence are approximately equal, although postpartum pulmonary embolism is associated with higher mortality rates.[47]

Prevention

Prophylactic anticoagulation should be considered for women at high risk for thromboembolism during pregnancy. Women with inherited thrombophilias that confer a high risk should be anticoagulated during pregnancy regardless of whether they have an antecedent history of thromboembolism. Women with a prior VTE that was related to a temporary risk factor (e.g., prolonged immobilization after injury) do not require anticoagulation during pregnancy. However, for women with a prior thromboembolic event related to pregnancy or estrogen-containing birth control pills and no thrombophilia, consideration may be given to anticoagulation during pregnancy.

Clinical Findings

The most common presenting symptom of pulmonary embolus is dyspnea, followed by pleuritic chest pain, apprehension, cough, syncope, and hemoptysis. Associated signs include tachypnea and tachycardia.

Diagnosis

Initial evaluation of the symptoms associated with pulmonary embolism usually consists of arterial blood gas measurement, chest radiograph, and electrocardiogram.

High-probability scans are indicative of pulmonary embolism in 88% of cases. Because of these limitations, spiral computed tomography (CT) pulmonary angiography has emerged as a useful, noninvasive modality for the detection of pulmonary embolism but is limited in the detection of small emboli.

Treatment

Treatment of pulmonary embolism is anticoagulation. The factors influencing anticoagulant choice [heparin vs. warfarin (Coumadin)] are the same as those for DVT. First-line therapy during pregnancy is adjusted dose unfractionated heparin or LMWH. Therapeutic anticoagulation should be continued for at least 4-6 months to prevent recurrence.

Septic Pelvic Thrombophlebitis

Essentials of Diagnosis

- Septic pelvic thrombophlebitis is thrombosis in the veins of the pelvis due to infection.
- It is associated with abdominal pain and high fever.
- CT or MRI can confirm the diagnosis.

Pathogenesis

Septic pelvic thrombophlebitis is thrombosis in the veins of the pelvis due to infection. The most important risk factor is cesarean section, especially if complicated by infection. In fact, almost 90% of cases occur after cesarean delivery.

Pelvic infection leads to infection of the vein wall and intimal damage. Thrombogenesis occurs at the site of intimal damage. The clot is then invaded by microorganisms. Both the uterine and ovarian veins may be involved, as well as the common iliac, hypogastric, and vaginal veins and the inferior vena cava. The ovarian vein is the most common site of septic thrombosis (40% of cases).[48-50]

Clinical Findings

The condition is suspected when fever persists in the puerperium despite adequate antibiotic therapy for aerobic and anaerobic organisms and no other discernible cause of fever. Abdominal pain and back discomfort are common presenting symptoms. Tachycardia and tachypnea may be present. Leukocytosis is usually present. Pelvic examination is often consistent with a normal postpartum examination and therefore not helpful in diagnosing this condition. Chest radiograph often reveals evidence of multiple, small septic emboli. CT or MRI may assist in the diagnosis of pelvic vein thrombosis and eliminate other pelvic causes, such as abscess.[51,52]

Complications

The serious complications associated with this condition are septic pulmonary emboli, extension of the venous clot in the pelvis, renal vein thrombosis, ureteral obstruction, and death.

Treatment

The mainstays are anticoagulation with heparin and broad-spectrum antibiotics (including coverage for anaerobes and common Enterobacteriaceae). Within 48-72 hours of initiation of heparin therapy, fever should resolve. Treatment usually is empirically continued for 7-10 days, although the optimal duration of therapy is not well defined.[52-54]

REFERENCES

1. Benz EJ. Disorders of hemoglobin. In: Kasper DL, Hauser SL, Jameson JL, Fauci AS, Longo DL, Loscalzo J (Eds). Harrison's Principles of Internal Medicine, 20th edition. Philadelphia: McGrawhill; 2018. pp. 690-98.
2. Rappaport VJ, Velazquez M, Williams K. MS Hemoglobinopathies in pregnancy. Obstet Gynecol Clin N Am. 2004;31:287-317.
3. Forget BG, Bunn HF. Classification of the disorders of hemoglobin. Cold Spring Harb Perspect Med. 2013;3:a011684.
4. Mohanty D, Colah RB, Gorakshakar AC, Patel RZ, Master DC, Mahanta J, et al. Prevalence of β-thalassemia and other haemoglobinopathies in six cities in India: a multicentre study. J Community Genet. 2013;4:33-42.
5. Shukla S, Singh D, Dewan K, Sharma S, Trivedi SS. Antenatal carrier screening for thalassemia and related hemoglobinopathies: a hospital-based study. J Med Soc. 2018;32:118-22.
6. Pauling L, Itano HA, Singer SJ, Wells IC. Sickle cell anaemia a molecular disease. Science. 1949;110:543-8.
7. Weatherall D, Akinyanju O, Fucharoen S, Olivieri N, Musgrove P. Inherited disorders of haemoglobin. In: Jamison DT, Breman JG, Measham AR, Alleye G, Claeson M, Evans V DB, et al. (Eds). Disease Control Priorities in Developing Countries, 2nd edition. Washington, DC: The World Bank and New York, HY: Oxford University Press; 2006. pp. 663-80.
8. Tuck SM, Studd JW, White JM. Pregnancy in sickle cell disease in the UK. Br J Obstet Gynaecol. 1983;90:112-7.
9. Rajab KE, Issa AA, Mohammed AM, Ajami AA. Sickle cell disease and pregnancy in Bahrain. Int J Gynaecol Obstet. 2006;93:171-5.
10. Smith JA, Espeland M, Bellevue R, Bonds D, Brown AK, Koshy M. Pregnancy in sickle cell disease: experience of the Cooperative Study of Sickle Cell Disease. Obstet Gynecol. 1996;87:199-204.
11. Al Jama FE, Gasem T, Burshaid S, Rahman J, Al Suleiman SA, Rahman MS. Pregnancy outcome in patients with homozygous sickle cell disease in a university hospital, Eastern Saudi Arabia. Arch Gynecol Obstet. 2009;280:793-7.
12. Afolabi BB, Iwuala NC, Iwuala IC, Ogcdengbe OK. Morbidity and mortality in sickle cell pregnancies in Lago, Nigeria: a case control study. J Obstet Gynaecol. 2009;29:104-6.
13. Sun PM, Wilbum W, Raynor BD, Jamieson D. Sickle cell disease in pregnancy: twenty years of experience at Grady Memorial Hospital, Atlanta, Georgia. Am J Obstet Gynecol. 2001;184:1127-30.
14. Serjeant GR, Loy LL, Crowther M, Hambleton IR, Thame M. Outcome of pregnancy in homozygous sickle cell disease. Obstet Gynecol. 2004;103:1278-85.
15. Chakravarty EF, Khanna D, Chung L. Pregnancy outcomes in systemic sclerosis, primary pulmonary hypertension, and sickle cell disease. Obstet Gynecol. 2008;111:927-34.
16. Powars DR, Sandhu M, Niland-Weiss J, Johnson C, Bruce S, Manning PR. Pregnancy in sickle cell disease. Obstet Gynecol. 1986;67:217-28.
17. Howard RJ, Tuck SM, Pearson TC. Pregnancy in sickle cell disease in the UK: results of a multicentre survey of the effect of prophylactic blood transfusion on maternal and fetal outcome. Br J Obstet Gynaecol. 1995;102:947-51.
18. Villers MS, Jamison MG, De Castro LM, James AH. Morbidity associated with sickle cell disease in pregnancy. Am J Obstet Gynecol. 2008;199:125.e1-5.
19. El-Shafei AM, Sandhu AK, Dhaliwal JK. Maternal mortality in Bahrain with special reference to sickle cell disease. Aust N Z J Obstet Gynaecol. 1988;28:41-4.
20. Serjeant GR, Hambleton I, Thame M. Fecundity and pregnancy outcome in a cohort with sickle cell haemoglobin C disease followed from birth. BJOG. 2005;112:1308-14.

21. Sickle Cell Society. Standards for the Clinical Care of Adults with Sickle Cell Disease in the UK. London: Sickle Cell Society; 2008.
22. Ataga KI, Moore CG, Jones S, Olajide O, Strayhom D, Hinderliter A, et al. Pulmonary hypertension in patients with sickle cell disease: a longitudinal study. Br J Haematol. 2006;134:109-15.
23. Gladwin MT, Sachdev V, Jison ML, Shizukuda Y, Plehn JF, Minter K, et al. Pulmonary hypertension as a risk factor for death in patients with sickle cell disease. N Engl J Med. 2004;350:886-95.
24. Clarkson JG. The ocular manifestations of sickle-cell disease: a prevalence and natural history study. Trans Am Ophthalmol Soc. 1992;90:481-504.
25. Sun D, Shehata N, Ye XY, Gregorovich S, De France B, Arnold DM, et al. Corticosteroids compared with intravenous immunoglobulin for the treatment of immune thrombocytopenia in pregnancy. Blood. 2016;128(10):1329-35.
26. Kong Z, Qin P, Wang X, Hou M. Recombinant human thrombopoietin: a novel therapeutic option for patients with immune thrombocytopenia in pregnancy [abstract]. Blood. 2014;124(21).
27. Patil AS, Dotters-Katz SK, Metjian AD, James AH, Swamy GK. Use of a thrombopoietin mimetic for chronic immune thrombocytopenic purpura in pregnancy. Obstet Gynecol. 2013;122:483-85.
28. Decroocq J, Marcellin L, Le Ray C, Willems L. Rescue therapy with romiplostim for refractory primary immune thrombocytopenia during pregnancy. Obstet Gynecol. 2014;124(2 Pt 2 Suppl 1);481-83.
29. NHS. (2021). NHS Sickle Cell and thalassaemia (SCT) screening programme: detailed information. (online) Available from https://www.gov.uk/topic/population-screening-programmes/sickle-cell-thalassaemia [Last accessed November, 2022].
30. Prevention of neural tube defects: results of the Medical Research Council Vitamin Study. MRC Vitamin Study Research Group. Lancet. 1991;338:131-7.
31. Lindenbaum J. Klipstein FA. Folic acid deficiency in sickle-cell anaemia. N Engl J Med. 1963;269:875-82.
32. Diav-Citrin O, Hunnisett L, Sher GD, Koren G. Hydroxyurea use during pregnancy: a case report in sickle cell disease and review of the literature. Am J Hematol. 1999; 60:148-50.
33. Byrd DC, Pitts SR, Alexander CK. Hydroxyurea in two pregnant women with sickle cell anemia. Pharmacotherapy. 1999;19:1459-62.
34. Foucan L, Bourhis V, Bangou J, Mérault L, Etienne-Julan M, Salmi RL. A randomized trial of captopril for microalbuminuria in normotensive adults with sickle cell anemia. Am J Med. 1998;104:339-42.
35. McKie KT, Hanevold CD, Hernandez C, Waller JL, Ortiz L, McKie KM. Prevalence, prevention, and treatment of microalbuminuria and proteinuria in children with sickle cell disease. J Pediatr Hematol Oncol. 2007;29:140-4.
36. RCOG. (2011). Management of Sickle Cell Disease in Pregnancy. RCOG Green-top Guideline No. 61. (online) Available from https://www.rcog.org.uk/media/nyinaztx/gtg_61.pdf [Last accessed November, 2022].
37. Fujimura K, Harada Y, Fujimoto T, Kuramoto A, Ikeda Y, Akatsuka J, et al. Nationwide study of idiopathic thrombocytopenic purpura in pregnant women and the clinical influence on neonates. Int J Hematol. 2002;75(4): 426-33.
38. Van Veen JJ, Nokes TJ, Makris M. The risk of spinal haematoma following neuraxial anesthesia or lumbar puncture in thrombocytopenic individuals. Br J Haematol. 2010;148(1):15-25.
39. Loustau V, Dcbouverie O, Canoui-Poitrine F, Baili L, Khellaf M, Touboul C, et al. Effect of pregnancy on the course of immune thrombocytopenia: a retrospective study of 118 pregnancies in 82 women. Br Haematol. 2014;166(6):929-35.
40. Michel M, Novoa MV, Bussel JB. Intravenous anti-D as a treatment for immune thrombocytopenic purpura (ITP) during pregnancy. Br J Haematol. 2003;123(1):142-46.

41. Tannetta DS, Hunt K, Jones CI, Davidson N, Coxon CH, Ferguson D, et al. Syncytiotrophoblast extracellular vesicles from pre-eclampsia placentas differentially affect platelet function. PLoS One. 2015;10(11): e0142538.
42. Kohli S, Ranjan S, Hoffmann J, Kashif M, Daniel EA, Al-Dabet MM, et al. Maternal extracellular vesicles and platelets promote preeclampsia via inflammasome activation in trophoblasts. Blood. 2016;128(17): 2153-64.
43. Creasy RK, Resnick R, Iams JD, Lockwood CJ, Moore TR (Eds). Creasy and Resnick's Maternal-Fetal Medicine: Principle and Practice, 6th edition. Philadelphia, PA: Saunders/Elsevier; 2009.
44. American College of Obstetricians and Gynecologists; Task Force on Hypertension in Pregnancy. Hypertension in pregnancy. Report of the American College of Obstetricians and Gynecologists' Task Force on Hypertension in Pregnancy. Obstet Gynecol. 2013;122(5):1122-31.
45. Sibai BM. Diagnosis, controversies, and management of the syndrome of hemolysis, elevated liver enzymes, and low platelet count. Obstet Gynecol. 2004;103:981-91.
46. Mao M, Chen C. Corticosteroid therapy for management of hemolysis, elevated liver enzymes, and low platelet count (HELLP) syndrome: a meta-analysis. Med Sci Monit. 2015;21:3777-83.
47. Le Fevre ML; U.S. Preventive Services Task Force. Low-dose aspirin use for the prevention of morbidity and mortality from preeclampsia: U.S. Preventive Services Task Force recommendation statement. Ann Intern Med. 2014;161:819-26.
48. Riely CA. Acute fatty liver of pregnancy. Semin Liver Dis. 1987;7(1):47-54.
49. Moatti-Cohen M, Garrec C, Wolf M, Boisseau P, Galicier L, Azoulay E, et al. French Reference Center for Thrombotic Microangiopathies. Unexpected frequency of Upshaw-Schulman syndrome in pregnancy-onset thrombotic thrombocytopenic purpura. Blood. 2012;119(24):5888-97.
50. Scully M. Thrombotic thrombocytopenic purpura and atypical hemolytic uremic syndrome microangiopathy in pregnancy. Semin Thromb Hemost. 2016;42(7):774-9.
51. Scully M, Thomas M, Underwood M, Watson H, Langley K, Camilleri RS, et al. Collaborators of the UK TTP Registry. Thrombotic thrombocytopenic purpura and pregnancy: presentation, management, and subsequent pregnancy outcomes. Blood. 2014;124(2):211-19.
52. Jiang Y, McIntosh JJ, Reese JA, Deford CC, Kremer Hovinga JA, Lämmle B, et al. Pregnancy outcomes following recovery from acquired thrombotic thrombocytopenic purpura. Blood. 2014;123(11):1674-80.
53. Martin JN Jr, Bailey AP, Rehberg JF, Owens MT, Keiser SD, May WL. Thrombotic thrombocytopenic purpura in 166 pregnancies: 1955-2006. Arn J Obstet Gynecol. 2008;199:98-104.
54. McMinn JR, George JN. Evaluation of women with clinically suspected thrombotic thrombocytopenic purpura-hemolytic uremic syndrome during pregnancy. J Clin Apher. 2001;16:202-09.

CHAPTER 10

Neurological Disorders in Pregnancy

Prabhat Agrawal

■ INTRODUCTION

Many neurological diseases coexist with pregnancy. Changes in hemodynamics, blood volume, and hormonal influence on the vessel wall increase risk of bleeding from aneurysms and arteriovenous malformations during pregnancy and the postpartum period. Epilepsy may worsen in one-third of pregnant patients, and seizures are common during labor.

■ HEADACHE

Red Flag Signs in Headache

- Altered GCS
- Seizures
- Papilledema
- Neck stiffness
- Fever
- Trauma
- Focal deficits
- Worst headache of life.

Causes of Headache

A brief bedside history of headache accompaniments and examination in the form of blood pressure measurement and fundus examination can provide immense information about the headache being primary or secondary.

Hypercoagulability, hormonal changes, and anesthesia for labor are some of the factors contributing to the high incidence of secondary headaches during pregnancy.

Robbins et al., 10% of 140 pregnant women presenting with acute headache 35% had secondary headaches. Hypertensive disorders of pregnancy covered 51% of these cases (about 18% of total), with preeclampsia as the major cause, followed by [posterior reversible leukoencephalopathy syndrome (PRES) and eclampsia], reversible cerebral vasoconstriction syndrome (RCVS) and acute arterial hypertension. The history of lack of prior headaches, elevated blood pressure, and abnormalities at the neurologic examination are the main red flags for a secondary origin of an acute headache during pregnancy.

Management of Primary Headache

The safety of acute and prophylactic treatment of primary headache is important. Nonpharmacologic treatment should precede management. This is in the form of prevention of attack triggers such as diet and sleep disturbance. Preventable triggers such as excessive caffeine intake, psychiatric and pain comorbidities, and obesity should be identified and managed. Nonpharmacologic treatments, are highly recommended and include relaxation strategies, biofeedback, and cognitive-behavioral therapy.

While paracetamol seems to be the safest for acute treatment, prophylactic treatments

Flowchart 1: Classification of headache.

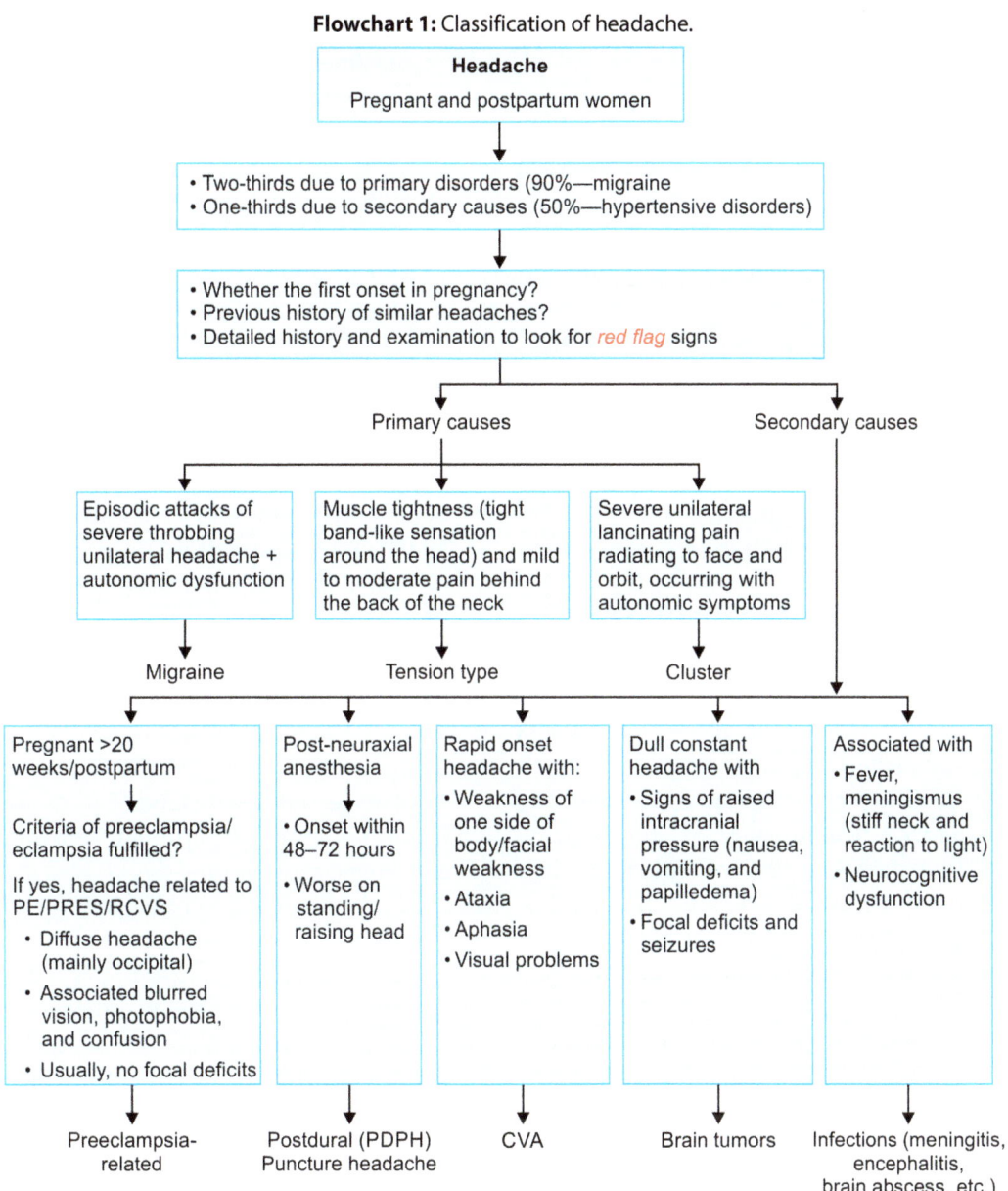

may be avoided or given with informed caution, providing a risk-benefit ratio.

Occipital and trigeminal pericranial nerve blocks are a treatment used for migraine, cluster headache, and other headache disorders as an acute therapy as well as for short-term prevention and are appealing to use in pregnancy because of their peripheral administration and presumed safety.

■ MIGRAINE

- Prevalence in pregnancy—2%
- Linked to hormonal fluctuation

- Increases risk of ischemic stroke in women
- Increased adverse events in pregnancy [preeclampsia, preterm births, venous thromboembolism (VTE), and myocardial infarction (MI)]
- Three types—(1) migraine with aura, (2) migraine without aura, and (3) chronic
- *Management:*
  - First line—paracetamol and antiemetics
  - Second line—aspirin and nonsteroidal anti-inflammatory drugs (NSAIDs) → (avoid after 30 weeks)
  - Third line—sumatriptan and opioids
- Avoid ergot alkaloids in pregnancy.

CEREBROVASCULAR DISEASES

- Includes transient ischemic attacks (TIA), strokes (ischemic and hemorrhagic), and anatomical abnormalities (aneurysms and malformations)
- Stroke in pregnant women—50% ischemic and 50% hemorrhagic
- Risk factors—10% antepartum, 40% intrapartum, and 50% postpartum
  - General R/F—age, obesity, hypertension, smoking, thrombophilias, cardiac disease, and sickle cell disease
  - *Specific to pregnancy:* Hypertensive disorders of pregnancy, gestational diabetes mellitus (GDM), cesarean section, obstetrical hemorrhage, amniotic fluid embolism (AFE), and gestational trophoblastic diseases (GTDs)
- *Cerebral venous thrombosis:* 2% pregnancy-related strokes, associated with preeclampsia, sepsis, and thrombophilias
  - *Clinical features:* Headache, neurological deficits, and seizures
  - Late pregnancy and puerperium are the times of greatest risk
  - Diagnosed with MR venography
  - Management includes anticonvulsants for seizures, heparinization (efficacy controversial), antimicrobials if septic thrombophlebitis is suspected and fibrinolytic therapy for women failing systemic anticoagulation
- Risk of stroke recurrence is low, and previous ischemic stroke is not a contraindication to pregnancy
- Hemorrhagic stroke can be differentiated from an ischemic stroke only on imaging
- Systolic hypertension control important for the prevention of stroke
- 80% subarachnoid hemorrhage caused by rupture of Berry's aneurysm.

POSTERIOR REVERSIBLE ENCEPHALOPATHY SYNDROME

- A distinctive clinical and imaging syndrome characterized by acute headache, visual impairment, seizures, and altered sensorium.
- Disordered cerebral autoregulation and endothelial dysfunction.
- *Causes:* Elevated blood pressure (preeclampsia/eclampsia syndromes)
- Occasional focal deficits may be found.
- Imaging shows bilateral parieto-occipital hypodensities.
- Typical signs of PRES are best detected by T2- weighted and fluid-attenuated inversion recovery (FLAIR) MRI, which is the golden standard. CT scans only reveal 50% of the lesions
- Common findings are symmetric edema involving the white matter of the posterior regions of the cerebral hemispheres. Bilateral parieto-occipital hypodensities are the classic findings.

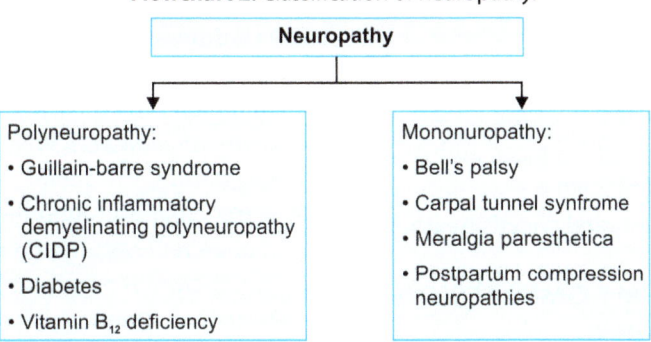

Flowchart 2: Classification of neuropathy.

GUILLAIN–BARRÉ SYNDROME

- Acute demyelinating rapidly progressive disorder
- Immune mediated. Triggers such as infections [*Cytomegalovirus (CMV)*, Epstein-Barr virus (EBV), Zika, and *Campylobacter*), immunization, and surgery
- *Clinical features:* Progressive symmetric ascending weakness, areflexic paralysis, and associated autonomic dysfunction
- Severe respiratory muscle weakness in 30% of women
- *Management:* Supportive, intensive care unit (ICU) admission for respiratory, cardiac, and hemodynamic monitoring, bladder bowel care, deep vein thrombosis (DVT) prophylaxis, enteral nutrition, intravenous immune globulin (IVIG), and plasma exchange beneficial if begun within 1–2 weeks of motor symptoms
- Guillain-Barré syndrome (GBS) is not an indication for lower (uterine) segment cesarean section (LSCS)
- Anesthetic issues to be considered (autonomic instability and avoid succinylcholine)
- Most patients recover completely within months to 1 year
- Mortality rate is 5% mainly due to pulmonary complications and arrhythmias.

BELL'S PALSY

- Facial nerve inflammation, often associated with herpes zoster (HSV) or zoster virus
- Four-fold increased prevalence in pregnant women
- *Clinical features:* Abrupt painful onset, maximum by 48 hours, asymmetric facial expression, and weakness in eye closure, can be associated with hyperacusis and loss of taste
- Recovery slightly worse in pregnant women (50%)
- *Management:* Facial muscle massage, eye protection against corneal laceration, and prednisone 1 mg/kg for 5 days.

CARPAL TUNNEL SYNDROME

- Most frequent mononeuropathy in pregnancy
- *Clinical features:* Burning, numbness, or tingling of thumb, index, and middle fingers of hand, bilateral in 80%
- *Management:* Wrist splints, occasional steroid injections, and surgical decompression.

MERALGIA PARESTHETICA

- Sensory neuropathy
- Lateral femoral nerve compression at the inguinal ligament
- Dysesthesias in the upper and middle part of the lateral thigh
- Self-limiting and rarely needs treatment.

POSTPARTUM COMPRESSION NEUROPATHIES

Postpartum compression neuropathies is depicted in **Table 1**.

MISCELLANEOUS DISORDERS

Multiple Sclerosis

- Immune-mediated demyelinating disorder. Genetic susceptibility and likely environmental trigger
- *Clinical features:* Sensory loss, optic neuritis causing visual symptoms, asymmetric weakness, and ataxia
- Decreased relapse rates during pregnancy and vice versa in postpartum
- Slight increased risk of pregnancy complications
- Acute attacks treated with high-dose IV methylprednisolone
- Symptomatic relief and disease-modifying agents.

Myasthenia Gravis

- Autoimmune mediated neuromuscular disorder.
- Antibodies to acetylcholine receptors.
- *Clinical features:* Weakness and easy fatigability of facial, oropharyngeal, extraocular and limb muscles, and deep tendon reflexes preserved.
- *Exacerbations triggers:* Systemic diseases, infections, emotional upsets.
- *Management:* Oral pyridostigmine, IVIG, or plasma exchange in the crisis.
- *Concerns in pregnancy:* No increased risk of adverse outcomes but avoid magnesium sulfate (curariform action), muscle relaxants with general anesthesia, and aminoglycosides.
- *Neonatal effects:* Due to transplacental passage of antibodies. Transient symptoms include feeble cries, poor suckling, and respiratory distress.

CONCLUSION

Neurological disorders generally have a good prognosis for both mother and neonate. Cerebral venous sinus thrombosis is common in postpartum patients. Brain tumors invariably enlarge during pregnancy because of estrogen and progesterone receptors on tumor cells. Although research related to neurologic

TABLE 1: Postpartum compression neuropathies.

Nerve	Compression site	Symptom–sign
Femoral (L2–L4)	Under Inguinal ligament	• Due to prolonged hip flexion • Difficulty climbing stairs • Weakness in knee extension
Obturator (L2–L4)	Lateral wall of the pelvis	• Weak adductors, Groin pain • Sensory loss in the inner thigh
Common peroneal (L4–5; S1–2)	Head of fibula	• Pressure from stirrups at head of fibula • Causes foot drop

disease in pregnancy is growing, but further research is needed.

REFERENCES

1. Cunningham FG, Leveno K, Bloom S, Spong C, Dashe J, Hoffman B, et al. Williams Obstetrics, 25th edition. McGraw Hill/Medica; 2018.
2. In: James D, Steer PJ, Weiner CP, Gonik B, Robson SC (Eds). High Risk Pregnancy management options, 5th edition. United Kingdom: Cambridge University Press; 2018.

MULTIPLE CHOICE QUESTIONS

1. All are true regarding migraine in pregnancy except for?
   a. Linked to hormone levels
   b. Most common cause of primary headache disorder in pregnancy
   c. No increased risk of ischemic stroke
   d. Ergotamine derivatives should be avoided

   Ans: c

2. A 30-year-old pregnant woman at 26 weeks of gestation presents to the emergency room with complaints of incapacitating throbbing unilateral headache with visual symptoms for 6 hours. Now she has altered sensorium. Her husband gives a history of similar headache episodes for the past 4 years that were relieved with medications. What should be done next?
   a. Only symptomatic management as a patient has had similar episodes
   b. Symptomatic management coupled with comprehensive neurological evaluation
   c. Defer evaluation for the postpartum period
   d. None of the above

   Ans: b

3. The most frequent presentation of cerebral venous thrombosis is?
   a. Headache
   b. Convulsions
   c. Visual symptoms
   d. Fever

   Ans: a

4. All are true regarding stroke in pregnancy except for?
   a. Women with preeclampsia undergoing general anesthesia are at higher risk of stroke compared to neuraxial anesthesia
   b. Previous ischemic stroke is a contraindication to pregnancy
   c. Risk of stroke recurrence in pregnancy is low if preventative factors are modified
   d. Differentiation of ischemic from hemorrhagic stroke is possible only with imaging

   Ans: b

5. The most common cause of subarachnoid hemorrhage in pregnancy is?
   a. Trauma
   b. Infection
   c. Ruptured Berry's aneurysm
   d. Coagulopathy

   Ans: c

6. Multiple sclerosis relapse rate during pregnancy:
   a. Increases during pregnancy and decreases postpartum
   b. Decreases during pregnancy and increases postpartum
   c. Remains unchanged
   d. Decreases in pregnancy and postpartum

   Ans: b

7. A 25-year-old G2P1 at 30 weeks gestation presents with weakness of bilateral legs that rapidly ascended to thighs in

few days. On examination deep tendon reflexes were absent. Which of the following is not true regarding this condition?
a. Poor and partial recovery in the maximum women
b. Immune-mediated disorder
c. Mortality in such patients is mainly due to pulmonary complications
d. Commonly associated with infections and immunization

Ans: a

8. A 22-year-old G1P0 + 0 at 38 weeks of gestation presents with a history of weakness and easy fatigability of lower and upper limbs on doing daily household chores for past 6 months. She now complains of severe headache since yesterday evening. On examination: BP—170/116, urine albumin +2, deep tendon reflexes present. All should be done except for?
a. Urgent blood pressure control
b. Magnesium sulphate prophylaxis to prevent seizures
c. Induction of labor
d. Close observation and respiratory support if needed during labor and delivery

Ans: b

9. All are true regarding Bell's palsy in pregnancy except:
a. Pregnant women carry a four-fold increased risk of having Bell's palsy
b. Maximum weakness is by 48 hours
c. Excellent recovery in pregnant women
d. Bilateral palsy is a prognostic marker for incomplete recovery

Ans: c

10. The most frequent mononeuropathy in pregnancy involves which nerve?
a. Median
b. Obturator
c. Common peroneal
d. Femoral

Ans: a

CHAPTER 11: Hypertensive Disorders in Pregnancy

Parul Sinha, Garima Gupta

INTRODUCTION

- Most common medical complications of pregnancy.
- Affects 7–15% of all gestations.
- Leading cause of maternal mortality.
- About 19% of maternal deaths were attributed to hypertensive disorder in pregnancy in developed countries (WHO, 2014).
- Incidence of preeclampsia was found to be 10.3%.
- The incidence of eclampsia is 1.9% antepartum >50% and postpartum 13%.
- Maternal mortality attributed to eclampsia is 4–6%.
- Hypertensive disorders of pregnancy are the spectrum of disorders ranging from already existing chronic hypertension in pregnancy to complex multisystem disorder such as preeclampsia leading to complication hemolysis, elevated liver enzymes, low platelet count (HELLP) syndrome, acute renal failure, pulmonary edema, stroke, and left ventricular failure.
- According to *International society for study of hypertension in pregnancy (ISSHP)* hypertensive disorders divided into groups as shown in **Flowchart 1**.

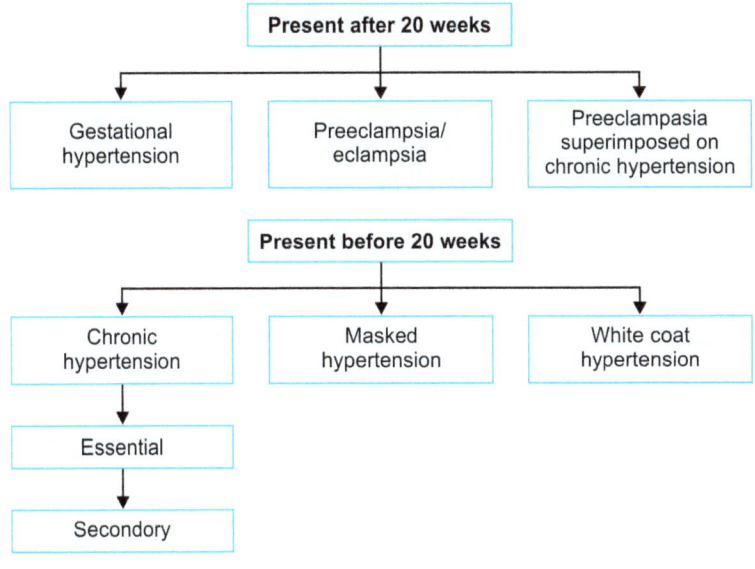

Flowchart 1: Classification of hypertensive disorders.[1]

TABLE 1: Types of hypertensive disorders.[2]

Types of hypertensive disorders	Definition
Prepregnancy or at <20 weeks	
• Chronic hypertension	• Hypertension detected prepregnancy or before 20 weeks' gestation.
• Essential	• Hypertension without a known secondary cause
• Secondary	• Hypertension with a known secondary cause (e.g., renal disease).
• White-coat hypertension	• sBP ≥140 and/or dBP ≥90 mm Hg when measured in the office or clinic, and BP <135/85 mm Hg using HBPM or ABPM readings
• Masked hypertension	• BP that is <140/90 mm Hg at a clinic/office visit, but ≥135/85 mm Hg at other times outside the clinic/office
Prepregnancy or a ≥20 weeks	
• Gestational hypertension	• Hypertension arising de novo at ≥20 weeks' gestation in the absence of proteinuria or other findings suggestive of preeclampsia
• Transient gestational hypertension	• Hypertension arising at ≥20 weeks' gestation in the clinic, which resolves with repeated BP readings

• Preeclampsia de novo	• Preeclampsia (de novo) is gestational hypertension accompanied by one or more of the following new onset conditions at ≥20 weeks' gestation:
	  – Proteinuria
	  – Other maternal end-organ dysfunction, including:
	    - Neurological complications (e.g., eclampsia, altered mental status, blindness, stroke, clonus, severe headaches, or persistent visual scotomata)
	    - Pulmonary edema
	    - Hematological complications (e.g., platelet count <150,000/μL, DIC, hemolysis)
	    - AKI (such as creatinine ≥90 μmol/L or 1 mg/dL)
	    - Liver involvement (e.g., elevated transaminases such as ALT or AST >40 IU/L) with or without right upper quadrant or epigastric abdominal pain)
	    - Uteroplacental dysfunction (e.g., placental abruption, angiogenic imbalance, fetal growth restriction, abnormal umbilical artery Doppler waveform analysis, or intrauterine fetal death)

(AKI: acute kidney injury; ALT: alanine transaminase; AST: aspartate transaminase; ABPM: ambulatory blood pressure monitoring; dBP: diastolic blood pressure; DIC: disseminated intravascular coagulation; HBPM: home blood pressure monitoring; sBP: systolic blood pressure)

■ DEFINITIONS

Types of hypertensive disorders are defined in **Table 1 and Table 2**.

■ BLOOD PRESSURE MEASUREMENT

- Blood pressure measurement is the most important clinical test to diagnostic hypertensive disorders of pregnancy (HDP).
- Blood pressure (BP) assessment is to be done with utmost care and proper technique.
- Mercury manometer periodically standardized is the ideal equipment to be used.
- The position of the pregnant mother especially after 20 weeks of gestation should be either in the sitting position or

TABLE 2: The classification of hypertensive disorders of pregnancy according to different organizations.[2]

	ACOG	ISSHP	NICE
Chronic hypertension	BP >140/90 mm Hg, predating the pregnancy or before 20 weeks	BP >140/90 mm Hg, predating the pregnancy or before 20 weeks	BP >140/90 mm Hg, present at the booking visit or before 20 weeks or if the woman is already taking antihypertensive medication when referred to maternity services
Gestational hypertension	New onset hypertension and >140/90 mm Hg after 20 weeks gestation in the absence of features of PE	New onset hypertension and >140/90 mm Hg after 20 weeks gestation in the absence of features of PE	>140/90 mm Hg after 20 weeks gestation without significant proteinuria
Preeclampsia (PE)	New onset hypertension >140/90 mm Hg, after 20 weeks gestation, with at least one of the following: • Proteinuria >300 mg per 24 hour urine collection or protein to creatinine ratio 0.3 or dipstick reading of +2 • Renal insufficiency (serum creatinine of 1.1 mg/dL or doubling of serum creatinine concentration • Thrombocytopenia pc <100 × 10^9/L • Impaired liver function (elevated liver enzymes to twice the upper limit of normal) • Pulmonary edema • New onset headache or visual symptom	New onset hypertension >140/90 mm Hg, after 20 weeks gestation, with at least one of the following: • Proteinuria (protein to creatinine ratio >30 mg/mmol • Acute kidney injury (creatinine >90 µmol >1 mg/dL) • Hematological complication pc <1.5 lac/µmol DIC, hemolysis • Liver involvement (elevated transaminase level at >40 IU/L • Neurological complication • Uteroplacental complications (fetal growth restriction)	New onset hypertension >140/90 mm Hg after 20 weeks gestation with at least one of the following: • Proteinuria (protein to creatinine ratio >30 mg/mmol or albumin to creatinine ratio of >8 m/mmol/L or >1 g/L +2 on dipstick testing • Renal insufficiency (creatinine >90 µmol/mL and >1.02 mg/dL • Hematological complications (pc 1.5 lac DIC, hemolysis • Liver involvement (elevated transaminase level >40 IU/L • Neurological complication, • Uteroplacental dysfunction (fetal growth restriction, abnormal umbilical artery Doppler waveform analysis stillbirth)

(ACOG: American College of Obstetricians and Gynecologists; DIC: disseminated intravascular coagulation; ISSHP: International society for study of hypertension in pregnancy; NICE: National Institute for Health and Care Excellence)

left lateral position with the zero level at the level of the heart.
- Any forearm left/right can be used to tie the cuff of the appropriate size.
- In absence of mercury manometer, calibrated aneroid equipment may be used.

PROTEINURIA

- Significant proteinuria is urinary excretion of >300 mg protein in a 24 hour period.
- Once significant proteinuria is established, further quantification is not required as proteinuria does not have prognostic value from management point of view.
- However, if proteinuria is absent, pregnant woman with hypertension still requires frequent monitoring.
- The HDP Gestosis scientific group recommends the following methods till further research findings are out:
  • Urinary dipstick method (visual/by automated device)
  • Spot urine protein: creatinine (P/C) ratio.

ETIOPATHOGNESIS

Hypertensive disorders are more likely to develop in women with following characteristics:
- Exposed to chorionic villi for the first time.
- Exposed to superabundance of chorionic villi (multifetal pregnancy or molar pregnancy).
- Though chorionic villi are essential but need not be intrauterine (preeclampsia may develop in abdominal pregnancy).
- Having preexisting conditions associated with endothelial cell activation or inflammation such as diabetes, obesity, cardiovascular disease, and renal disease.

TWO STAGE HYPOTHESIS

Stage 1

Faulty endovascular trophoblastic remodeling.

In normal pregnancy endovascular trophoblastic tissue invades spiral arteries initiated at 12 weeks and completed by 16th week.

Advantage

- Converts high resistance vessels into low resistance vessels.
- Become resistant to effects of vasomotor agents.
- However, in preeclampsia this trophoblastic invasion is incomplete (does not reach myometrial portion)
- Also arteries maintain their response to vasomotor agents.

Stage 2

- Amenable to modification by preexisting conditions like diabetes obesity Cardiovascular disease
- Conversion of this uteroplacental maladaptation to maternal systemic syndrome of preeclampsia.

IMMUNOLOGICAL FACTORS (FLOWCHART 2)

- Loss of maternal tolerance to paternally derived placental and fetal antigens.
- Paternal antigen load if increased, e.g., molar pregnancy.
- Th1 action more than Th2 action.
- In normal pregnancy there is type 2 bias (type 2 helper cells action more than type 1).

Extravillous trophoblast early in pregnancy has low expression of human leukocyte antigens (HLA)-G in case of preeclampsia.

Flowchart 2: Immunological factors.[3]

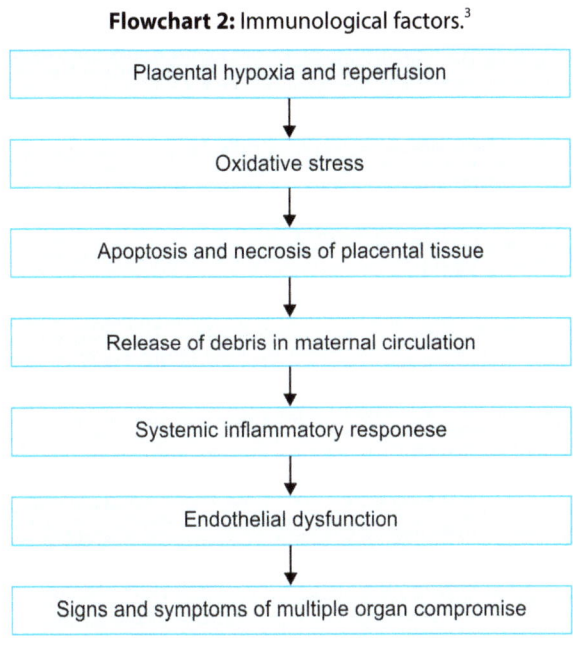

Fig. 1: Pathology of hypertensive disorders.

GENETIC FACTORS

- Preeclampsia is a multifactorial polygenic disorder.
- Incidence of preeclampsia in daughters of preeclamptic mother is 20–40%.
- Incidence in sisters of preeclampsia women is 11–37%.
- In twins 22–47%.
- Hundreds of genes have been studied.
- Because of complex phenotypic expression it is doubtful that a one single gene is responsible.

PATHOLOGY

Pathology of hypertensive disorders is depicted **Figure 1**.

TABLE 3: Prevention of hypertensive disorders.[3]

BP level	BP (mm Hg) dBp*	Next BP	Actions — Contact maternity care provider	Ongoing BP monitoring
Very high	≥105	Sit quietly for 5 min, measure BP again, and send in readings	Contact maternity unit within **4 hours**	Daily
High	90–104		Contact care-provider within **24 hours**	Daily
High-normal	86–89		If repeat BP still high-normal, contact care-provider within **24 hours**	Daily
Normal	81–85	As planned	As planned	As planned
Low-normal	75–80	• If not taking BP medication, continue as planned • If taking BP medication, sit quietly for 5 min, measure BP again, and send in readings	• If not taking BP medication and feeling well, no action required • If taking BP medication and repeat BP still low-normal or low, contact care-provider within 24 hours • Regardless of whether BP medication is being taken, if feeling unwell (such as dizzy), contact care-provider within **4 hours**	• As planned if not taking BP medication and feeling well • Daily if taking BP medication, or as instructed by care provider if antihypertensive therapy is changed
Low	<75			

(BP: blood pressure; dBP: diastolic blood pressure)
*If at any time, sBP is ≥155 mm Hg, BP should be considered very high and actions taken accordingly.

■ PREVENTION (TABLES 3 AND 4)

- Unless there are contraindications, all women should exercise in pregnancy to reduce the likelihood of gestational hypertension and preeclampsia.
- For women with low dietary intake of calcium (<900 mg/day), oral calcium supplementation of at least 500 mg/day is recommended.
- Women should not receive low-molecular-weight heparin*, vitamins C or E, or folic acid for preeclampsia prevention.

Women at Increased Risk of Preeclampsia

Recommendations

- Low-dose aspirin is recommended to be taken at bedtime, preferably before 16 weeks and discontinued by 36 weeks.
- After multivariable screening, aspirin should be given at a dose of 150 mg/night.
- After screening with clinical risk factors and BP, aspirin should be given at a dose of 100–162 mg/day.

TABLE 4: Maintenance therapy and suggested dose titration of antihypertensive therapy for nonurgent control of hypertension in pregnancy (modified from Magee, et al., 2020).[3]

First-line	Caution	Low*	If BP not controlled	Medium	Dosage (mg) If BP not controlled on medium dosage	High†	Maximum
Labetalol	• Contraindicated with poorly-controlled asthma • May cause neonatal bradycardia and hypoglycaemia and warrants newborn screening	100 mg three to four times/day	→ Proceed to medium dose of same low-dose medication	200 mg three to four times/day	→ Consider ADDING another low-dose medication rather than going to a high dose of the same medication(s), for a maximum of 3 medications	300 mg three to four times/day →	1200 mg/day
Nifedpine PA or MR	Contraindicated with aortic stenosis	10 mg two to three times/day		20 mg two to three times/day		30 mg two to three times/day →	120 mg/day
Nifedipine XL or LA		30 mg once/day		30 mg two times/day *or* 60 mg once/day		30 mg each morning and 60 each evening →	120 mg/day
Methyldopa	May cause maternal depression	250 mg three to four times/day	→	500 mg three to four times/day		750 mg three times/day →	2250 mg/day

(LA: long-acting; MR: modified release; PA: prolonged action; XL: extended release).
*Starting doses are higher than generally recommended for adults given more rapid clearance in pregnancy.
†When a medication is at high (or maximum) dosage, consider using a different medication to treat any severe hypertension that may develop

Exercise

To achieve these reductions, women must undertake at least 140 minutes per week of moderate-intensity exercise, such as brisk walking, water aerobics, stationary cycling with moderate effort, resistance training, carrying moderate loads, and household chores such as gardening or washing windows. Typically during these activities, a person can talk but not sing, and notices that their heart rate has increased.

Exercise is contraindicated in all women with established preeclampsia, and relatively contraindicated in women with gestational hypertension but among those without contraindications, there are no significant adverse effects of exercise in pregnancy.

Calcium

Calcium administered from 20 weeks' gestation is effective in decreasing preeclampsia risk when administered at high (1.5–2.5 g/day) or low dose (<1 g/day) and to women at high or low risk of preeclampsia, but only among populations with low baseline intake of calcium (<900 mg/day).

SEVERE HYPERTENSION MANAGEMENT

Prevention of seizures $MgSO_4$ administration is depicted in **Table 5 and Figure 2**.

HELLP SYNDROME

Mississippi classification
- Class I (severe thrombocytopenia) pc <50,000.
- Class II (moderate thrombocytopenia) pc 50,000–100,000.
- Class III (mild thrombocytopenia) pc 100,000–150,000 and aspartate transaminase (AST) >40 IU/L.
- Stabilize the patient, give antihypertensive and $MgSO_4$ for seizure prophylaxis.
- The lowest observed value of platelets occurs after 23 hours of delivery.
- The disease may achieve peak intensity during first 2 days after delivery including downward trend in hematocrit.
- With supportive care alone 90% of patients with HELLP syndrome will have platelet count 1lac/mm^3 and are versed trend in liver enzyme within 7 days of delivery.
- Platelets are given when platelet count is below 50,000/mm^3.
- After delivery the platelet count will reach nadir at in 24–48 hours but will rapidly increase after 3rd day postpartum.
- An upward trend in platelet and downward trend in liver enzymes should be apparent by 4th postpartum day in patients recovering without complication.
- Plasmapheresis has a dramatic effect on the course of disease and is life-saving procedure in patients who follow a relentless course of deterioration despite conventional therapy.
- The use of corticosteroids for improvement in platelet count is not recommended.
- Timing of delivery In hypertensive disorder of pregnancy **(Table 6)**.

TABLE 5: Prevention of seizures $MgSO_4$ administration.

Regimen	Loading dose	Maintenance dose
Pritchard's	20 mL of 20% (4 g) slow in 3–5 min; +10 mL of 50% (5 g) deep IM* on each buttock (10 g)	10 mL of 50% (5 g) deep IM on alternate buttock every 4 h
Dhaka	4 g IV + (20%) given over 15 min and 2 g as 50% solution given IM in each buttock	2.5 g as 50% solution IM on alternate buttock every 4 h
Zuspan	4 g IV (20%) in 100 mL fluid given over 15 to 20 min	1 g/h in 100 mL fluid IV
Sibai	6 g IV over 20 min	2 g IV infusion

*IM = Intramuscular; †IV = Intravenous

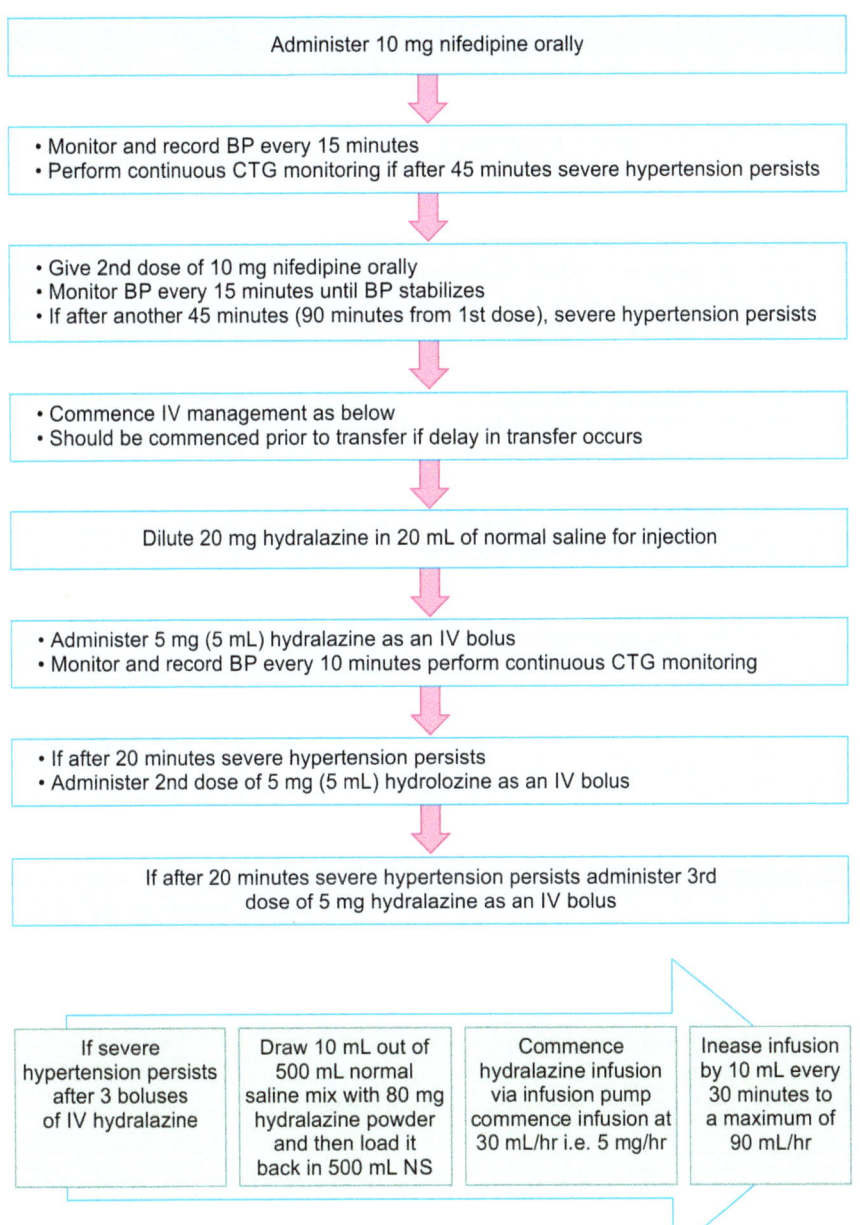

Fig. 2: Management of severe hypertension.[2]

■ CONCLUSION

- HDP results in multi systemic affection with profound implications for both the mother and the baby.
- Early recognition of the signs and symptoms is important in preventing its complications.
- Timely delivery is crucial for maternal and fetal well-being.

TABLE 6: Recommendations for timing of birth.[2]

Gestational age	Preeclampsia	Gestational hypertension	Chronic hypertension
Previability	Termination of pregnancy should be discussed		
Viability to 33^{+6} weeks	Expectant management should be considered, but only in hospitals where very preterm infants and sick mothers can be cared for	Expectant care is recommended unless there is an indication for birth	Expectant care is recommended unless there is an indication for birth
34^{+0} to 36^{+6} weeks	At 34^{+0} to 36^{+6} weeks, initiation of delivery should be discussed as it decreases maternal but increases neonatal risk, particularly where antenatal corticosteroids are not prescribed		
$\geq 37^{+0}$ weeks	Initiation of delivery is recommended	Women who reach 40^{+0} weeks should be offered delivery Women at 37^{+0} to 39^{+6} weeks may be offered delivery	Women who reach 40^{+0} weeks should be offered delivery Initiation of delivery may be offered at 38^{+0} to 39^{+6} week

REFERENCES

1. Brown MA, Magee LA, Kenny LC, Karumanchi SA, McCarthy FP, Saito S, et al. The hypertensive disorders of pregnancy: ISSHP classification, diagnosis & management recommendations for international practice. Pregnancy Hypertens. 2018;13:291-310.
2. Hoffman B, Casey B, Spong C, Cunningham FG, Dashe J, Leveno K. Williams obstetrics, 26th edition. India: McGraw-Hill Education; 2022.
3. Arias F. Arias' Practical Guide to High-Risk Pregnancy and Delivery: A South Asian Perspective, 5th edition. Gurgaon: Elsevier; 2019.

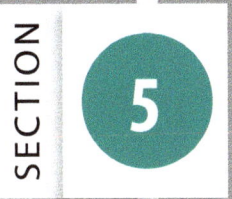

General

- **Multiple Births**
  Priyankur Roy, Athulya Shajan

- **Isoimmunization in Pregnancy**
  Rekha Rajendrakumar

- **Bleeding in Pregnancy**
  Sayamstuti Pattanaik

- **Bad Obstetric History in Pregnancy**
  Umme Ruman

- **Assisted Reproductive Technology Pregnancy—Are They Different?**
  Neharika Malhotra

CHAPTER 12

Multiple Births

Priyankur Roy, Athulya Shajan

■ INTRODUCTION

Multiple pregnancy rates have been largely fueled by infertility treatments. Evolving infertility treatments to optimize outcomes have lowered the rates of higher order multifetal births. Twin fetuses result from fertilization of two separate ova, which yields dizygotic/fraternal twins and are like any other pair of siblings from a genetic perspective.[1]

Less often a single fertilized ovum divides to create monozygotic/identical twins. This postzygotic mutation is a teratogenic event and has higher risk of discordant malformations and a 12-fold increased risk of congenital heart diseases.[2,3] The incidence of splitting increases 2 to 5-fold in pregnancies conceived with assisted reproductive technology (ART). This may be due to specimen handling, growth media or sperm deoxyribonucleic acid (DNA) microinjection.[4] The outcome in multiple gestations depends on when the division occurs.[5]

Division occurring after first 72 hours of fertilization gives rise to a dichorionic diamniotic (DCDA) pregnancy with two embryos—two amnions and two chorions, with two separate placentas or a single large fused placenta. Division between the 4th–8th day results in an monochorionic diamniotic (MCDA) twin pregnancy and between 8th and 14th day results in an monochorionic monoamniotic (MCMA) pregnancy (chorion and amnion differentiated). Although very rare, division beyond 14 days leads to conjoint MCMA twins (embryonic disc differentiated).

■ FACTORS AFFECTING TWINNING (FIG. 1)

Frequency varies between races and ethnic groups; highest recorded in Nigeria (1 in every 20 births) and lowest in Japan (1 in 1,300). This may be attributed to racial variations in follicle stimulating hormone (FSH) levels. Advancing maternal age increases the risk, probably due to higher FSH levels in response to impending ovarian failure and increased ART pregnancies.[6] Twinning also increases with parity. History of twinning in the family especially on the maternal side is a determinant of twinning.[7] Taller and heavier women had a higher twinning rate 25–30% greater than short, nutritionally deprived women. Higher rate of DCDA twins has been reported in women who conceive within 1 month after stopping oral contraceptive pills (OCP's).[8] ART increased multifetal gestations by 30%, but after American Society of Reproductive Medicine (ASRM) revised their age-related guidelines, younger women <35 years are encouraged for single embryo transfer

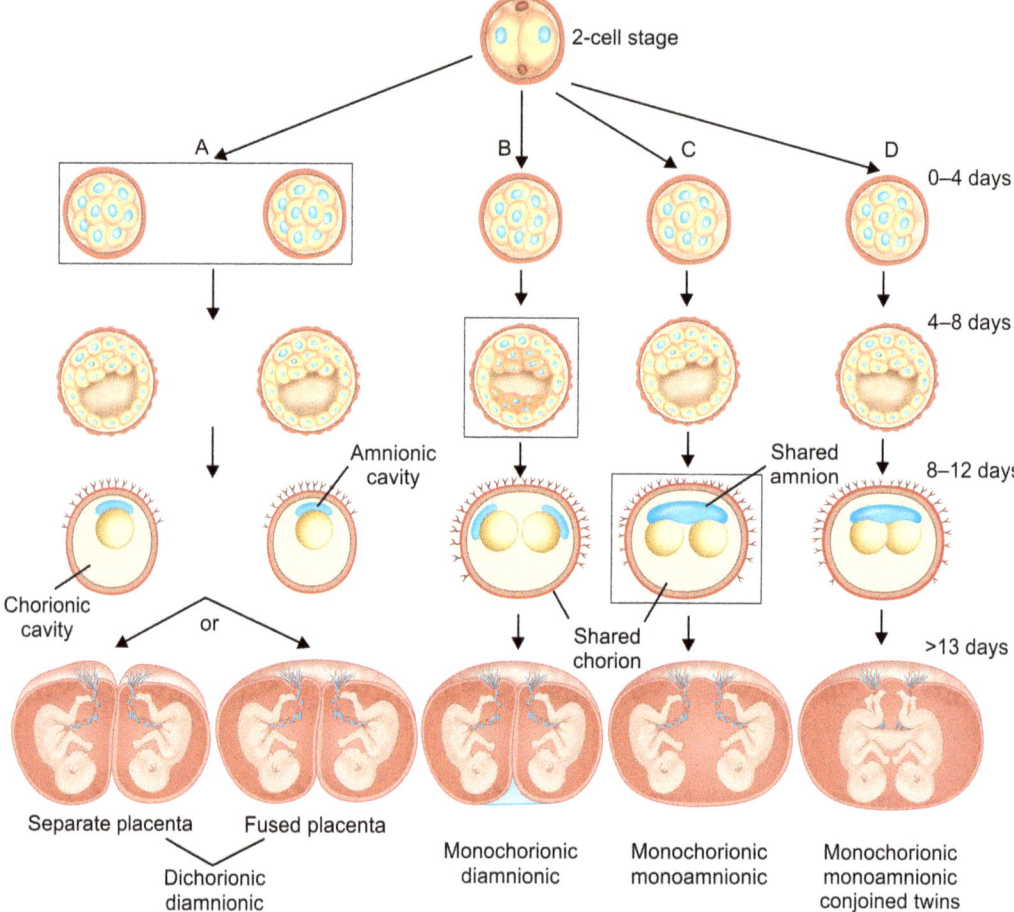

Fig. 1: Classification of twins based on chorionicity and amniocity.

regardless of embryo stage, and thus, higher order pregnancies have declined.

■ COMPLICATIONS[9]

Antenatal Maternal Complications

First Trimester

1. Hyperemesis [elevated β-human chorionic gonadotropin (β-HCG) levels]
2. Spontaneous miscarriage (16 times more risk in monochorionic twins).

Second Trimester

1. Hypertensive disorders (3–4 times increased risk of pre-eclampsia)
2. Hyperglycemia in pregnancy (elevated human placental lactogen (HPL) and other placental hormones)
3. Anemia (dimorphic anemia)
4. Valvular heard disease—decompensation
5. Increased risk of skin manifestations and obstetric cholestasis.

Third Trimester

1. Preterm labor (50% of women with twin pregnancies give birth by 36 weeks)
2. Polyhydramnios [Monochorionic (MC) twins with twin to twin transfusion syndrome (TTTS)]

3. Pressure symptoms
4. Breathing difficulty (increased cardiac output 20% more than singleton pregnancy, increased stroke volume, reduced vascular resistance)
5. Edema of lower limbs [pressure on iliac veins and inferior vena cava (IVC)]
6. Obstructive uropathy
7. Varicose veins
8. Antepartum hemorrhage
   a. Placenta previa
   b. Abruption.

Intrapartum and Postpartum Complications

First Stage
1. Malpresentations and malpositions
2. Premature preterm rupture of membranes (PPROM)
3. Abruptio
4. Prolonged/dysfunctional labor (inertia of overdistension)
5. Requiring augmentation with oxytocin
6. Cord prolapse.

Second Stage
1. Operative vaginal delivery
2. Internal podalic version (IPV) and breech extraction (second of twin)
3. Placental abruption in second of twin
4. Cord entanglement and its complications (in MCMA twins)
5. Cesarean section.

Third Stage
1. Atonic postpartum haemorrhage (PPH) (inertia due to overdistension, prolonged labor, and large placental bed)
2. Retained products.

Postpartum
1. Secondary PPH
2. Subinvolution
3. Venous thromboembolism
4. Lactation difficulties
5. Postpartum depression.

Fetal Complications

Antepartum
1. Vanishing twin may get resorbed or is seen as fetus papyraceus during delivery (**Fig. 2**).
2. Congenital anomalies (higher risk of discordant malformations and congenital heart diseases)
3. Discordancy (>20% difference in birth weight/>20 mm difference in abdominal circumference (AC) or >8 mm discordance in biparietal diameter (BPD) between twins)
4. Prematurity—spontaneous or iatrogenic
5. Intrauterine Growth Restriction (IUGR) (2 times more in Dichorionic (DC) and four times increased risk with MC)—may be due to crowding, uteroplacental insufficiency, or abnormal placentation

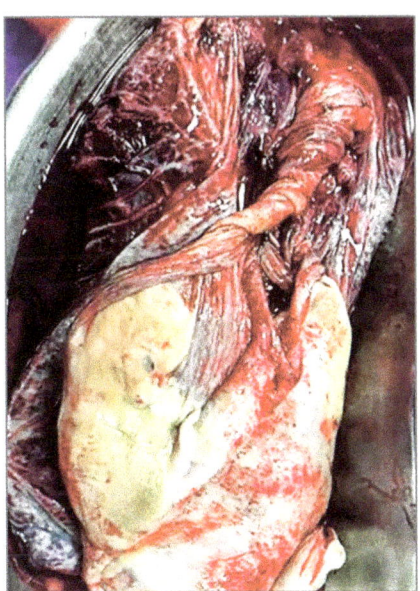

Fig. 2: Fetus papyraceus.

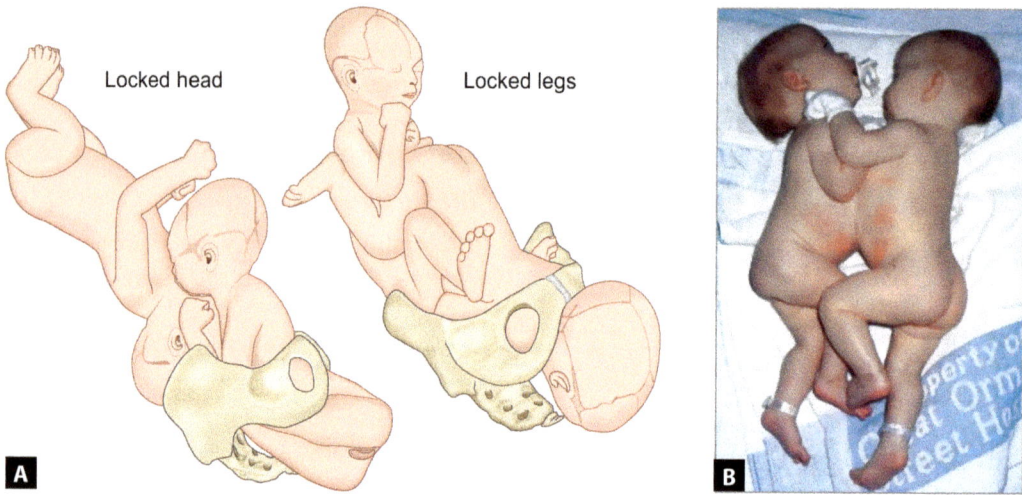

Figs. 3A and B: (A) Interlocking twins; (B) Conjoint twins.

6. Single fetal demise—due to anomalies/cord entanglement/placental insufficiency/abruption, requires more careful surveillance and magnetic resonance imaging (MRI) in MC twins
7. Complications unique to MC twins—congenital anomalies, TTTS, twin reversed arterial perfusion sequence (TRAPS), twin anemia-polycythemia sequence (TAPS), conjoint twins, perinatal mortality, interlocking twins **(Figs. 3A and B)**.

Intrapartum

1. Preterm labor
2. PPROM
3. Cord prolapse
4. IPV and breech extraction (second of twin)
5. Abruption of second of twin.

■ CASE SCENARIO–1

Mrs. X diagnosed to have DCDA twins, now at 37 weeks with no known comorbidities reports with lower abdominal pain for 4 hours. P/A-contractions+, F1-cephalic, Non-stress test (NST-reactive), ultrasound was done to confirm the lie of both babies and the placenta was upper segment anterior. Per vaginal exam-cervix soft, fully effaced, 3 cm dilated, head at 0 station, pelvis adequate.

■ DIAGNOSIS OF DCDA TWINS

History and physical examination:
1. Maternal age
2. Parity
3. Body mass index (BMI)
4. Family history of twins
5. Recent use of ovulation induction drugs or gonadotrophins
6. Pregnancy conceived on ART.

Late in first trimester two heartbeats may be separately heard, more distinctly with a handheld Doppler. In second and third trimester, uterus appears overdistended, about 5 cm greater than expected. Palpating two fetal heads in different quadrants oints to a diagnosis of twins, but palpation may be challenging if one twin overlies the other or if the woman is obese or if there is hydramnios.

Diagnosis of DCDA twins:
1. *Number of gestational sacs* in the first trimester is useful to determine chorionicity in the early part of the first trimester because during early gestation, the amnion would be closely applied to the embryo and a definite amniotic cavity may not be visible. If *two separate gestational sacs are seen*, it means there are two chorionic cavities and is therefore dichorionic.
2. *Number of placental masses:* If two placental masses are distinctly seen, it is dichorionic.
3. *Discordant sex:* Definitely DCDA.
4. *Twin peak/lambda sign:* Examining the point of origin of the dividing membrane on the placental surface for the twin peak or lambda sign helps determine the chorionicity in pregnancies with a single placental mass, or two placentas lying side by side. Twin peak sign is characteristic of dichorionic pregnancy and is due to the lifting of the chorion, i.e., chorionic tissue intervening between the two layers of the inter twin membrane at the placental base. On ultrasonography (USG) we see an isoechoic triangular projection of trophoblastic tissue. The absence of the sign does not exclude dichorionicity.
5. *Thickness and number of layers on the intertwin membrane:* By high resolution ultrasound it is now possible to determine the number of layers on the inter twin membrane. Four layers indicate dichorionicity. The membrane thickness gives a clue to chorionicity. A hyperechoic membrane with a thickness >2 mm can be considered as dichorionic. Membrane thickness assessment becomes unreliable beyond 26 weeks as the membranes get thinned out.
6. *Placental examination:* Adjacent amnions are separated by a chorion, it could be dizygotic or monozygotic but more commonly dizygotic twinning.

Differential Diagnosis
1. Full bladder
2. Polyhydramnios
3. Macrosomia
4. Fibroid with pregnancy
5. Ovarian mass with pregnancy
6. Abruptio
7. Mass arising from any other pelvic structures.

Management
1. Review antenatal records
2. Admit the patient to labor room
3. Check hemoglobin, group Rh, and routine ANC investigations.

First Stage
1. Keep her hydrated.
2. Establish IV access.
3. Keep crossmatched blood ready.
4. Senior obstetrician, assistant, 2 neonatologists, and an anesthetist must be available.
5. Labor ultrasound machine.
6. Two delivery sets.
7. Monitor pulse rate, BP, RR, SpO_2 and contractions, augment with oxytocin if necessary.
8. Continuous cardiotocogram (CTG) monitoring
9. Per-vaginal exam every 4 hours to assess the progress of labor.

Second Stage
1. Delivery of the first twin is completed like a singleton pregnancy and cord is clamped. *There is no sufficient evidence*

or recommendations on delayed cord clamping and is usually not practiced in twin. Intertwin delivery interval normally does not exceed 30 minutes.[10]

Delivery of second of twin
1. Palpate the abdomen to find the lie and presentation, ultrasound also may be used, and if there is excess bleeding suggestive of abruptio, delivery of the second twin should be expedited with instrumentation.
2. If second twin is vertex – once engaged, oxytocin augmentation can be done and membranes may be ruptured and delivered.
3. If it is breech presentation, an assisted breech delivery is performed.
4. If transverse lie, try external version and if it is unsuccessful, IPV and breech extraction. Cesarean done is IPV is unsuccessful and is the os is closed.
5. After delivery of second twin two clamps are applied to the cord of the second twin. Cord blood samples may help confirm the zygosity and DNA fingerprinting can be used for a more definitive diagnosis.
6. Perineal laceration or episiotomy is sutured.

Third Stage
1. One should actively manage the third stage in twin pregnancies-controlled cord traction, uterine massage, and uterotonics.
2. Once the signs of placental separation are visible, deliver the placenta in toto
3. Examine the placenta for the number of layers in the intertwin membrane.
4. Episiotomy is given is sutured in layers.

Fourth Stage
1. Monitor pulse rate, BP, RR, and SpO_2.
2. Watch for bleeding and palpate the uterus to make sure it is contracted.
3. Initiate breast feeding for both babies.
4. Encourage the mother to pass urine.

■ CASE SCENARIO–2

Mrs. X, 30-year-old primipara, IVF pregnancy was diagnosed to have MCDA twins by first trimester ultrasound. At 24 weeks, ultrasound showed absent urine in the fetal bladder, an single deepest pocket (SDP) of 1.5 cm and reversal of flow in umbilical artery in twin A and twin B had an SDP of 8.5 cm.

Diagnosis—MCDA twins with TTTS Quintero stage 3; Diagnosis is by ultrasound with Doppler:
1. *Number of gestational sacs:* If only one sac is seen it implies a monochorionic twin. MCDA twins may appear as one sac in early gestation as they share a common chorionic cavity.
2. *Number of placental masses:* If only a single placental mass is seen one cannot be sure if it is monochorionic or a fused dichorionic placenta.
3. *Discordant sex:* Definitely DCDA.
4. Twin peak/lambda sign: The absence of the sign does not exclude dichorionicity.
5. *Thickness and number of layers on the intertwin membrane:* A hyperechoic membrane with a thickness <2 mm it is considered monochorionic. Membrane thickness assessment becomes unreliable beyond 26 weeks as the membranes get thinned out.

■ TWIN TO TWIN TRANSFUSION SYNDROME[11]

It develops due to unbalanced deep A-V anastomosis. Blood is transfused from the twin on the arterial side that (donor) to its recipient sibling on the venous side (recipient).

This slow and continuous donation of blood from one fetus into the other continues over weeks to months, making the donor anemic and growth restricted. In contrast, the recipient develops polycythemia and circulatory overload, which manifests as hydrops. The donor twin becomes pale, and the recipient sibling becomes plethoric.

Also due to the imbalance in blood flow, there is oligoamnios in the donor and polyhydramnios in the recipient twin. If the heart failure, severe hypervolemia, and hyper viscosity are not identified and promptly treated, it may lead to severe hyperbilirubinemia and kernicterus in the neonatal period. There are two types of TTTS—obligatory and facultative. Obligatory TTTS is due to imbalance in vascular communications where there is at least one deep A-V anastomoses, with unidirectional flow with or without superficial anastomoses. If superficial anastomoses are present, the unidirectional flow is countered to some extent and thereby the risk of developing T'TTS is much lesser (15%). If counter directional flow is absent in the presence of a deep A-V anastomosis, the risk of TTTS is higher (61%).

Facultative TTTS occurs due to selective cardiac dysfunction or pump failure in one twin. The median age at diagnosis of TTTS is 21-29 weeks. The ultrasound markers that help with diagnosis are:
1. An MC gestation is the first predictor (<10 weeks)
2. Discordance in NT between the two twins (11 – 13^{+6} weeks scan)
3. Folding of the intertwin membrane (15-17 weeks)
4. Poor growth of one twin on serial ultrasound
5. Absence of superficial A-A anastomosis in color Doppler from 14 weeks.

The following sonographic findings suggest the diagnosis of TTTS:
1. MC gestation
2. Polyhydramnios (SDP >8 cm) in one sac and oligoamnios (SDP <2 cm) in the other[12]
3. Discrepancy between umbilical cord sizes
4. Cardiac dysfunction and hydramnios in the recipient twin
5. Abnormal umbilical artery or ductus venous Doppler velocimetry.

One should assess the cardiovascular function of MC twins with echocardiography. Cardiac function is measured by the Doppler myocardial performance index. It is the global ventricular function and is calculated for each ventricle.

■ QUINTERO STAGING SYSTEM

Stage I: Polyhydramnios (largest vertical pocket >8 cm in one sac) and oligoamnios (largest vertical pocket <2 cm in the other twin) and urine is seen in the fetal bladder of the donor twin.

Stage II: Stage I and urine is not visible within the donor bladder.

Stage III: Stage II with abnormal Doppler studies of the umbilical artery, ductus venous, or umbilical vein.

Stage IV: Stage III and ascites or frank hydrops in either twin.

Stage V: Demise of either fetus.

All stages are further sub-divided into A and B. A is when superficial A-A anastomoses present and in B superficial A-A anastomoses is absent.

The Quintero staging system predicts the fetal prognosis. The recipient's outcome is generally worse than the donor's. Acute TTTS happens quickly, typically after 30 weeks of pregnancy. It can also happen during labor in a vaginal birth, or after the cord of the first

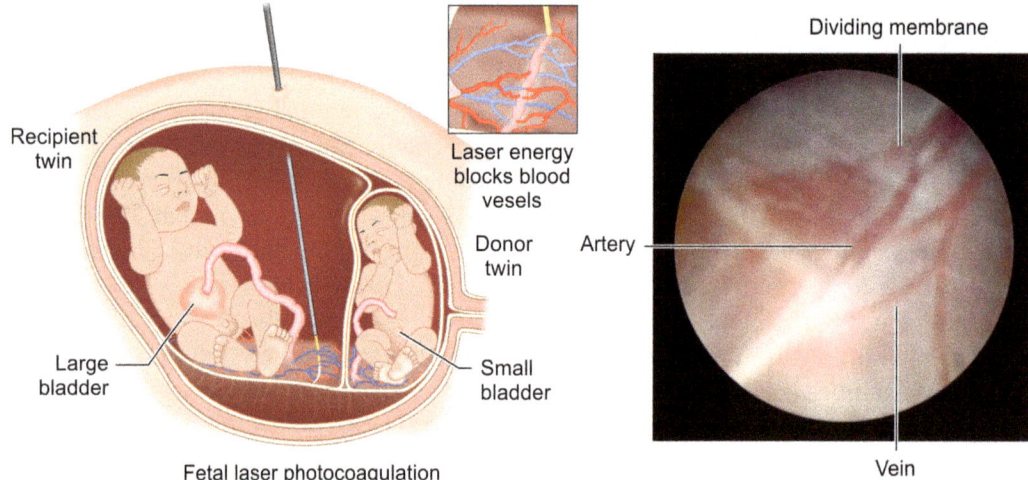

Fig. 4: Fetoscopic laser occlusion of chorioangiopagus vessel (FLOC) procedure.

baby is clamped. Also occurs in cases of single fetal demise.

Several therapies are used for TTTS. These include[13]:
1. *Serial amnio reduction:* If the amniotic fluid index (AFI) is >40 or the SDP >12; (Target—AFI being 15).
2. *Septostomy:* One step procedure; by creation of a communication in the dividing amniotic membrane using 20–22 G needle.
3. *Selective feticide* of the recipient twin by bipolar/laser coagulation of the cord.
4. *Laser ablation of vascular anastomoses:* Fetoscopic laser occlusion of chorioangiopagus vessel (FLOC) is now the preferred method for management between 16–26 weeks of gestation **(Fig. 4)**. The procedure is conducted under regional or local anesthesia. Tocolysis and prophylactic antibiotics are used. It is the only treatment option, which targets the underlying pathology (of unilateral arteriovenous anastomosis (AVAs)) and involves ultrasound-guided insertion of a 3-mm trocar in to the recipient sac at right angles to the donor's longitudinal axis to allow the operator to visualize the intertwin membrane and AVAs. A fetoscope and laser fiber (an Nd-YAG or diode laser at 40-60 Watts) is introduced through the trocar and anastomoses are coagulated under direct fetoscopic vision.

Techniques for coagulation include:

The selective sequential technique—avoiding the A-A and V-V anastomoses.

The non-selective technique—coagulating all vessels crossing the membrane to ensure none—is missed. Missed anastomoses are the most common cause of recurrence and morbidity, with recurrent TTTS occurring in up to 14% of pregnancies treated with FLC and can be associated with or without TAPS.

The equatorial laser dichorionization (known as the Solomon technique) involves completing an initial selective coagulation and then coagulating a dividing line across the vascular equator.[10] Fetoscopic laser occlusion of chorioangiopagous vessel (FLOC) is used to treat Quintero stage II or above.

The maternal complications include:
- Pain secondary to amniotic fluid leaking in to the peritoneal cavity.
- Bleeding, chorioamnionitis, preterm labor, and PPROM.
- Abruption and maternal thromboembolism are rare complications.

Fetal complications include:
- Early, especially in the first 6 days, single and double intrauterine death (IUD) and TAPS.
- Late complications are recurrent or reversed TTTS and late TAPS.
- Delivery is recommended between 34–36 weeks' gestation or earlier if there are any concerns.[10]

A TRAP sequence is caused by an abnormal, large A-A anastomotic channel accompanied by a V-V anastomosis. When the arterial pressure in one twin exceeds that of the other, deoxygenated blood from the umbilical artery of that twin (called pump/donor twin) is shunted via this A-A anastomosis to the recipient twin. The minimal oxygen in this deoxygenated blood is extracted by the recipient's lower limb (through the iliac vessels). Further deoxygenated blood reaches the upper body so heart and upper body develop poorly and results in failure of head growth (acardius acephalus) or a partially developed head with identifiable limbs (acardius myelacephalus) or failure of any recognizable structure to form (acardius amorphous). Blood then flows back via umbilical vein and a V-V anastomosis takes it back to the pump twin.

Thus, blood flow in all four umbilical vessels is reversed as a consequence of the pressure difference. The pump twin, therefore, develops high output cardiac failure, hydrops, polyhydramnios or dies. The mortality of the pump twin is as high if untreated and the recipient is never viable.[14]

In case of monochorionic twins elective delivery at 36 weeks is recommended due to increased risk of unexplained fetal death even in seemingly uncomplicated cases despite fetal surveillance.

MCMA twins are delivered by elective caesarean section (CS) at 32–34 weeks. Indications for elective CS in twins are[15]:
1. 1st twin non-vertex and <1.5 g
2. MCMA twins
3. TTTS
4. Conjoined twins at term
5. Severe IUGR with abnormal Doppler in one or both fetus
6. Obstetric indications
7. IVF pregnancy.

Single fetal demise may be due to:
1. Placental insufficiency
2. Abruption
3. Congenital anomalies
4. TTTS
5. Cord entanglement (MCMA twins).

The prognosis for the surviving twin depends on the chorionicity, gestational age at the time of the demise, and the time between the demise and delivery of the surviving twin. First trimester loss is usually inconsequential (vanishing twin). If the loss is in the second or third trimesters, then chorionicity determines the outcome.

DC twins usually pose no problems and can be managed conservatively but require antepartum surveillance and is delivered at 36–37 weeks. Later in gestation, it could theoretically trigger coagulation defects in the mother therefore a baseline coagulation profile is indicated.

Single fetal demise (SFD) in MC twins: Morbidity in the monochorionic twin survivor is due to vascular anastomoses. The demise of one twin causes sudden hypotension in the other. Sudden exsanguination of the survivor due to this fall in BP carries a 15% risk of death and 25% risk of neurologic handicap or ischemic multiorgan injury such as injury. The survivor may become anemic and might need an intrauterine transfusion. If SFD occurs before 24 weeks of gestation, consider delivering the mother if it is an MC twin because the risks to the co-twin far exceeds the possible benefits of continuing the pregnancy. Most cases of a single fetal death in twin pregnancy involve monochorionic placentation.

Beyond 24 weeks, the pregnancy is best terminated as soon as the survivor attains lung maturity and is capable of extrauterine survival, till then serial scans must be done to look for growth, and fetal anemia as well as close antepartum fetal surveillance is mandatory NST and biophysical profile (BPP). Ultrasound cannot detect neurological changes in the surviving twin. Recently, fetal medicine centers offer an MRI of the fetal brain to look for changes, at around 28 weeks of gestation, or at least 3–4 weeks after the demise, whichever is later.

SFD: It is much rarer compared to the chronic form of TTTS. The overall mortality is as high as 70%. The incidence of cerebral palsy and neurological abnormalities are high in survivors.

MULTIFETAL PREGNANCY REDUCTION (FIG. 5)

In some cases of higher-order multifetal gestation, the number of fetuses is reduced to two or three to improve the survival of the remaining fetuses. Selective reduction is early pregnancy intervention. It can be performed, transvaginally, or transabdominally, but the transabdominal route is usually easiest and

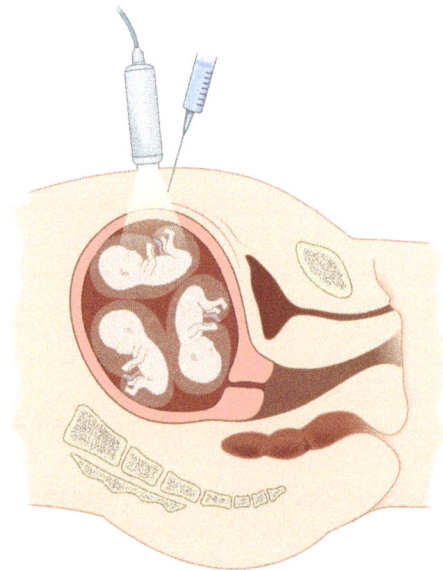

Fig. 5: Multifetal pregnancy reduction.

preferred by most fetal medicine specialists. The fetuses to be reduced have to be carefully chosen by detailed anatomic evaluation. It is better to avoid the fetus overlying the cervix, as it increases the risk of abortion. Transabdominal fetal reductions are typically performed between 10–13 weeks because most spontaneous abortions have already occurred, the remaining fetuses are large enough to be evaluated by ultrasound, the amount of fetal tissue remaining after the procedure is less, and the risk of aborting the entire pregnancy as a result of the procedure is low. The smallest fetuses and anomalous fetuses are chosen for reduction. Potassium chloride is then injected into the heart or thorax of each selected fetus under ultrasound guidance, taking care not to enter or traverse the sacs of fetuses selected for retention. Needle is maintained in the same position until fetal cardiac activity ceases for 2–3 minutes. A maximum of two fetuses are reduced in one sitting. The optimum fetal number following multifetal pregnancy reduction (MFPR) would be twins, as they have significantly better outcome compared to triplets or higher order pregnancies.[16]

Karyotyping by chorionic villous sampling (CVS) or amniocentesis should be done in high-risk cases. One of the MC pairs should not be reduced as the risk of co-twin death is very high due to the vascular connections.

Complications associated with MFPR:
1. Abortion of the remaining fetuses
2. Abortion of the wrong (normal) fetus(es)
3. Retention of genetic or structurally abnormal fetuses after a reduction in number
4. Damage without death to a fetus
5. Preterm labor
6. Discordant or growth-restricted fetuses
7. Maternal infection, hemorrhage due to retained products of conception after the procedure.

■ KEY POINTS

Antenatal examination of twin gestations involves a variety of diagnostic tools, each one of which has its differential role in the assessment of twins' health status. It is a fact that twin gestations represent a challenging reality of modern obstetrics, especially in the era of assisted reproduction. A significant proportion of twin gestations is associated with the advent of assisted reproduction techniques and therefore couples encounter additional stress to reassure wellbeing of the pregnancy. Management of complications due to multifetal pregnancy is a Catch-22 scenario sometimes for the clinicians, timely decisions are a must for the better outcome of the pregnancy.

■ REFERENCES

1. Hoekstra C, Zhao ZZ, Lambalk CB, Willemsen G, Martin NG, Boomsma DI, et al. Dizygotic twinning. Hum Reprod Update. 2008;14(1):37-47.
2. Devoe LD. Antenatal fetal assessment: multifetal gestation-an overview. Semin Perinatol. 2008;32:281-7.
3. Lee YM, Cleary-Goldman J, Thaker HM, Simpson LL. Antenatal sonographic prediction of twin chorionicity. Am J Obstet Gynecol. 2006;195:863-7.
4. Bora SA, Papageorghiou AT, Bottomley C, Kirk E, Bourne T. Reliability of transvaginal ultrasonography at 7-9 weeks' gestation in the determination of chorionicity and amnionicity in twin pregnancies. Ultrasound Obstet Gynecol. 2008;32:618-21.
5. Audibert F, Gagnon A, Genetics Committee of the Society of Obstetricians and Gynaecologists of Canada, Prenatal Diagnosis Committee of the Canadian College of Medical Geneticists. Prenatal screening for and diagnosis of aneuploidy in twin pregnancies. J Obstet Gynaecol. 2011;33:754-67.
6. Linskens IH, de Mooij YM, Twisk JW, Kist WJ, Oepkes D, van Vugt JM. Discordance in nuchal translucency measurements in monochorionic diamniotic twins as predictor of twin-to-twin transfusion syndrome. Twin Res Hum Genet. 2009;12:605-10.
7. Sepulveda W, Wong AE, Casasbuenas A. Nuchal translucency and nasal bone in first-trimester ultrasound screening for aneuploidy in multiple pregnancies. Ultrasound Obstet Gynecol. 2009;33:152-6.
8. Maymon R, Rosen H, Baruchin O, Herman A, Cuckle H. Model predicted Down syndrome detection rates for nuchal translucency screening in twin pregnancies. Prenat Diagn. 2011;31:426-9.
9. Wright D, Syngelaki A, Staboulidou I, Cruz Jde J, Nicolaides KH. Screening for trisomies in dichorionic twins by measurement of fetal nuchal translucency thickness according to the mixture model. Prenat Diagn. 2011;31:16-21.
10. Madsen HN, Ball S, Wright D, Tørring N, Petersen OB, Nicolaides KH, et al. A reassessment of biochemical marker distributions

in trisomy 21-affected and unaffected twin pregnancies in the first trimester. Ultrasound Obstet Gynecol. 2011;37:38-47.
11. Ng D, Bouhlal Y, Ursell PC, Shieh JT. Monoamniotic monochorionic twins discordant for noncompaction cardiomyopathy. Am J Med Genet A. 2013;161:1339-44.
12. Pettit KE, Merchant M, Machin GA, Tacy TA, Norton ME. Congenital heart defects in a large, unselected cohort of monochorionic twins. J Perinatol. 2013;33:457-61.
13. Agarwal K, Alfirevic Z. Pregnancy loss after chorionic villus sampling and genetic amniocentesis in twin pregnancies: a systematic review. Ultrasound Obstet Gynecol. 2012;40:128-34.
14. Bekiesinska-Figatowska M, Herman-Sucharska I, Romaniuk-Doroszewska A, Jaczynska R, Furmanek M, Bragoszewska H. Diagnostic problems in case of twin pregnancies: US vs. MRI study. J Perinat Med. 2013;11:1-7.
15. Hoffmann C, Weisz B, Yinon Y, Hogen L, Gindes L, Shrim A, et al. Diffusion MRI findings in monochorionic twin pregnancies after intrauterine fetal death. AJNR Am J Neuroradiol. 2013;34(1):212-6.
16. Arora D, Arora R, Sangthong S, Leelaporn W, Sangratanathongchai J. Universal screening of gestational diabetes mellitus: prevalence and diagnostic value of clinical risk factors. J Med Assoc Thail. 2013;96:266-71.

CHAPTER 13

Isoimmunization in Pregnancy

Rekha Rajendrakumar

INTRODUCTION

Isoimmunization in pregnancy is a condition that happens when a pregnant woman's blood protein is incompatible with the baby's, causing her immune system to react and destroy the baby's blood cells.

What causes isoimmunization in pregnancy? When the proteins on the surface of the baby's red blood cells (RBCs) are different from the mother's protein, the mother's immune system produces antibodies that fight and destroy the baby's cells. Red cell destruction can make the baby anemic well before birth. Although the Rh(D) protein is the most common one, several other proteins can cause this problem, including among proteins Kell, anti-C, ABO, anti-E antibodies, Kidd, Duffy, and others. Incidence of Rh isoimmunization has fallen steeply from 15–16% to 1%.

RH ISOIMMUNIZATION IN PREGNANCY

Epidemiology of Rh Isoimmunization in Pregnancy

Globally, the Basque population (of Spain) has the highest incidence of Rh negativity (30–35%).[1] Otherwise,
- European whites: 15–16 %
- African Americans: 8%
- Black Africans: 4%
- China: 1%
- Asians: 2% or less
- Almost nil in Japan.

Incidence

Reported incidence of fetomaternal hemorrhage (FMH) varies by volume threshold:
- 0.2 per 1,000 births for fetal blood loss >150 mL
- 0.9 per 1,000 births for fetal blood loss >80 mL
- 3 per 1,000 births for FMH ≥30 mL.

Incidences of massive FMH are about 1 in 1,000 births leading to approximately 14 % of fetal health.

Pathophysiology

The two most common systems for blood group classification are:[2]
1. *ABO system*: Groups A, B, AB, O antigen (Ag)
2. *Rhesus system:* C, c, D, d, E, e, and G.[1] The D antigen is considered to be the most potent and immunogenic (aka *Rh factor*) and accounts for 95% of all the Rh factor damage **(Fig. 1)**.

Etiology of Rh Isoimmunization

Rh alloimmunization occurs by one of two mechanisms mentioned here:
1. As a result of mismatched blood transfusion
2. Rh negative pregnancy incompatibility (after FMH between mother and an incompatible fetus).

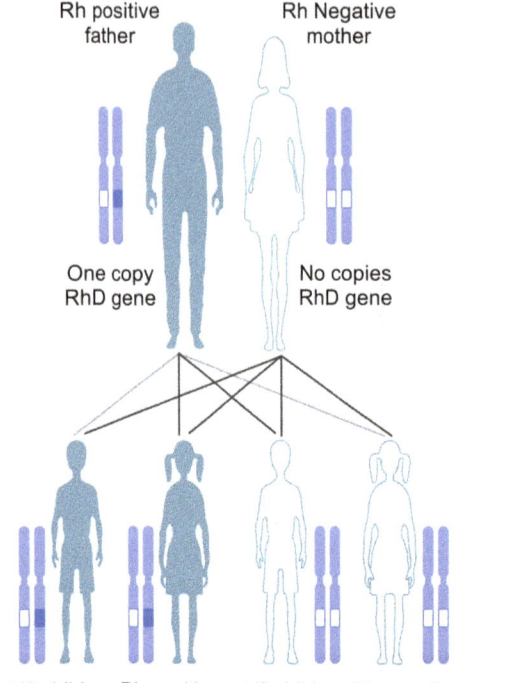 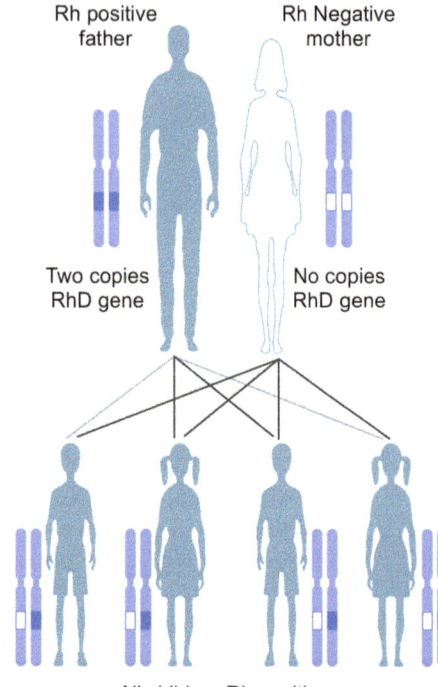

Fig. 1: Description of Rh factor inheritance probability.
Source: US National Library of Medicine. Modified by Focus I.T.

Fetomaternal Hemorrhage and Rh incompatibility

The amount of fetal blood necessary to produce Rh incompatibility varies, but as little as 0.05–0.1 mL of Rh+ cells in maternal circulation can cause isoimmunization.[1] Studies have suggested that up to 30% of persons (nonresponders) with Rh negative blood never develop Rh incompatibility even when challenged with large volumes of Rh+ blood.[3]

Nonresponders: Not all "at risk" Rh negative become isoimmunized. The chance is only 1 in 12, even in those who have had two Rh positive babies.

Following are the reasons:
- Inborn inability to respond to the Rh-antigenic stimulus
- Associated ABO group incompatibility decreases incidence of Rh incompatibility
- Variation in the strength of Rh antigenic stimulus depends on the Rh genotype of the fetal blood, e.g., Cde/cde genotype
- Volume of the fetal blood entering maternal circulation (0.05 mL is considered as critical sensitizing volume)

Incidence has reduced to a very great extent because of:
- Increased awareness among patients and doctors
- Multiparity has reduced.
- Strict administration of Rh anti-D immunoglobulin.
Male to female fetus ratio = 13.1–1.

Fetomaternal hemorrhage and Rh incompatibility: Fetomaternal hemorrhage may occur during pregnancy (10–30%) or delivery

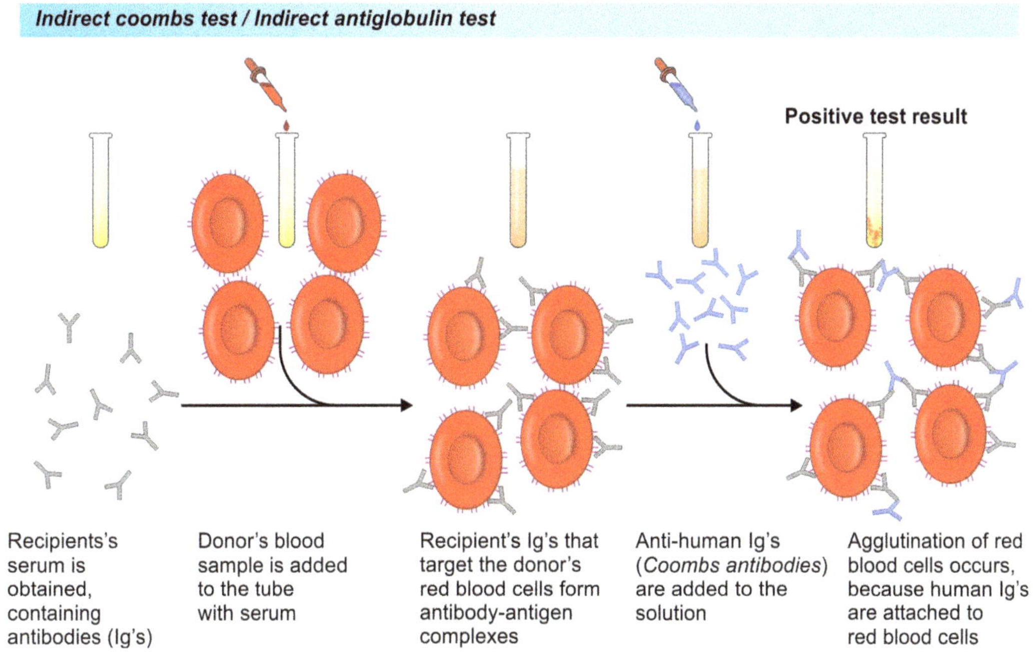

Indirect coombs test / Indirect antiglobulin test

Positive test result

| Recipients's serum is obtained, containing antibodies (Ig's) | Donor's blood sample is added to the tube with serum | Recipient's Ig's that target the donor's red blood cells form antibody-antigen complexes | Anti-human Ig's (*Coombs antibodies*) are added to the solution | Agglutination of red blood cells occurs, because human Ig's are attached to red blood cells |

Fig. 2: An overview of Indirect Coomb's test.

(70–90%).[3] Fetal RBCs have been detected in the maternal blood in all three trimesters (7, 16, and 29% respectively) without an apparent predisposing factor.[1] The initial maternal response to Rh sensitization is low levels of immunoglobulin (IgM antibodies). These are confined to maternal circulation being unable to cross the placental barrier. Within 6 weeks to 6 months, IgG antibodies are formed [as demonstrated in Indirect Coomb's Test (ICT)] **(Fig. 2)**. These are able to cross the placenta and destroy fetal Rh positive cells. Therefore, firstborn infants with Rh positive blood type are not affected. The short period of first exposure of mother to fetal RBCs is insufficient for production of significant IgG antibodies response.

Hemolytic Disease of the Newborn—Clinical Scenario

- Hydrops fetalis
- Icterus gravidarum neonatorum
- Congenital anemia of the newborn.

Sequence of in Utero Events (Fig. 3)

- Maternal IgG enters fetal circulation via placenta
- Destruction of fetal red cells (hemolysis) occurs
- When cell destruction exceeds production, severe *fetal anemia* occurs [hematocrit (HCT) <30%]
- Hydrops fetalis occurs when the HCT falls below 15%. Heart failure eventually results, with ascites, edema, and pericardial effusion—*erythroblastosis fetalis,* often resulting in fetal death shortly before or after birth.
- Extramedullary erythropoiesis is stimulated and immature erythroblasts are produced.
- Hepatosplenomegaly occurs
- Heme is formed and converted to bilirubin—*fetal hyperbilirubinemia.*
- Heme and bilirubin, both are neurotoxic, but effectively cleared by placenta and metabolized by the mother.

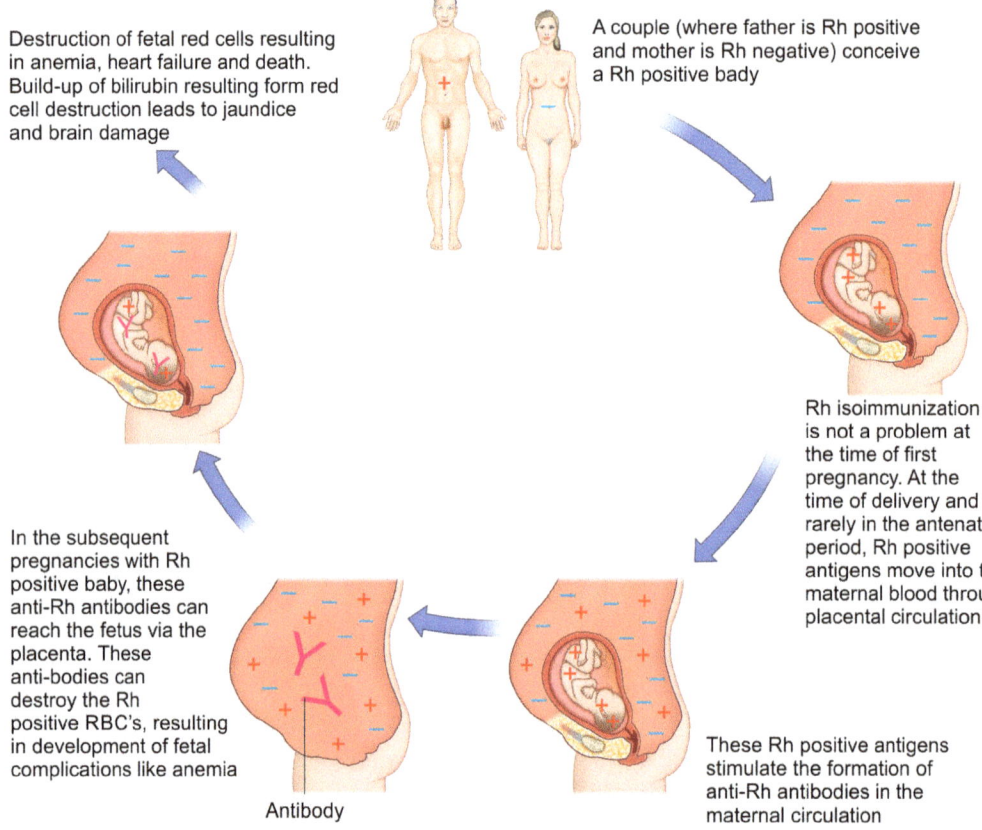

Fig. 3: Pathophysiology of Rh isoimmunization - Sequence of in utero events.

Rh Sensitization Risk

The risk and severity of sensitization response increases with each subsequent pregnancy involving an ABO compatible fetus with Rh positive blood. Without prophylaxis, this risk is 16% after two deliveries.

- 1.5–2% occur antepartum
- 7% within 6 months of delivery
- 7% manifest early in second pregnancy. With prophylaxis, the risk drops to 0.1%.

Rh sensitization risk depends on the three main factors:
1. Volume of transplacental hemorrhage
2. Extent of the maternal immune response
3. Concurrent presence of ABO incompatibility (protective—risk drops to 1.5–2%).[1]

Rh incompatibility is only of medical concern for females who are pregnant, or plan to get pregnant in future.

Rosette Test

Rosette test is depicted in **Figure 4**.

Acid Elution Test

Kleihauer count: To note the volume of fetal blood in maternal circulation. Dark refractile bodies per 50 low-power fields. If there are 80 fetal cells in 50 low-power fields in maternal peripheral films, it represents a transplacental hemorrhage of 4 mL of fetal blood.

Management

The 4-step laboratory procedure:
1. Rosette fetal RBC screen for FMH

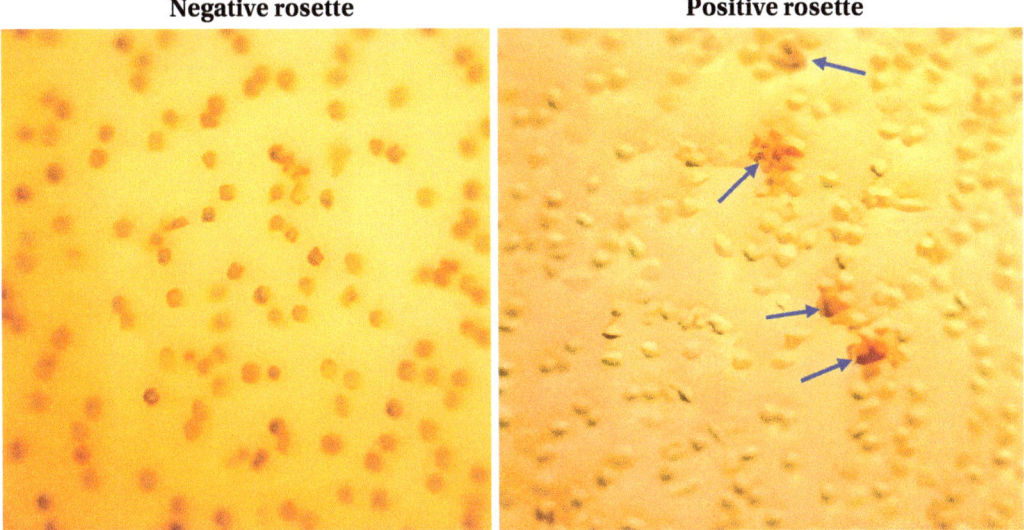

Fig. 4: Rosette test.

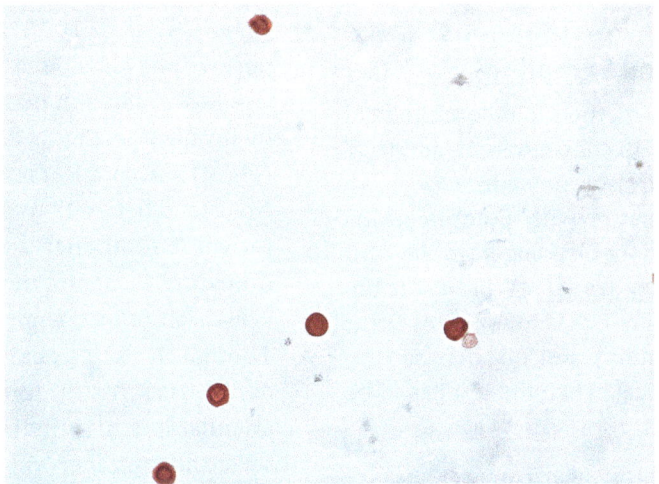

Fig. 5: Acid elution test.

2. If positive, acid elution (Kleihauer-Betke) test to quantify the RBCs in maternal circulation **(Fig. 5)**
3. Estimate the *volume of FMH* (50 × % fetal RBCs)
4. Calculate the dose of Rh IgG to be given within 72 hours of delivery.

Invasive Tests for Fetal Assessment of Hemolysis: Amniocentesis

Amniocentesis is depicted in **Figure 6**.

Spectrophotometry Charts

Spectrophotometry charts is depicted in **Figure 7**.

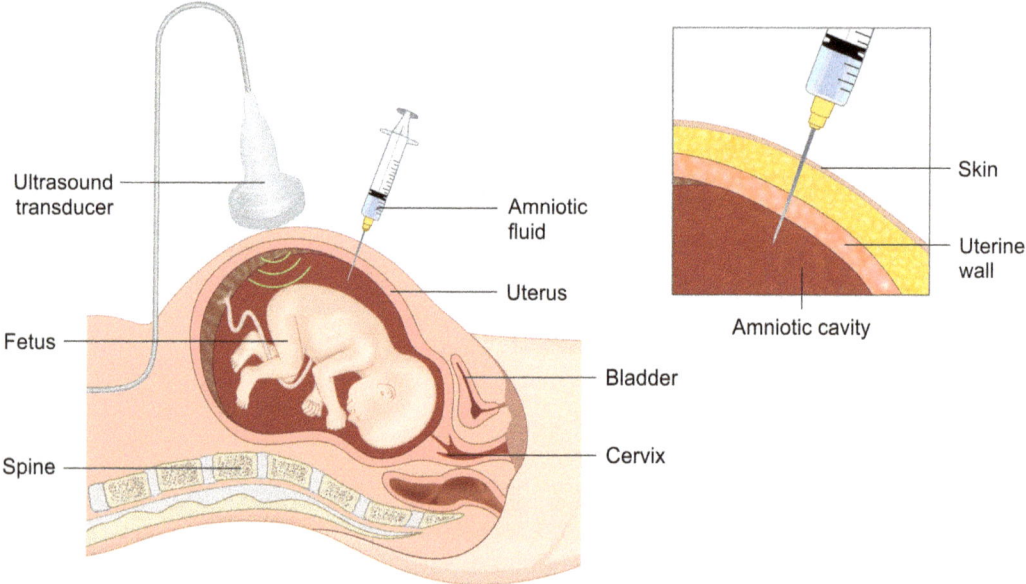

Fig. 6: Amniocentesis—Diagnostic test during pregnancy.

Cordocentesis (Percutaneous Umbilical Blood Sampling)

- It is a reliable method to determine fetal blood group, Hb concentration, and HCT directly, but invasive procedure.
- Rarely associated with complications such as infection, bleeding from the cord puncture site, transient bradycardia, FMH (which can worsen fetal alloimmunization), and fetal demise.
- It is not practical, when the test has to be repeated.

Noninvasive Test—Middle Cerebral Artery Doppler Velocimetry

- Accurate and noninvasive screening tool for detecting moderate to severe fetal anemia.
- By measuring and monitoring peak systolic velocity (PSV) in the fetal middle cerebral artery (MCA), the noninvasive prediction of fetal anemia due to Rh isoimmunization could be significantly improved.
- A sensitivity of 100% and a 12% false positive rate for anemia.
- Use has resulted in up to 80% reduction in invasive testing (i.e., amniocentesis **(Fig. 6)** and cordocentesis).
- Not useful before 18 weeks of gestation—reticuloendothelial system (RES) too immature to hemolyze enough cells to cause significant anemia.[4]
- Though it is a reliable noninvasive clinical test for the prediction of fetal anemia, it is not a reliable predictor of severe anemia after 35 weeks' gestational age (GA).[5]
- Found to be similar[6] or better than amniotic fluid OD450 nm in prediction of anemia **(Fig. 7)**.

Normal Versus Abnormal MCA-PSV (Peak Systolic Velocimetry)

Normal versus abnormal MCA-PSV (peak systolic velocimetry is depicted in **Figure 8**.

CHAPTER 13: Isoimmunization in Pregnancy

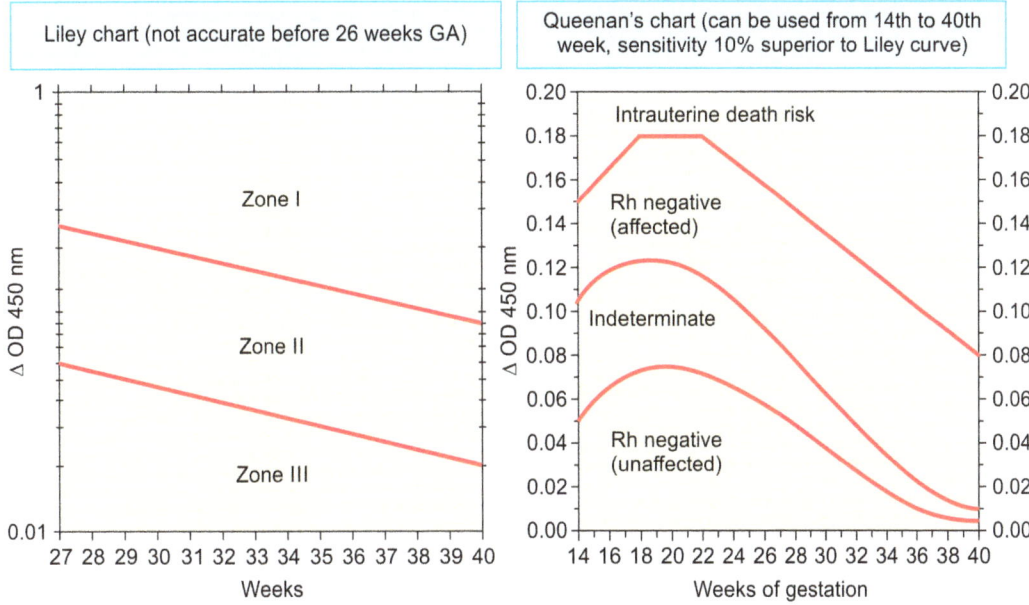

Fig. 7: Spectrophotometric charts—amniocentesis and checking optical density (OD) 450 to check bilirubin level in amniotic fluid. (GA: gestational age)

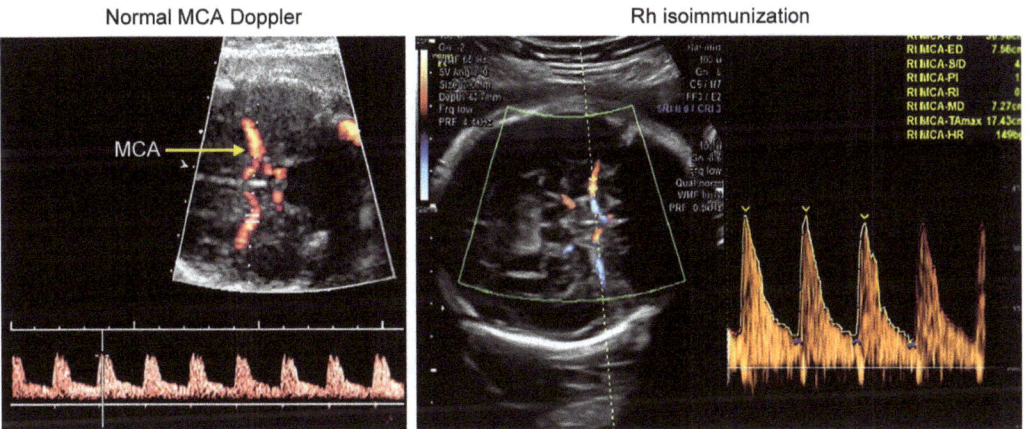

Fig. 8: Normal v/s abnormal MCA-PSV (peak systolic velocimetry). (MCA: middle cerebral artery)

Middle Cerebral Artery Doppler (MCAD) Findings in Rh Isoimmunization

- Elevated MCA-PSV
- The fetal MCA correlates well with the Hb concentration and HCT
- This method is based on the fact that anemic fetuses have an increased blood flow velocimetry secondary to anemia and hyperdynamic circulation.
- The advantages of studying the MCA rather than other vessels are that it allows

Flowchart 1: Interpretation of MCA doppler velocimetry for further management.

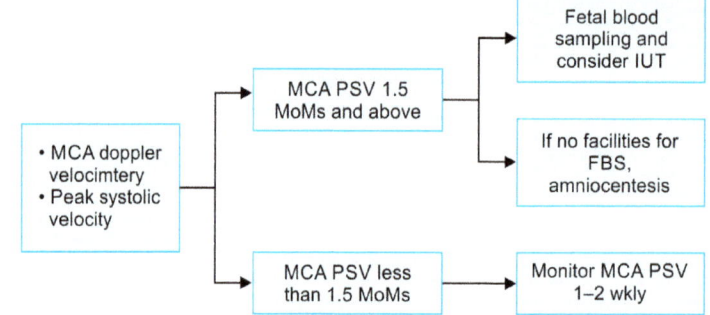

(FBS: fetal blood sampling; IUT: intrauterine transfusion; MCA: middle cerebral artery; MoM: multiples of median; PSV: peak systolic velocity)

measurements of velocity without angle correction because in the axial plane, the angle of insonation of the MCA is close to 0 degree, improving reproducibility.

Results of MCAD Velocimetry[7]

Inference (Flowchart 1)

Unaffected/mildly affected fetus: Normal middle cerebral artery Doppler (MCAD). Doppler is repeated monthly. Deliver at or near term after lung maturity. Low risk of intra uterine fetal demise (IUFD).

Moderately affected: MCAD about 1.5 multiples of median (MoM). Repeat 1–2 weekly. Deliver after lung maturity. Enhancement of lung maturity may be necessary.

Severely affected: MCAD >1.55 MoM or has frank evidence of fetal hydrops. Fetus needs help to attain lung maturity before delivery. high risk of IUFD.

There was a significant association (indirect relationship) between MoM of MCA and MoM Hb—more the former, lesser was the latter.

Management (Flowcharts 2 and 3)

Potentially Sensitizing Events

- Abortion/ectopic pregnancy
- Abdominal/pelvic trauma
- External cephalic version
- Intrauterine fetal demise
- Vaginal bleeding/antepartum hemorrhage (placenta previa, abruptio)
- Multiple gestation
- Manual removal of the placenta
- Cesarean delivery
- Prior invasive procedures (amniocentesis, chorion villous sampling)
- Prior blood transfusion
- All previous pregnancies, outcomes, intervention (history of hydrops = 90% chance recurrence).

Intrauterine Blood Transfusion

Intrauterine blood transfusion[2] **(Fig. 9)** is the recommended treatment for severe (hemolytic) anemia in utero.

- Typically carried out between 18 and 35 weeks GA
- May be given intraperitoneal or intravascular
- O RhD negative packed cells with HCT of 80% is used.
- Amount to be transfused in milliliter is (GA-20) × 10 where GA >20 weeks.

Precautions during Delivery

- Ensure consultation with neonatologist

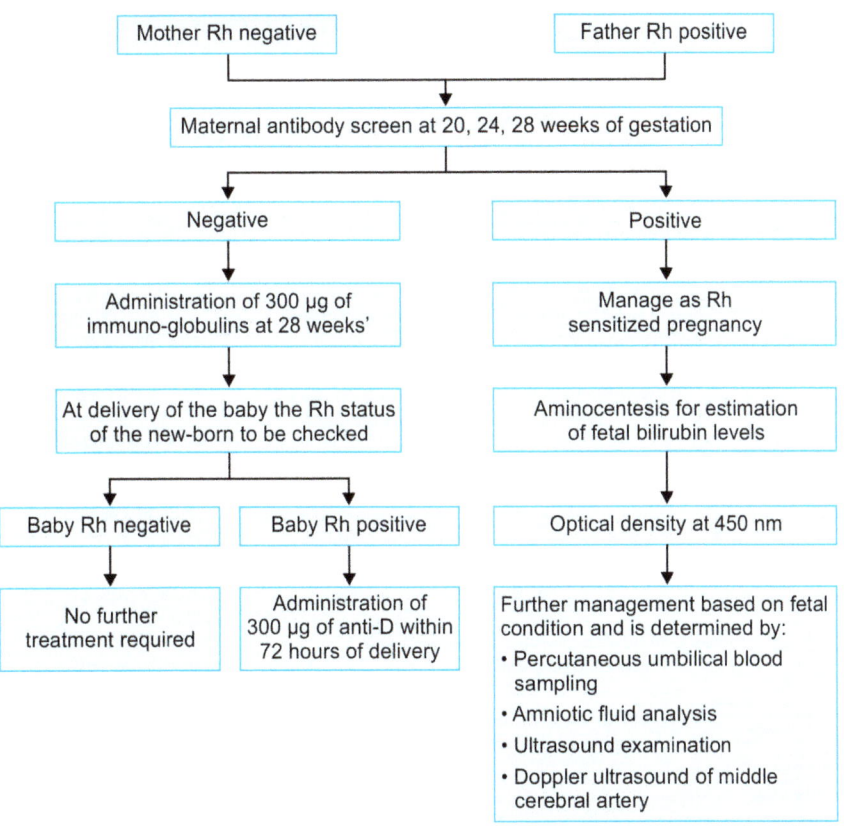

Flowchart 2: Overall management of Rh incompatible pregnancy.

- Gentle handling of the uterus during antepartum hemorrhage (APH) and third stage of labor.
- Do not give oxytocics at delivery of anterior shoulder.
- If manual removal of placenta is required, do that gently.
- During CS, try not to spill blood into the peritoneal cavity.
- Manual removal of placenta (MRP) should not be done as routine during lower segment cesarean section (LSCS).
- If blood transfusion is indicated, use Rh-negative blood only.
- Early clamping of umbilical cord is indicated.
- Leave a long length of cord, about 15–20 cm, if exchange transfusion needed.

Postpartum Anti-D dose to the Mother

- If newborn is Rh positive and normal FMH expected, administer 300 μg of anti-D
- The normal amount of fetal blood that enters the maternal circulation is <0.5 mL.[8]
- 300 mcg dose of Rh IgG given will neutralize nearly 30 mL whole fetal blood (or 15 mL Rh+ fetal RBCs).
- If more fetomaternal hemorrhage is expected than the standard one, then management is guided by the estimated volume of FMH determined by the four-step laboratory tests to determine the

Flowchart 3: Management of sensitized Rh Negative pregnancy.

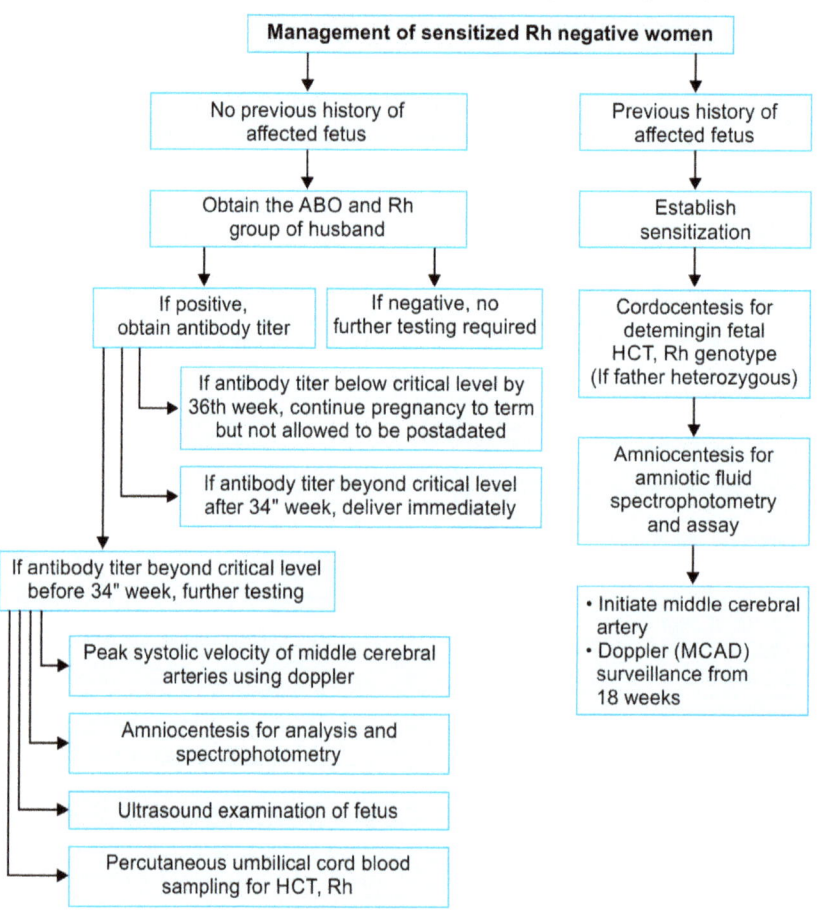

dose of Rh IgG to be administered than routine standard dose of 300 microgram.

NICU Care

- Send cord samples for—ABO/Rh typing, Direct Coomb's test **(Fig. 10)**, Hb, bilirubin levels, and peripheral smear.
- If baby is Rh negative, no further intervention.
- An urgent exchange blood transfusion is indicated in moderate to severely affected neonates.
- Phototherapy for mild affected one.

Anti-D dose Recommended in Different Obstetric Events

- *Abortion/ectopics:* Up to 5% chance of sensitization, 50 µg is recommended.
- *Invasive fetal procedure:* Up to 11% of sensitization, dose of 300 µg is recommended.
- *Antepartum hemorrhage:* 300 µg stat, to be repeated 12 weeks later if pregnancy lasts that long.
- *External cephalic version:* Up to 6% chance of sensitization. Dose is 300 µg.
- *Term delivery:* 300 µg.

Uterus
Placenta
Site of blood transfusion through the umbilical vein in the placenta
Umbilical arteries
Umbilical cord
Umbilical vein
Placenta
Maternal vessels
Intrauterine transfusion

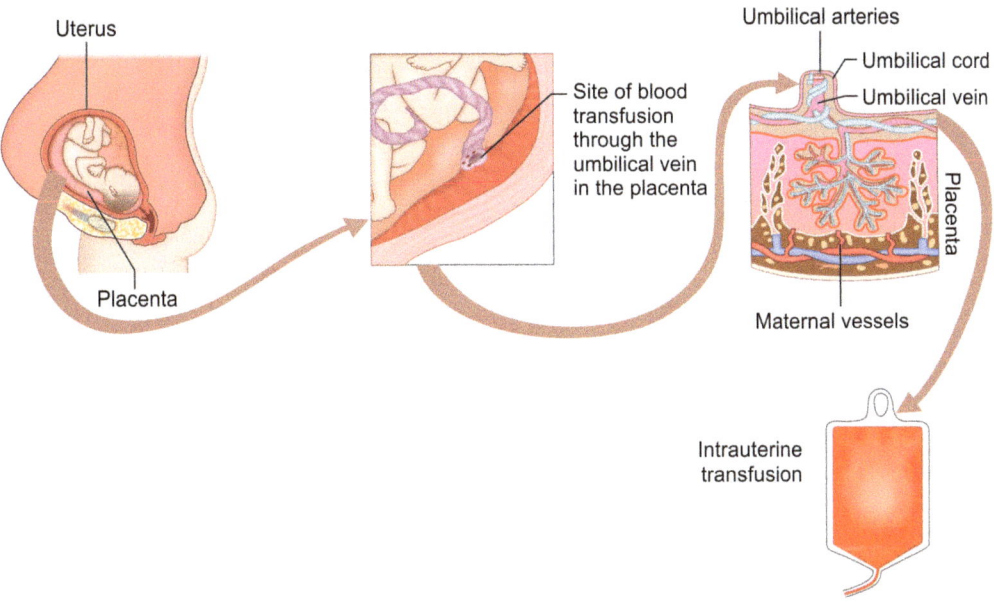

Fig. 9: Intrauterine blood transfusion.

Direct coombs test/direct antiglobulin test

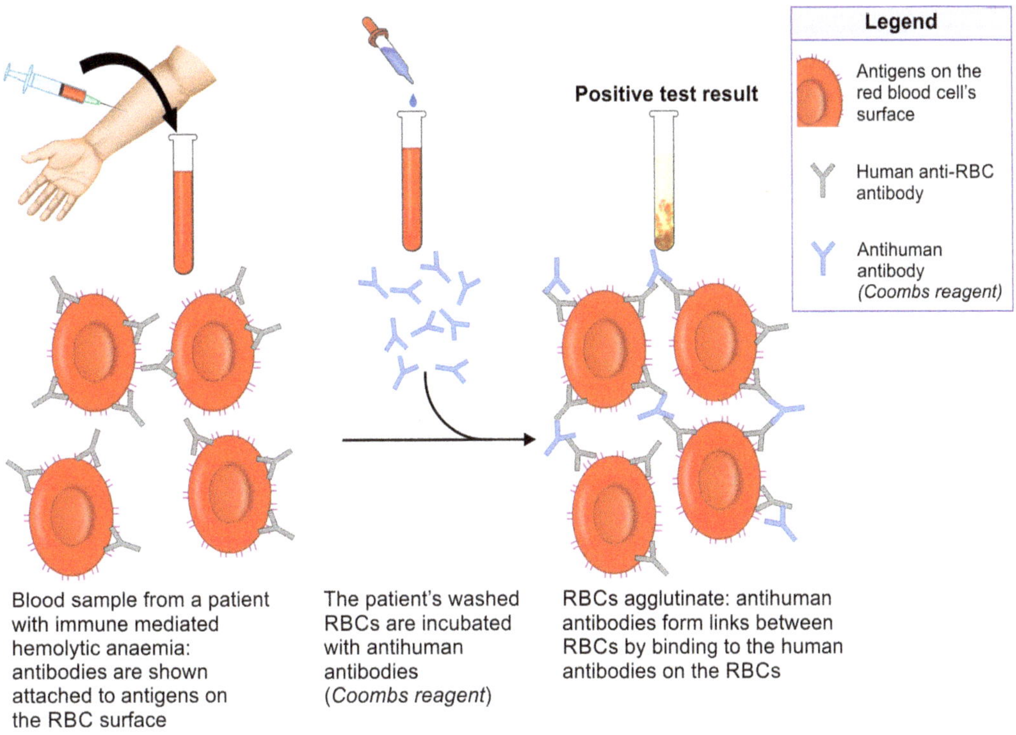

Legend
Antigens on the red blood cell's surface
Human anti-RBC antibody
Antihuman antibody (Coombs reagent)
Positive test result
Blood sample from a patient with immune mediated hemolytic anaemia: antibodies are shown attached to antigens on the RBC surface
The patient's washed RBCs are incubated with antihuman antibodies (Coombs reagent)
RBCs agglutinate: antihuman antibodies form links between RBCs by binding to the human antibodies on the RBCs

Fig. 10: An overview of Direct Coomb's test.

Problems in Our Setting

- High cost of the immunoglobulin
- Lack of resources to adequately investigate and monitor fetus in utero
- Lack of doctor and patient awareness about antenatal prophylaxis
- Low turnout for antenatal clinics—missed cases
- Poor documentation of prior sensitizing events
- Loss of case notes.

FOGSI-ICOG RECOMMENDATIONS FOR GOOD CLINICAL PRACTICE

Recombinant anti-D is safe and non-immunogenic.

RECENT ADVANCES

- Noninvasive fetal RhD genotyping (from fetal cell-free DNA in maternal circulation)[9]
- Point-of-care-tests (POCT), i.e., rapid tests for determining Rh status[10]
- A lower 50 µg dose preparation of Rh IgG for use following first trimester abortions[3]
- Concept of partial D and weak D antigens (usually test positive, but can also form anti-Rh antibodies).[11]

THINGS YET TO DO IN INDIA

- An Indian survey suggest only 10–20% doctors prescribe prophylaxis after medical termination, miscarriage, or ectopic pregnancy. Antenatal and postpartum prophylaxis awareness needs attention among service providers, young girls, and mothers. All nonsensitized Rh negative women should be given prophylaxis to avoid risk of sensitization in mid, late pregnancy, or postpartum.
- Efforts on improving FMH testing precision and awareness should be made.
- Instead of gluteal muscle, anti-D should be injected in deltoid or the anterolateral thigh to avoid delayed absorption.

RECOMMENDATIONS

- Advocacy for partnership by government and nongovernmental organizations (NGOs) to help subsidize the cost of the immunoglobulin.
- Special insurance cover for Rh-negative women to ensure ease of procurement when needed.
- Premarital counseling.

First trimester	Second trimester	Third trimester
Events	*Events*	*Events*
Significant bleeding during threatened abortion, spontaneous miscarriage, medical termination, surgical termination, ectopic pregnancy, vesicular mole, chorion biopsy, embryo reduction	All patients should be tested for Rh sensitization at the time of registration and again at 28 weeks.	Amniocentesis, abruptio placentae, blunt trauma, intrauterine fetal death, external cephalic version, placenta previa with bleeding
Prophylaxis:	*Prophylaxis:*	*Prophylaxis:*
A dose of 50–100 µg should be given	All nonsensitized (Rh –ve women with Rh +ve partner) should be given 100 µg anti-D at 28 weeks and at 34 weeks or a single dose of 300 µg at 28 weeks	300 µg (equivalent to 15 mL of fetal RBCs) should be given. For every additional 0.5 mL of fetal RBCs a dose of 10 µg should be given

Postpartum prophylaxis: Every Rh(D) negative mother who has delivered a Rh(D) positive baby irrespective of mode of delivery (normal or cesarean section) should be given 300 µg of anti-D dose within 72 hours of delivery.

- Creation of special fora/groups for Rh-negative people where potential Rh-negative spouses can be met.

Kell Antigen System

Also known as Kell–Cellano system, is a human blood group system, that is, group of antigens on the human RBC surface which are important determinants of blood type and are targets for autoimmune or alloimmune diseases which destroy RBCs. The Kell antigens are K, k, Kp^a, Kp^b, Js^a, and Js^b.[12]

Kell antigens are important in transfusion medicine, autoimmune hemolytic anemia, and hemolytic disease of the newborn (HDN) following transplacental hemorrhage (anti-Kell). Anti-K is the next most common immune red cell antibody after those in the ABO and Rh system. Anti-K typically presents as IgG class alloantibody. Individuals lacking a specific Kell antigen may develop antibodies against Kell antigens when transfused with blood containing that antigen. Following the formation of anti-K, subsequent blood transfusions may result in hemolysis because of the antibodies. Individuals without K antigens(K_0) who have formed an antibody to a K antigen, must be transfused with blood from donors who are also K_0 to prevent hemolysis.

Anti-c Isoimmunization

It is the third most common cause of severe hemolytic disease of the newborn (HDN). Rh disease is the most common and anti-Kell is the second most common cause of severe HDN. The c-antigen (little c) is part of the Rh blood group system. Anti-c antibody develops in individuals sensitized through previous exposure and is associated with acute and delayed hemolytic transfusion reactions as well as HDN. It occurs more commonly in women who are Rh D negative. A Rhc negative mother can become sensitized by RBC Rhc antigens by her first pregnancy with a Rhc positive fetus. The mother can make IgG anti-Rhc antibodies, which are able to pass through the placenta and enter the fetal circulation.[13] If the fetus is Rhc positive alloimmune hemolysis can occur leading to HDN. This is similar to Rh disease.

ABO Blood Group System

The classification of human blood based on the inherited properties of erythrocytes as determined by the presence or absence of the antigens A and B, which are carried on the surface of the red cells. A, B, and O blood groups were first identified by Austrian immunologist Karl Landsteiner in 1901.[14] He received the *Nobel Prize in Physiology or Medicine* in 1930 for this discovery.[15]

A mismatch (very rare in modern medicine) in this, or any other serotype, can cause a potentially fatal adverse reaction after a transfusion, or an unwanted immune response to an organ transplant.[16]

ABO blood group incompatibilities between the mother and child do not usually cause HDN because antibodies to the ABO blood groups are usually of the IgM type, which do not cross the placenta. However, in an O-type mothers with type A or B fetus, IgG ABO antibodies are produced and the baby can potentially develop ABO HDN with milder hemolysis compared to Rh incompatibility and rarely requires intervention. ABO incompatibility as a result of high titer maternal IgG anti-A and anti-B antibodies can cause prolonged neonatal jaundice and anemia associated with spherocytosis.

Anti-E Alloimmunization

The anti-RhE antibody can be naturally occurring, or arise following immune sensitization after a blood transfusion or pregnancy. The anti-RhE antibody is an antibody directed against the E antigen in the Rh blood group system and is quite common especially in the Rh genotype CDe/Cde. Anti-E is implicated in hemolytic transfusion reactions and hemolytic disease and anemia of the fetus and the newborn. It usually only causes a mild hemolytic disease. Only a few reports of pregnancy loss due to anti-E are described.[17] Unlike anti-D alloisoimmunization, anti-E titer is less sensitive in detecting severity of hemolysis in the subsequent pregnancy.

■ REFERENCES

1. Roman AS. Late pregnancy complications. In: Decherney AH, Nathan L, Laufer N, Roman AS (Eds). Current Diagnosis and Treatment: Obstetrics and Gynaecology, 11th edition. United States: McGraw-Hill Companies Inc; 2013. pp. 250-66.
2. Saxena R (Eds). Bedside Obstetrics and Gynaecology, 1st edition. New Delhi: Jaypee Brother Medical Publishers (P) Ltd; 2010. pp. 105-20.
3. Salem L, Singer KR. (2022). Rh Incompatibility. [online]. Available from http://emedicine.medscape.com/article/797150 [Last accessed November, 2022].
4. Scheier M, Hernandez-Andrede E, Carmo A, Dezerenyz V, Nicholaides KH. Prediction of fetal anemia in rhesus disease by measurement of fetal middle cerebral artery peak systolic velocity. Ultrasound Obstet Gynecol. 2004;23:432-6.
5. Zimmermann R, Durig P, Carpenter RJ Jr, Mari G. Logitudinal measurement of peak systolic velocity in the fetal middle cerebral artery for monitoring pregnancies complicated by red cell alloimmunization: A prospective multicentre trial with intention to treat. Br J Obstet Gynaecol. 2002;109:746-52.
6. Pessel C, Tsai MC. The Normal Pueperium. In: Decherney AH, Nathan L, Laufer N, Roman AS (Eds). Current Diagnosis and Treatment: Obstetrics and Gynaecology, 11th edition. United States: McGraw-Hill Companies Inc; 2013. pp. 190-213.
7. Bullock R, Martin WL, Coomarasamy A, Kilby MD. Prediction of fetal anemia in pregnancies with red-cell alloimmunization: comparism of middle cerebral artery peak systolic velocity and amniotic fluid OD450. Ultrasound Obstet Gynecol. 2005;25:331-4.
8. Onwuhafua JA. Pregnancy in Rhesus Negative Women in Kaduna, Northern Nigeria. Trop J Obstet Gynaecol. 2004;21(1):21-3.
9. Kolialexi A, Tounta G, Mavrou A. Noninvasive fetal RhD genotyping from maternal blood. Expert Rev Mol Diagn. 2010;10(3):285-96.
10. National Bioproducts Institute NPC. Rapidtest®Rh Test kit. [online]. Available from https://www.nbisa.org.za/index.php/products/30-products/71-diagnostics [Last accessed November, 2022].
11. Gonsorcik VK, Teruya J. (2018). Rh Typing. [online]. Available from https://emedicine.medscape.com/article/1731214-overview [Last accessed November, 2022].
12. Smart E, Armstrong B. Blood group systems. ISBT Science Series. 2008;3(2):68-92.
13. Hackney DN, Knudtson EJ, Rossi KQ, Krugh D, O'Shaughnessy RW. Management of pregnancies complicated by Anti c isoimmunization. Obstet Gynecol. 2004;103(1):24-30.
14. ISBT. Red Cell Immunogenetics and Blood Group Terminology. [online]. www.isbtweb.org [Last accessed November, 2022].
15. Anthea M, HopkinsJ, McLaughlin CW, Johnson S, Warner MQ, LaHart D, Wright JD. Human Biology and Health. Englewood Cliffs, New Jersey, USA: Prentice Hall; 1993.
16. Muramatsu M, Gonzalez HD, Cacciola R, Aikawa A, Yaqoob MM, Puliatti C. ABO incompatible renal transplants: Good or bad? World J Transplant. 2014;4(1):18-29.
17. Joy SD, Rossi KQ, Krugh D, O'Shaughnessy RW. Management of pregnancies complicated by anti-E alloimmunization. Obstet Gynecol. 2005;105(1):24-8.

CHAPTER 14

Bleeding in Pregnancy

Sayamstuti Pattanaik

■ BLEEDING IN EARLY PREGNANCY

Introduction[1-9]

Vaginal bleeding is seen in 20–25% of women in first trimester. In early pregnancy, it is associated with adverse antenatal complications, such as preterm births, small for gestational age (SGA) fetuses, and low birth weight (LBW) babies. Progesterone, produced by corpus luteum, is an immunomodulatory molecule that promotes pregnancy. Progesterone supplementation has shown long-term effects on fetal growth. The differential diagnosis for early pregnancy bleeding may be nonobstetric, bleeding from a viable intrauterine gestation, miscarriages, and ectopic gestation. The nonobstetric causes include vaginitis, cervicitis, cervical polyp, malignancy, cervical ectropion, etc. Various obstetric causes include implantation bleed, miscarriage, ectopic and molar pregnancy, etc.

History and Clinical Examination

Early pregnancy requires emergent attention. Menstrual history and previous ultrasonography (USG) can tell the period of gestation and the site of pregnancy. Amount of vaginal bleeding and pain associated has to be taken onto consideration. If pain and amount of bleeding is higher, it can indicate more toward an abortion. Signs and symptoms of hypovolemia due to blood loss should be evaluated. Vital signs indicating hemodynamic instability or peritoneal signs on physical examination require emergent attention. A per-speculum examination can help identify nonobstetric causes of bleeding, such as vaginitis, cervicitis, or a cervical polyp. If products of conception are visible on speculum examination, incomplete abortion is diagnosed and treatment offered accordingly.

Laboratory Testing[10-12]

Hemoglobin

Monitoring of baseline level.

β-Human Chorionic Gonadotropin

Beta-human chorionic gonadotropin (β-hCG) can be detected in the plasma as early as eighth day postovulation. Quantification of β-hCG is highly informative in early pregnancy. In a viable intrauterine pregnancy, initial β-hCG levels of <1,500 mIU/mL, 1,500–3,000 mIU/mL, or >3,000 mIU/mL will increase over 48 hours by at least 49%, 40%, or 33%, respectively. A slower rate of increase indicates an abortion or ectopic gestation. Around 10 weeks of gestation, the β-hCG levels plateau or decrease, after which USG examination done serially is the ideal diagnostic modality.

Progesterone

A prominent way of differentiating between an early viable or nonviable pregnancy is measurement of serum progesterone levels, especially when USG is inconclusive. A single progesterone test with a level <6 ng/mL (19.1 nmol/L) considerably excludes viable pregnancy.

RH Incompatibility

- Rh factor test to be done at first visit or the time of presentation.
- Rho(D) immunoglobulin is given within 72 hours to Rh-negative mothers with any trauma, ectopic gestation or uterine aspiration and curettage.
- Rho(D) immunoglobulin is to be given within 72 hours of early gestational loss (risk of alloimmunization in this condition is around 1.5–2%).

Ultrasonography

The embryonic events of early pregnancy that are detectable on ultrasound generally occurs in a stepwise hierarchy. Any deviation from these predictable stepwise patterns should raise alarm toward early pregnancy loss. The various USG findings seen across various entities indication first trimester abortion are:

- *Gestational sac:*
  - Mean sac diameter of ≥25 mm and absence of embryo
  - Absence of embryo with cardiac activity ≥14 days after USG showing gestational sac without yolk sac
- *Yolk sac:* Absence of embryo with cardiac activity ≥11 days after USG showing gestational sac without yolk sac
- Crown rump length of embryo ≥7 mm without cardiac activity.

Pregnancy of Unknown Location

With pregnancy test being positive and USG not showing intrauterine or ectopic gestation, it may be termed as pregnancy of unknown location. It can be a diagnostic nightmare as it may have a similar increase in β-hCG levels. Hence, mandating the serial monitoring of β-hCG level and USG. Close charting of vitals and symptoms in stable patients is of utmost regard. They should also be counseled regarding warning signs of ectopic pregnancy.

Molar Pregnancy

Least common of the causes for early pregnancy bleed found in 0.1–0.2% of the all pregnancies. It may be life-threatening rarely with excessive uterine bleeding or during evacuation. Intraperitoneal bleeding may be found in cases of perforating mole and may warrant an exploratory laparotomy. Various clinical presentations may include excessive nausea and vomiting, minimal bleeding per vaginum, and passage of grape like structures. On clinical examination, we may find uterus being larger than the gestational age, presence of anemia, and preeclampsia in few cases. Very rarely, features of thyrotoxicosis may be found. USG reveals absence of fetus and "snow storm appearance" which is gold standard for diagnosis.

Treatment may include suction and evacuation and regular follow-up for ruling out persistent trophoblastic disease and neoplastic conversion to gestational trophoblastic tumor.

The algorithm for evaluation of first trimester bleed has been detailed in **Flowchart 1**.

Management[13,14]

In incomplete abortion, watchful waiting is required as majority of the patients

Flowchart 1: Algorithm for evaluation of first trimester bleed.

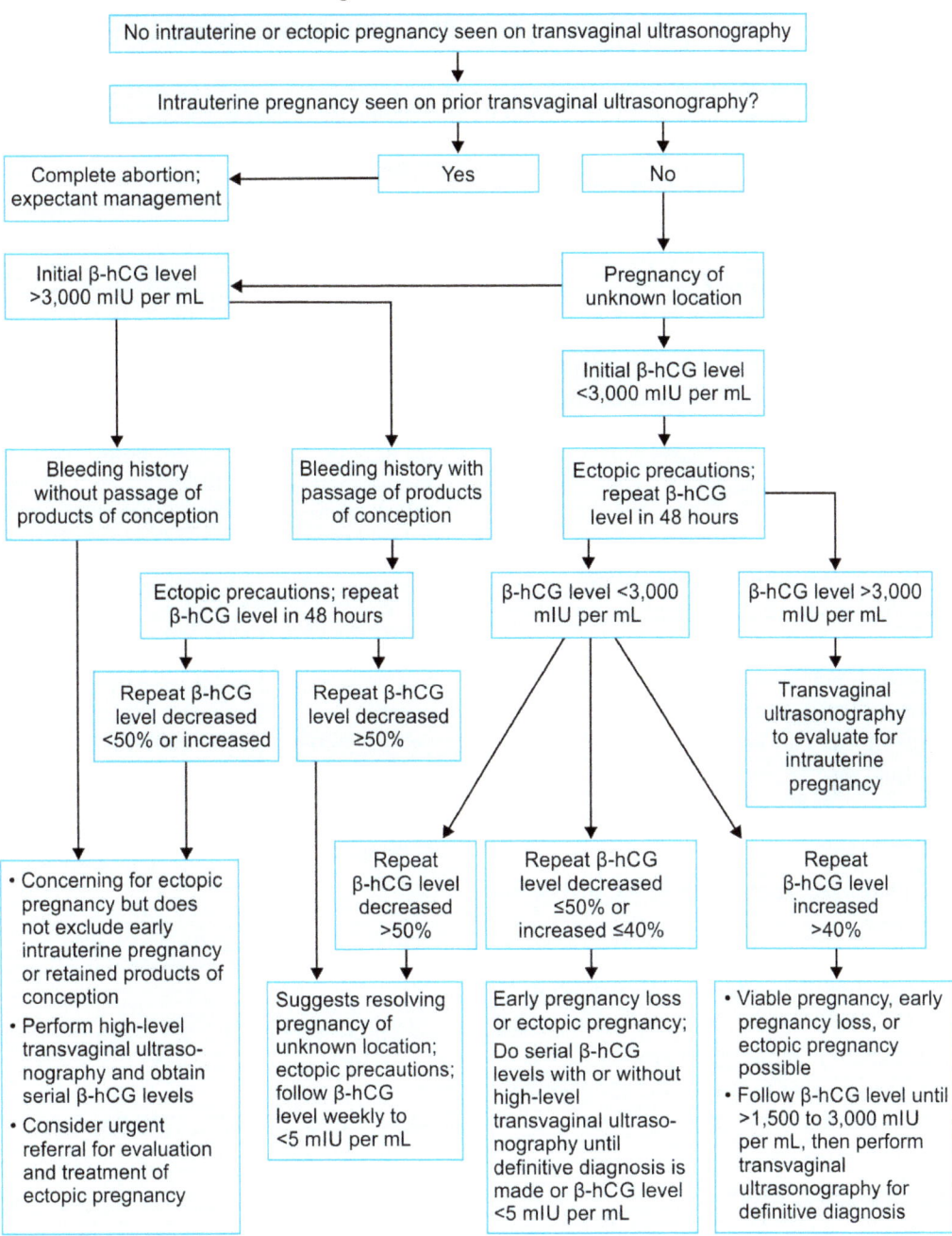

(β-hCG: beta-human chorionic gonadotropin)

will completely expel within a period of 3–4 weeks.

However, patients choosing watchful waiting over uterine aspiration are prone to experience longer days of vaginal bleed and more chances of emergency surgical management. Patients also have an option of medical management.

Medical Management

Review of various meta-analyses suggests that the best regimen is 200 mg oral mifepristone followed by 800 µg of vaginal misoprostol after 24 hours. Success rates registered with above regimen are up to 84% versus with just misoprostol alone (67%).

Uterine Curettage and Aspiration

It is the preferred surgical intervention for first trimester loss. Vacuum aspiration leads to lesser pain and blood loss during procedure and shorter hospital stay. Choice of anesthesia can be tapered as per patient requirement.

Follow-up

Complete evacuation can be evaluated by the following:
- Products of conception seen on examination or after uterine aspiration
- USG shows absence of an intrauterine pregnancy compared to previous scans
- Drop in β-hCG levels by at least 50% within 2 days or 85–87% at 7 days.

Ectopic Pregnancy

Ectopic pregnancy is one of the common causes of early pregnancy bleed. Risk factors include previous ectopic pregnancy, pelvic inflammatory disease, exposure to diethylstilbestrol, etc.

BOX 1: Management of ectopic pregnancy.

Conservative approach: Conditions
- Serum β-hCG <1,000 mIU/mL and decreasing
- Ectopic/adnexal mass <3 cm or not detected
- Mild/moderate pain or bleeding
- Embryonic cardiac activity absent
- Tubal rupture absent
- Follow-up of patient and availability of resources

Methotrexate: Conditions
- Cardiac activity of embryo not seen
- Serum β-hCG <2,000 mIU/mL
- Ectopic mass ≤3.5 cm
- Absence of contraindications (hematologic disorder; hepatic dysfunction, renal, or pulmonary disorders; immunosuppression; peptic ulcers; lactation; sensitivity to methotrexate; and alcoholics)
- Patient follow-up possible and proper access to healthcare
- Stable vitals and less symptoms
- Unruptured ectopic gestation

Surgical management: Conditions
- Advanced ectopic gestation (higher β-hCG level, huge mass, and cardiac activity of embryo)
- Contraindications for conservative approach or use of methotrexate
- Patient follow-up not possible or cannot access healthcare
- Uncertainty of diagnosis
- Unstable vitals or signs of shock or hemoperitoneum

(β-hCG: beta-human chorionic gonadotropin)

Management of ectopic pregnancy is given in **Box 1**.

■ BLEEDING IN LATE PREGNANCY

Vaginal bleeding in the later stages of pregnancy (>26 weeks period of gestation) warrants for increased maternal and fetal morbidity and mortality. Emergency delivery of fetus is called for in women with first episode of bleeding in <29 weeks of gestation and more than and equal to three episodes of antepartum hemorrhage. Prompt recognition of life-threatening hemorrhage, absolute causes, maternal-fetal distress, and emergent obstetric care and referral and availability of intensive care unit are important for proper management of such bleeding.

Recognition

Later in pregnancy the cervix ripens leading to tissues becoming elastic and friable. Minimal trauma like intercourse or per vaginal intervention may lead to spotting or minimal bleeding per vaginum. Cervical polyps, cervicitis, carcinoma cervix, etc., are other causes of late pregnancy bleeding. Mucus mixed with blood and little amount of self-limiting bleeding may be seen toward later part of term gestation. Major and minor reasons for bleeding per vaginum can be differentiated by an extensive history, proper USG, and adequate pelvic examination. Long-term and short-term observations may be required after admission and evaluation. Signs and symptoms for major vaginal bleeding toward later term include a sudden gush of bright red blood, passage of clots, or bleeding with pain and cramps. Effective resuscitation with fluids and/or blood products may be required in cases of shock wherein we find tachycardia and hypotension which may be found late in a pregnant lady.

Etiologic Factors

The most common causes of second and third trimester bleeding are placenta previa, abruptio placentae, rupture of uterus, vasa previa, etc. Other causes are mentioned in **Table 1**. The etiological factors are broadly classified into abnormal placentation causes and uteroplacental traumatic causes.

TABLE 1: Risk factors for vaginal bleeding in late pregnancy.[15-17]

Abnormal placentation	Uteroplacental trauma
Placenta previa: • Advanced maternal age (>40 years) • Chronic hypertension • Multiparity • Multiple gestations • Previous cesarean delivery • Tobacco use • Uterine curettage • Previous uterine surgery • Cocaine use • History of placenta previa • Chronic hypertension • In vitro fertilization and ART	Placental abruption: • Chronic hypertension • Domestic violence • Multiparity • Preeclampsia • Previous abruption • Short umbilical cord • Sudden decompression of an overdistended uterus • Thrombophilias • Tobacco, cocaine, or methamphetamine use • Trauma: blunt abdominal or sudden deceleration • Unexplained elevated maternal AFP level • Uterine fibroids
Vasa previa: • In vitro fertilization • Low-lying and second trimester placenta previa • Multiple gestation • Succenturiate-lobed and bilobed placenta • Velamentous cord insertion	Uterine rupture: • Abnormal placentation • Uterine surgeries • Induction of labor (prostaglandins) • Connective tissue disorders • Non-European ethnicity • Any injury or trauma • TOLAC • Anomalies of the uterus
Invasive placenta: • Previous gynecological procedure • Increased maternal age • Placenta previa • Hypertension (chronic/gestational) • Female fetus	

(AFP: alpha-fetoprotein; ART: assisted reproductive technology; TOLAC: trial of labor after cesarean delivery)

Placenta Previa

When the endocervical os is covered by the placenta in any degree it is called as placenta previa. The incidence of placenta previa has been on increasing trend due to increased commission of lower segment cesarean section (LSCS). Various risk factors include previous placenta previa, advanced maternal age, multiparity, drug abuse, maternal smoking, previous uterine surgeries, etc. Placenta previa commonly presents as painless and bright red per vaginal bleed which may or may not be accompanied by cramping. Placenta previa are commonly associated with vasa previa, and thus transvaginal USG can differentiate between the two.

Vasa Previa[18]

Vasa previa is a condition in which the blood vasculature of the fetus is not protected by umbilical cord or the placenta and is present in the amniotic membranes and throughout the cervix (=2 cm) with an increased risk of rupture with ruptured membranes. Vasa previa is believed to arise from early placenta previa near the cervix that degenerates and leaves only open blood vessels. It is a rare condition, seen in 1 per 2,500 births. Various risk factors are placenta previa, multiple gestations pregnancies, and placenta with a succenturiate lobe, bilobed placenta, or with velamentous insertion. Typical presentation includes painless vaginal bleeding, ruptured membranes, and fetal distress (fetal bradycardia) or intrauterine fetal death. Bleeding vasa previa leads to loss of blood from fetal-placental circulation and lead to fetal hypovolemia and fetal demise. Hence, antenatal USG is mandatory to detect this entity. Emergency LSCS and fetal-maternal resuscitation is the standing pillar for management of hemorrhage due to vasa previa.

Placental Invasiveness (Percreta, Increta, and Accreta)

Incidence of invasive placentation has increased due to rise in LSCS rates in present clinical scenario. Other risk factors include concomitant placenta previa, previous uterine surgery, previous invasive placentation history, and assisted reproductive techniques. Patient may present intra- and postpartum hemorrhage and specifically prolonged third stage of labor. Previously undiagnosed invasive placentation may lead to severe blood loss up to 3–4 liters and mandates aggressive resuscitation and massive transfusion. Fertility-preservation maneuvers, such as uterine artery embolization, may not always be feasible, and hysterectomy and emergency may be the need of the hour to save the mother and untoward consequences.

Abruptio Placentae[19]

In this condition, we see a premature separation of the placenta from the endometrium, and subsequent loss of fetal perfusion. Risk factors include increased age of mother, African race, multiparity, smoking of cigarettes, chorioamnionitis or any other intrauterine infection, any recent trauma, chronic hypertension, drug abuse, or intake of alcohol in pregnancy. Patient may present with vaginal bleed associated with severe pain abdomen, tenderness of uterine fundus, and uterine contractions (tetanic). The degree of placental separation corresponds poorly with the degree of vaginal bleed. Abruptio placentae is greatly diagnosed clinically. USG is important but has a poor sensitivity for abruptio placentae. Management includes expedited delivery in view of fetal distress with preparedness for handling of consumption coagulopathy, which is a dreaded known complication that may occur and availability of intensive care unit is important to handle disseminated intravascular coagulation.

■ SUMMARY

To reduce maternal morbidity and mortality, antepartum hemorrhage requires a detailed and strict of assessment for fetal distress, abnormalities in placentation, and signs of maternal distress and shock. Recognition of concealed hemorrhage like abruptio placentae or ruptured uterus and any other peripartum bleeding is of utmost importance. Availability of resources, infrastructure, and blood bank services are required for maternal resuscitation, rehabilitation, and targeted blood transfusion. Knowledge and skill of the doctor along with emergency department preparedness are of utmost importance to manage and save lives.

■ REFERENCES

1. Everett C. Incidence and outcome of bleeding before the 20th week of pregnancy: prospective study from general practice. BMJ. 1997;315(7099):32-4.
2. Hasan R, Baird DD, Herring AH, Olshan AF, Jonsson Funk ML, Hartmann KE. Association between first-trimester vaginal bleeding and miscarriage. Obstet Gynecol. 2009;14(4):860-7.
3. Al-Memar M, Vaulet T, Fourie H, Bobdiwala S, Saso S, Farren J, et al. Early-pregnancy events and subsequent antenatal, delivery and neonatal outcomes: prospective cohort study. Ultrasound Obstet Gynecol. 2019;54(4):530-7.
4. Sun L, Tao F, Hao J, Su P, Liu F, Xu R. First trimester vaginal bleeding and adverse pregnancy outcomes among Chinese women: from a large cohort study in China. J Matern Fetal Neonatal Med. 2012; 25(8):1297-301.
5. Yang J, Hartmann KE, Savitz DA, Herring AH, Dole N, Olshan AF, et al. Vaginal bleeding during pregnancy and preterm birth. Am J Epidemiol. 2004;160(2):118-25.
6. Yang J, Savitz DA. The effect of vaginal bleeding during pregnancy on preterm and small-for-gestational-age births: US National Maternal and Infant Health Survey, 1988. Paediatr Perinat Epidemiol. 2001;15(1):34-9.
7. Williams MA, Mittendorf R, Lieberman E, Monson RR. Adverse infant outcomes associated with first-trimester vaginal bleeding. Obstet Gynecol. 1991;78(1):14-8.
8. Bever AM, Pugh SJ, Kim S, Newman RB, Grobman WA, Chien EK, et al. Fetal growth patterns in pregnancies with first-trimester bleeding. Obstet Gynecol. 2018;131(6):1021-30.
9. Malassine A, Frendo JL, Evain-Brion D. A comparison of placental development and endocrine functions between the human and mouse model. Hum Reprod Update. 2003;9(6):531-9.
10. Barnhart KT, Guo W, Cary MS, Morse CB, Chung K, Takacs P, et al. Differences in serum human chorionic gonadotropin rise in early pregnancy by race and value at presentation. Obstet Gynecol. 2016;1 28(3):504-11.
11. Barnhart KT, Sammel MD, Rinaudo PF, Zhou L, Hummel AC, Guo W. Symptomatic patients with an early viable intrauterine pregnancy: HCG curves redefined. Obstet Gynecol. 2004;104(1):50-5.
12. Verhaegen J, Gallos ID, van Mello NM, Abdel-Aziz M, Takwoingi Y, Harb H, et al. Accuracy of single progesterone test to predict early pregnancy outcome in women with pain or bleeding: meta-analysis of cohort studies. BMJ. 2012;345:e6077.
13. Luise C, Jermy K, May C, Costello G, Collins WP, Bourne TH. Outcome of expectant management of spontaneous first trimester miscarriage: observational study. BMJ. 2002; 324(7342):873-5.
14. Butts SF, Guo W, Cary MS. Predicting the decline in human chorionic gonadotropin in a resolving pregnancy of unknown location. Obstet Gynecol. 2013;122(2 pt 1):337-43.

15. Pivano A, Alessandrini M, Desbriere R. A score to predict the risk of emergency caesarean delivery in women with antepartum bleeding and placenta praevia. Eur J Obstet Gynecol Reprod Biol. 2015; 195:173-6.
16. Frank J, Baeseman Z, Leeman L, Chapter C. Vaginal bleeding in late pregnancy. In: Leeman L, Quinlan JD, Dresang LT (Eds). ALSO: Advanced Life Support in Obstetrics Provider Manual, 8th edition. Leawood, Kansas: American Academy of Family Physicians; 2017. pp. 1-14.
17. Baldwin HJ, Patterson JA, Nippita TA, Torvaldsen S, Ibiebele I, Simpson JM, et al. Antecedent of abnormally invasive placenta in primiparous women: risk associated with gynecologic procedures. Obstet Gynecol. 2018;131(2):227-33.
18. Silver RM. Abnormal placentation: placenta previa, vasa previa, and placenta accreta. Obstet Gynecol. 2015;126(3):654-68.
19. Jain V, Chari R, Maslovitz S, Farine D, Bujold E, Gagnon R, et al. Guidelines for the management of a pregnant trauma patient. J Obstet Gynaecol Can. 2015;37(6):553-74.

CHAPTER 15

Bad Obstetric History in Pregnancy

Umme Ruman

BACKGROUND

- Bad obstetric history (BOH) implies previous unfavorable fetal outcome in terms of two or more consecutive spontaneous abortions, early neonatal deaths, stillbirths, intrauterine fetal deaths, intrauterine growth retardation, and congenital anomalies. It is mostly referred to those whose further pregnancy outcome is likely to be affected by pervious pregnancy events.[1]
- When the neonatal loss is due to fever, diarrhea, and any medical comorbidities, it is not referred as the same.
- In women with BOH, the underlying contributing factor is pinpointed in only about 40-50% cases and the rest are clubbed under "unexplained" group in spite of detailed evaluation.
- The worldwide incidence of BOH is said to be around 1-2%. But it also varies widely across different geographical areas. In the UK, recurrent pregnancy loss (RPL ≥3 consecutive early pregnancy losses <24 weeks of gestation) affects around 1-3% of pregnancies.[2]
- The updated draft guideline of the Royal College of Obstetricians and Gynaecologists (RCOG) states the pregnancy loss do not necessarily have to be consecutive to be defined as RPL. American Society of Reproductive Medicine (ASRM) defines RPL as two or more failed clinical pregnancies.[2] European Society of Human Reproduction and Embryology (ESHRE) defines as the loss of two or more pregnancies whether they are consecutive or not was not specified.[3]
- BOH may be occur due to still birth, growth restriction, prolonged labor, intrauterine death, and RPL.

Some common causes of BOH are given in **Table 1**.

PARENTAL GENETIC FACTORS

- In couples with BOH, percentages of chromosomal abnormality (CA) is found in 50% for couples. Individual variation ranges from 1 to 25%.
- Most frequently occurring CA is balanced translocation. Sex chromosomal mosaicism, inversions, and ring chromosomes are other chromosomal anomalies seen commonly. Chromosomal inversions and insertions are other variants of CA found in RPL. Reciprocal translocations are associated with 60% and Robertsonian translocation 40% in couples with history of RPL.
- Parental balanced structural chromosome rearrangement is associated with 2-4% of RPL. Single gene defects, for example, cystic fibrosis or sickle cell anemia, are rarely associated with RPL.[3] The most

TABLE 1: Causes of bad obstetric history.	
Parental genetic defects	25–47% of cases of habitual abortion

Anatomical	• Congenital
	  – Septate uterus
	  – Bicornuate uterus
	  – Arcuate uterus
	• Acquired
	  – Cervical incompetence
	  – Myoma
	  – Intrauterine adhesions

Endocrine	• Thyroid disorder • Uncontrolled DM • PCOS • Hyperprolactinemia • Hyperandrogenism • Luteal phase defect • Obesity

Immunological	5–15% causes.
	• Acquired: Antiphospholipid antibody
	• Inherited:
	  – Protein C deficiency
	  – Protein S deficiency
	  – Antithrombin deficiency
	  – Activated protein C deficiency
	  – Prothrombin gene mutation
	  – Hyperhomocystinemia

Infection	• Primary infection caused by toxoplasma, rubella, CMV, and HSV • Syphilis • Bacterial vaginosis • Ureaplasma urealyticum • Chlamydia trachomatis

(CMV: cytomegalovirus; DM: Diabetes mellitus; HSV: herpes simplex virus; PCOS: polycystic ovarian syndrome)

prevalent abnormality of spontaneous abortion is chromosomal aneuploidy.[4] Balanced structure chromosome abnormalities in any of parents is also prone to cause BOH.

- In couples with two or more miscarriage these abnormalities frequently seen between 3 and 6%.[5]

ANATOMICAL FACTOR[6]

- Women with RPL have a 3.2–6.9% higher probability of having a major uterine anomaly. An arcuate uterus found in 1.0–16.9% of them. Bicornuate as well as septate uterus are found to have a negative impact on pregnancy in shape of miscarriage. Ample studies are yet needed to set individual criteria to diagnose the arcuate, septate, and bicornuate uteri.
- The ESHRE/ESGE classification of müllerian anomalies published on 2021 is the most commonly used and standardized classification of uterine anomalies.
- Evidence says that, after metroplasty, 65–85% of patients with bicornuate or septate uteri have a successful pregnancy. It is also seen that without surgery 59.5% of the patients with such anomalies have a successful subsequent pregnancy. No case control or cohort study are yet demonstrate the comparison between live birth rate with uterine anomaly with or without surgery. More studies are required to confirm the benefits of metroplasty.
- Acquired uterine malformations such as fibroids, polyp, and uterine adhesions have been found in RPL. There is evidence that removal of fibroids distorting uterine cavity increases live birth rate.
- Cervical insufficiency is associated with RPL commonly in mid trimester.
- Hydrosalpinx can increase risk of pregnancy loss and treatment can reduce the same.

ENDOCRINE FACTOR[7]

Polycystic Ovarian Syndrome

- Polycystic ovarian syndrome (PCOS) is the most common cause of anovulatory infertility in the developed countries. It is the most commonly identified abnormality among women with recurrent miscarriage. This occurs in 40% women with PCOS and the causes behind commonly found are obesity, hyperinsulinemia, insulin resistance, hyperhomocysteinemia, hyperandrogenemia, high levels of plasminogen activator inhibitor-1 factor, elevated levels of luteinizing hormone (LH), and poor endometrial receptivity. Weight loss and metformin plays pivotal role in management.

Thyroid Disorder

- Approximately 0.1–0.4% of pregnancies are affected by hyperthyroidism. Untreated hyperthyroidism in pregnancy poses risks of spontaneous miscarriage, thyroid storm, congestive heart failure, preeclampsia, fetal growth restriction, preterm delivery, and increased perinatal morbidity or mortality. Pregnancy outcome in patients who are treated for overt Graves' hyperthyroidism.
- Hypothyroidism is more prevalent (7%) during pregnancy. It is significantly associated with RPL in <20 weeks of gestation. The most common cause of hypothyroidism in pregnancy is chronic autoimmune thyroiditis. When thyroid-stimulating hormone (TSH) levels >6 mIU/mL, it is more seen to be associated with still birth. Endemic iodine deficiency, previous radioactive iodine therapy, and thyroidectomy are being other prevalent causes. It needs to be treated during pregnancy otherwise mostly leads to untoward pregnancy complications, and it is detrimental on fetal neurocognitive development, and impaired fertility. Both overt hypothyroidism and subclinical thyroid dysfunction can have negative effects on fetal and maternal outcome.
- Autoimmune thyroid disease is the most frequent cause of hypothyroidism in women of reproductive age. With an approximate prevalence of 10–15%, thyroid antibody is found to be associated with recurrent abortions. Therefore, thyroid autoantibodies may be employed as a marker for high risk pregnancies.

Uncontrolled Diabetes Mellitus

- Up to 1% of all pregnancies Type 1 and Type 2 diabetes mellitus. Poorly controlled diabetes prior and during pregnancy causes lethal embryonic malformations. It also increases the risk of spontaneous abortion, preterm labor, hypertensive disorders, and operative deliveries.
- Insulin resistance plays a fundamental role in the ovarian androgen excess and might promote miscarriage by increasing circulating testosterone concentration and hyperhomocysteinemia. Latter alters endometrial blood flow and vascular integrity causing raised oxidative stress in vascular endothelium causing early pregnancy loss.
- First aim should be control of blood sugar during the preconceptional period as well-controlled diabetes mellitus is less likely to be a cause of BOH.

Hyperprolactinemia

- Prolactin plays important role in female reproduction mainly for its role in ovulation.

- Transient hyperprolactinemia is associated with unexplained infertility and RPL.
- One study revealed that subnormal basal serum prolactin concentration poses increased risk of miscarriage in a subsequent pregnancy in women with RPL.

Luteal Phase Defect

- RPL is often associated with decreased levels of. Progesterone creates a preferable milieu for the embryo during the implantation window.
- Progesterone also helps in maintaining early pregnancy. It helps in proliferation and differentiation of stromal cells, enhances uterine receptivity through the locally acting growth factors modulation, and it regulates cytokine production in maternal fetal interface.
- Luteal phase defect is generally perceived as suboptimal production of progesterone by the corpus luteum resulting in inadequate endometrial maturation to allow proper placentation. This may occur in up to 35% of women with RPL.

■ IMMUNOLOGICAL FACTORS

- Antiphospholipid antibody syndrome (APLS) can be primary in absence of autoimmune disease or it can be secondary to autoimmune diseases like systemic lupus erythematosus (SLE). Latter comprises 40% of the cases.[8] Genetic risk factors increases the risk of antiphospholipid antibody (APLA)-associated thrombosis, such as coagulation factor mutations. HLA-DR7, DR4, DRw53, DQw7, and C4 null alleles have been reported to be associated with APLS. APLA formation associated with infections such as *Borrelia*, *Treponema*, human immunodeficiency virus (HIV), *burgdorferi* and *Leptospira*.[9] Many drugs, including chlorpromazine, procainamide, quinidine, and phenytoin, can induce APLA production. Merely, low level of APLA may also be found.
- Pregnancy loss is common in patients with APLS, especially in the second half of pregnancy. Three blood markers lupus anticoagulant, anticardiolipin and anti-beta-2-glycoprotein-I antibodies are found in APLS associated with previous pregnancy loss, history of thrombosis, and SLE are risk factors for adverse pregnancy-related outcomes and pregnancy losses in APLS.[10] The pregnancy-related complications in APLS include preeclampsia, placental insufficiency, abruptio placentae, HELLP syndrome (Hemolysis, Elevated Liver enzymes, Low Platelet count), fetal distress, premature birth, and intrauterine growth retardation.[11]

■ INFECTIOUS CAUSES[12]

- Infections caused by TORCH [toxoplasma gondii, rubella virus, cytomegalovirus (CMV), herpes simplex virus (HSV), and others agents like chlamydia trachomatis, *Treponema pallidum*, *Neisseria gonorrhoeae*, HIV, etc.] are the major causes of BOH.
- Most cases of toxoplasmosis are asymptomatic or mild and influenza-like symptoms. It can cause fulminating life-threatening symptoms as pneumonia and encephalitis in immune-compromised patients. Spontaneous abortion or stillbirth are commonly seen due to primary infection. Intrauterine infection may cause congenital toxoplasmosis characterized ocular and neurological manifestations.

- Maternal CMV is the most common viral infection in perinatal period and is the leading cause of congenital CMV infection. The incidence of congenital CMV ranges from 0.5 to 3.0% in all live births. Primary HSV infection during first half of pregnancy is associated with increased frequency of spontaneous abortion, stillbirth, and congenital malformation.
- Rubella infection mostly affects baby who receives with this virus during the first trimester. The rubella virus readily crosses the placenta and affect fetus during gestation.
- Chlamydia is seen to be associated with women with three or more recurrent miscarriage.

DIAGNOSIS OF BAD OBSTETRIC HISTORY

- *History:* A detailed obstetric history is important:
  - Gestational age at which abortion occur—T1-genetic and endocrine, T2-anatomical cause
  - Consanguinity
  - *Previous pregnancy performance:* Preterm labor, premature rupture of membrane, prolonged labor, malpresentation, Rh isoimmunization, and history of congenitally malformed baby
  - Drug and environmental exposure
  - Family history of thrombotic events, pregnancy losses, or complications
  - History of infertility
  - Symptoms of metabolic disorders and autoimmune disorders
  - Review the previous medical records and any investigation results. Any recurrent or nonrecurrent causes of pregnancy loss should be identified to make a management plan to reduce or modify the risks in the current or future pregnancies
- Physical examination
- Investigations **(Table 2)**.

TABLE 2: Investigations for bad obstetric history.

Factors	Investigations
Parental genetic defect	Parental karyotyping
Anatomical	2D or 3D ultrasonography, hysterosalpingography, sonohysterosalpingography, MRI, CT scan, laparoscopy, and hysteroscopy
Endocrine	Serum TSH, FT4, FT3, antithyroid antibody, 75 g OGTT, HbA1C, serum prolactin, free testosterone, free androgen index, and serum DHEA
Immunological	Antiphospholipid antibody, lupus anticoagulant, anticardiolipin antibody, anti-DNA antibody, protein C and protein S measurement
Infective	TORCH panel, chlamydia, endometrial biopsy, cell culture, specific IgM, IgG, ELISA, and PCR

(DHEA: dehydroepiandrosterone; ELISA: enzyme-linked immunosorbent assay; FT3: free triiodothyronine; FT4: free thyroxine; HbA1C: hemoglobin A1C; IgG: immunoglobulin G; IgM: immunoglobulin M; OGTT: oral glucose tolerance test; PCR: polymerase chain reaction; TSH: thyroid-stimulating hormone)

MANAGEMENT

General Measures

- Proper counselling and tender loving care
- Lifestyle modification—healthy diet, regular exercise, optimization of body weight, and quitting smoking, alcohol, and recreational drugs

- High dose folic acid if maternal body mass index (BMI) ≥30
- Vitamin D supplementation is recommended in periconceptional period.[13]

Specific Measures

- *Chromosomal abnormality:*
  - Genetic counselling is helpful.
  - Preconceptional genetic testing (PGT) can be offered though not shown to increase total live birth rate.[14]
- *Anatomical abnormality:*
  - According to the ESHRE 2021 guidelines, surgical correction of uterine anomaly does not improve pregnancy. However, decisions must be individualized. Metroplasty, septum removal are the commonly performed surgical methods. There is evidence that septal resection reduces miscarriage rates, resulting in live birth rates. As it lacks evidence on safety and efficacy, this should be offered on individual basis.[15]
  - Live birth rate is shown in patients with fibroid that distorts uterine cavity, myomectomy improves live birth rate.[16]
- *Acquired thrombophilia:*
  - Aspirin and low molecular weight heparin shown to increase live birth rate in APLS.[17]
  - Recommendation is to start these medicines from first positive pregnancy test.
  - Low molecular weight heparin (LMWH) has a benefit of single daily administration and better safety profile than unfractionated heparin for thrombocytopenia and osteopenia.[18]
- *Immunological treatments:*
  - Evidence showed no improvement on immunotherapy according to systemic review and meta-analysis published in 2018.[19]
- *Endocrinological treatment:*
  - Optimization of endocrinological causes by hormonal replacement therapy like thyroxine (target TSH should be <4.0 mIU/L), insulin progesterone, and also some drugs such as insulin sensitizers as metformin, and bromocriptine in hyperprolactinemia have been shown to improve pregnancy rate.[20]
- *Male factor treatments:*
  - Still there is lack of evidence-based treatment for male factors. So lifestyle modification, advice on smoking, obesity, and excessive exercise to improve sperm DNA damage is emphasized.[4]
  - 2019 Cochrane review[21] emphasized on antioxidant supplementation in subfertile male suggested that it may improve live birth rates.
  - Management should be individualized.
- *Unexplained pregnancy loss treatments:*
  - In 2019, Cochrane review suggested that progesterone supplementation in these case may have a positive effect in further pregnancies.
  - In 2020, a meta-analysis,[22] live birth rate or continuing pregnancy outcome with progesterone versus placebo or no treatment which increased significantly from 71 to 75%.
  - Analysis from two trials; one exploring the use of vaginal micronized progesterone on live birth rates in RPL (PROMISE),[23] and one exploring threatened pregnancy loss (PRISM).[24]
  - This analysis showed a less but positive treatment effect dependent on the number of pregnancy losses.

The authors believed the double risk factors of early pregnancy that is bleeding and a history of one or more previous loss, identifies high-risk women where progesterone may bring positive results.[22]

CONCLUSION

Though many of causes remain unexplained, we should try to find the cause of BOH. Prompt management should be done keeping the emotional, social, and cultural belief of the women and her partner in mind. Patient should be counseled that even after diagnosis of RPL, 70% will achieve live birth in their subsequent pregnancy. Treatment should be individualized and evidence based. It can increase live birth rate and prevent recurrence of the sad incidents.

REFERENCES

1. Singh G, Sidhu K. Bad Obstetric history: a prospective study. Med J Armed Forces India. 2010;66(2):117-20.
2. Bhargavi AB, Sailatha R, Anuradha CR. Changing trends of causative factors in antenatal mothers with bad obstetric history: A retrospective study. Int J Reprod Contracept Obstet Gynecol. 2021;10: 3371-4.
3. Practice Committee of the American Society for Reproductive Medicine. Evaluation and treatment of recurrent pregnancy loss: a committee opinion. Fertil Steril. 2012;98:1103-11.
4. European Society of Human Reproduction and Embryology (ESHRE). (2022). Guideline on the management of Recurrent pregnancy loss. [online] Available from https://www.eshre.eu/Guidelines-and-Legal/Guidelines/Recurrent-pregnancy-loss.aspx. [Last accessed November, 2022].
5. Simpson JL, Elias S. Genetics in Obstetrics and Gynecology. Philadelphia, USA: Saunders; 2003. pp. 101-32.
6. Lim JH, Kim MH, Han YJ, Lee DE, Park SY, Han JY, et al. Cell-free fetal DNA and cell-free total DNA levels in spontaneous abortion with fetal chromosomal aneuploidy. PLoS One. 2013;8(2):e56787.
7. Franssen MT, Korevaar JC, Leschot NJ, Bossuyt PM, Knegt AC, Gerssen-Schoorl KB, et al. Selective chromosome analysis in couples with two or more miscarriages: case-control study. BMJ. 2005;331:137-41.
8. Sugiura-Ogasawara M, Ozaki Y, Katano K, Suzumori N, Mizutani E. Uterine anomaly and recurrent pregnancy loss. Semin Reprod Med. 2011;29(6):514-21.
9. Kaur R, Gupta K. Endocrine dysfunction and recurrent spontaneous abortion: an overview. Int J Appl Basic Med Res. 2016;6(2):79-83.
10. Levine JS, Branch DW, Rauch J. The antiphospholipid syndrome. N Engl J Med. 2002;346(10):752-63.
11. Arvieux J, Renaudineau Y, Mane I, Perraut R, Krilis SA, Youinou P. Distinguishing features of anti-beta-2 glycoprotein I antibodies between patients with leprosy and the antiphospholipid syndrome. Thromb Haemost. 2002;87(4):599-605.
12. Mohammad EAK, Salman YJ. Study of TORCH infections in women with Bad Obstetric History (BOH) in Kirkuk city. Int J Curr Microbiol App Sci. 2014;3(10):700-9.
13. Palacios C, Kostiuk LK, Pena-Rosas JP. Vitamin D supplementation for women during pregnancy. Cochrane Database Syst Rev. 2019;(7):CD008873.
14. Singh N, Rastogi K. Microbiology of recurrent pregnancy loss. In: Mehta S, Gupta B (Eds). Recurrent Pregnancy Loss. Singapore: Springer; 2018. pp. 129-36.
15. Akhtar MA, Saravelos SH, Li TC, Jayaprakasan K; Royal College of Obstetricians and Gynaecologists. Reproductive implications and management of congenital uterine anomalies. Scientific Impact Paper No. 62 November 2019. BJOG. 2020;127:e1-13.
16. Saravelos SH, Yan J, Rehmani H, Li TC. The prevalence and impact of fibroids and their treatment on the outcome of pregnancy in

women with recurrent miscarriage. Hum Reprod. 2011;26:3274-9.
17. Shi T, Gu ZD, Diao Q. Meta-analysis on aspirin combined with low-molecular-weight heparin for improving the live birth rate in patients with antiphospholipid syndrome and its correlation with d-dimer levels. Medicine (Baltimore). 2021;100(25):e26264.
18. Hamulyak EN, Scheres LJ, Marijnen MC, Goddijn M, Middeldorp S. Aspirin or heparin or both for improving pregnancy outcomes in women with persistent antiphospholipid antibodies and recurrent pregnancy loss. Cochrane Database Syst Rev. 2020;(5):CD012852.
19. Achilli C, Duran-Retamal M, Saab W, Serhal P, Seshadri S. The role of immunotherapy in in vitro fertilization and recurrent pregnancy loss: a systematic review and meta-analysis. Fertil Steril. 2018;110:1089-100.
20. Dong AC, Morgan J, Kane M, Stagnaro-Green A, Stephenson MD. Subclinical hypothyroidism and thyroid autoimmunity in recurrent pregnancy loss: a systematic review and meta-analysis. Fertil Steril. 2020;113:587-600.e1.
21. Smits RM, Mackenzie-Proctor R, Yazdani A, Stankiewicz MT, Jordan V, Showell MG. Antioxidants for male subfertility. Cochrane Database Syst Rev. 2019;(3):CD007411.
22. Coomarasamy A, Devall AJ, Brosens JJ, Quenby S, Stephenson MD, Sierra S, et al. Micronized vaginal progesterone to prevent miscarriage: a critical evaluation of randomized evidence. Am J Obstet Gynecol. 2020;223:167-76.
23. Coomarasamy A, Williams H, Truchanowicz E, Seed PT, Small R, Quenby S, et al. A randomized trial of progesterone in women with recurrent miscarriages. N Engl J Med. 2015;373:2141-8.
24. Coomarasamy A, Devall AJ, Cheed V, Harb H, Middleton LJ, Gallos ID, et al. A randomized trial of progesterone in women with bleeding in early pregnancy. N Engl J Med. 2019;380:1815-24.

CHAPTER 16

Assisted Reproductive Technology Pregnancy— Are They Different?

Neharika Malhotra

INTRODUCTION

Assisted reproductive technologies (ARTs) involve handling of eggs, sperms, or both gametes outside the body and include in vitro fertilization (IVF), intracytoplasmic sperm injection (ICSI), or use of donor gametes. Since the birth of first IVF baby Louis Brown in 1978, the use of ART has increased tremendously over last three decades with 5 million babies being born till date and around 1.5 million ART cycles each year in various centers. According to latest published report by the National ART Registry of India (NARI) there are 139 registered centers in our country conducting around 9,000 IVF and 24,000 ICSI cycles per year with average pregnancy rate of 38–41%.

In present scenario, ART contributes to 1–5% of all births[1] and 1 child in every classroom, i.e., 1 in 25 children is born with use of this technology. So almost every obstetrician today faces the challenge of managing an ART pregnancy.

PROBLEMS ASSOCIATED WITH ASSISTED REPRODUCTIVE TECHNOLOGY PREGNANCY

Women who have conceived with ART pose a unique challenge for the obstetrician as they usually have a variety of associated risk factors. These include older age, obesity, polycystic ovary syndrome (PCOS) and endocrinological problems, fibroids, ovarian cysts, uterine anomalies, and uniquely multiple pregnancy.

Today due to the fast paced lifestyle and more women opting to work there is a trend for delayed marriage and consequently late child bearing. According to latest Human Fertilisation and Embryology Authority (HFEA) data (2010), the average age of women undergoing IVF is 35 years. Elderly women conceived with IVF have a higher risk of preeclampsia, gestational diabetes, dysfunctional labor, obstetric hemorrhage, and operative delivery even when compared to age-matched controls.[2]

About 5–10% of these women might have underlying PCOS or other endocrinological problems. Pregnant women with PCOS have an increased risk of not only gestational diabetes but also pregnancy-induced hypertension (PIH), preeclampsia, preterm birth, and a higher perinatal mortality rate and neonatal intensive care unit (NICU) admissions for the offspring.

In pregnancies complicated by fibroid uterus, complications include abortions, preterm labor, malpresentations, antepartum and postpartum hemorrhage, operative deliveries, and degeneration of fibroid.

MULTIPLE PREGNANCY AND ASSISTED REPRODUCTIVE TECHNOLOGY

Since early phase of ART development, following the advent of hyperstimulation drugs to produce multiple oocytes and the practice to transfer of multiple embryo in order to improve pregnancy and live birth rate, there has been an increase in the rate of multiple pregnancy.

Most of the maternal and perinatal complications in ART pregnancies can be attributed to the multiple pregnancies. The incidence of twins is 20 times greater after superovulation and ART and higher order multiples are 100 times more common.[3] According to 2006 SART data, 49% of 2006 ART births were multiple gestation births. Maternal risk of multiple pregnancies include PIH, preeclampsia, preterm labor, increase in cesarean section rate, and difficulty in detecting congenital malformations, especially in three or more fetuses.

Neonatal complications includes increased mortality, low birth weight, very low birth weight, respiratory distress syndrome (RDS), necrotizing enterocolitis (NEC), intraventricular hemorrhage (IVH), twin-twin transfusion syndrome (TTTS), sepsis, long-term neurological sequel, etc.[4]

In vitro fertilization also increases the risk of monochorionic twins which have a worse obstetric outcome. Even studies comparing the outcome of IVF conceived twins with spontaneously conceived ones have found them to fare worse.[5]

OUTCOME OF SINGLETON ASSISTED REPRODUCTIVE TECHNOLOGY PREGNANCY

There is existing controversy whether ART singletons fare any different than spontaneous conceived ones because studies differ in their inclusion exclusion criteria as well as nature of comparison groups. But most studies conclude that IVF pregnancies are at more risk. They have a18-32% risk of miscarriages, mostly due to advanced age, PCOS, and other associated pathology. ART pregnancies also have 1 in 100 risk of having a heterotopic pregnancy. Apart from this, Jackson RA et al. in 2004[6] have reported an increased risk of preeclampsia and abruption in ART conceptions. ART pregnancies have a twofold risk of developing gestational diabetes.[7] Several studies have found an increased risk of placenta previa in singleton ART pregnancies.[8]

Apart from multiple pregnancy, there is an association between ART pregnancies and low birth weight babies. A large retrospective cohort study of >31,000 singleton IVF births in the US-Society of Assisted Reproductive Technology (SART) registry demonstrated that low birth weight was significantly more likely in singleton infants born after transfer of fresh embryos compared with infants born after transfer of frozen embryos.[9] The current evidence therefore suggests that ART births are at an increased risk of adverse perinatal outcomes in part because of absolute increases in multiple gestations and in part because of higher rates of low birth weight and preterm births among singleton infants conceived after assisted conception. Treatment with ART is also associated with increased risks of cardiovascular, musculoskeletal, urogenital, gastrointestinal defects, and cerebral palsy.[10] The increase in birth defects in singletons born after ART may be related with the hormonal treatment for infertility or the procedure itself, but the underlying cause of infertility and also play a role. Increased prevalence of autosomal and sex chromosomal aberrations are found in children born with ICSI due to the associated sperm abnormalities. ART pregnancies also have a small increased risk of imprinting disorders such as Angelman's and Beckwith-Wiedemann syndrome.

Specific IVF procedures have also been linked to the reproductive outcome. Blastocyst transfer is linked with a slight increase risk of preterm birth and congenital malformations. Recipients of oocyte donation even from a young donor are associated with 16–40% risk of PIH.[11]

ANTENATAL MANAGEMENT OF ASSISTED REPRODUCTIVE TECHNOLOGY PREGNANCY

Despite few guidelines available most experts worldwide believe that ART pregnancies should be managed in a high risk unit by an obstetrician with expertise and knowledge regarding the issues involved.

- Any woman conceived by ART should be evaluated for all the risk factors at the first visit itself and a plan of care should be devised accordingly.
- Couple should be counseled in advance regarding maternal and perinatal risks and increased risk of obstetric interventions such as induction of labor and cesarean delivery.
- Genetic counseling should be offered for men with male factor infertility regarding prevalence of chromosomal abnormalities.
- Identify parental karyotyping or Y microdeletion reports wherever available, especially in cases of male factor, recurrent implantation failures which can aid in counseling regarding future progeny.
- Make sure the woman is on folic acid supplementation at least 400 μg.
- During the first scan, usually 2 weeks after the beta-human chorionic gonadotropin (β-hCG) result documentation of the number of gestational sacs should be done.
- Even if intrauterine pregnancy is documented, adnexal region must be evaluated to rule out heterotopic pregnancy.
- Early diagnosis of any first trimester problems.
- There are reports of high false positives in serum screening for Down's syndrome and lower pregnancy-associated plasma protein A (PAPP-A) levels. History of IVF should be provided to the laboratory. In future, newer software's for risk calculation might become available for ART pregnancies.
- A good scan for fetal anomalies is a must and attention to soft markers for aneuploidies.
- All ART pregnancies should be monitored for preterm labor by transvaginal cervical length measurement at 16–20 weeks. At present there is substantial evidence of benefit with use of vaginal progesterone in prevention.
- Consider low-dose aspirin for mothers at high risk of preeclampsia to be started before 16 weeks of gestation.
- Screening for gestational diabetes should be done at 24–26 weeks of gestation.
- Increased vigilance-serial ultrasound scans/fetal monitoring in third trimester of pregnancy for fetal growth and well-being.
- Intrapartum electronic fetal monitoring should be offered.
- Discuss with the couple regarding induction of labor versus cesarean section at 36 weeks of gestation depending on maternal age, period of infertility, number of attempts, antenatal complications, and parental wishes.

COUNSELING AND SUPPORT

This group of women are very high strung and need a lot of mental and psychological support constantly. They have a fear in their mind of losing their pregnancy and so need to be tackled differently and patiently. Wherever possible, access to counselor should be provided.

CONCLUSION

Yes, ART pregnancies are different—they need special care and attention throughout their pregnancy starting from the first scan to postpartum period. Large majority of births from ART are not associated with any complications; however, there are increased maternal and perinatal risks for few mothers. It is still unclear whether the ART procedure itself or the underlying maternal factors such as age, parity, and subfertility lead to this increased risk. Continued research and audit of the reproductive performance are needed for optimal counseling and to find ways of reducing these adverse outcomes. ART units should develop strict policies regarding the number of embryos to be transferred to avoid complications related to multiple pregnancy.

There is a need to look at legal, ethical, moral boundaries for all practicing ART while always considering the future of the unborn child.

REFERENCES

1. Talaulikar VS, Arulkumaran S. Reproductive outcomes after assisted conception. Obstet Gynecol Surv. 2012;67:566-83.
2. Hayashi M, Nakai A, Satoh S, Matsuda Y, Adverse obstetric and perinatal outcomes of singleton pregnancies may be related to maternal factors associated with infertility rather than the type of assisted reproductive technology procedure used Fertil Steril. 2012;98:922-28.
3. https://www.sciencedirect.com/science/article/pii/S2666571922000093. Assisted reproductive technology or infertility: What underlies adverse outcomes? Lessons from the Massachusetts Outcome Study of Assisted Reproductive Technology 2022, F and S Reviews.
4. Kawwass JF, Badell ML. Maternal and fetal risk associated with assisted reproductive technology. Obstet Gynecol. 2018;132(3): 763-72.
5. Gui J, Ling Z, Hou X, et al. In vitro fertilization is associated with the onset and progression of preeclampsia. Placenta. 2020;89:50-57.

SECTION 6

Infections

- **Infections in Pregnancy**
  Ashwini Kale

- **Maternal Sepsis and its Management**
  Shazia Parveen, Ekta Tiwari, Shaheen Anjum

CHAPTER 17

Infections in Pregnancy

Ashwini Kale

■ INTRODUCTION

Viral infections during pregnancy are major cause of maternal and fetal morbidity and mortality. The infections can spread to neonate by transplacentally, perinatally, or postnatally. The clinical manifestations in neonate depend on viral agent and gestational age.

The knowledge about the ways the maternal-fetal interface and placenta interact with the maternal immune system may explain these findings. Once thought to be "immunosuppressed", the pregnant woman actually undergoes an immunological transformation, where the immune system is necessary to promote and support the pregnancy and growing fetus. When this protection is breached, as in a viral infection, this security is weakened and infection with other microorganisms can then propagate and lead to outcomes, such as preterm labor.

Perinatal outcomes from viral infections during pregnancy can range from no effect on pregnancy to loss by spontaneous abortion to fetal infection with resulting congenital viral syndromes. As there is no standard management of viral infections during pregnancy, expect for toxoplasmosis, rubella cytomegalovirus, herpes simplex, and HIV (TORCH) infections. These guidelines allow for a diagnosis of infection, no treatment or preventative strategy is available to prevent adverse pregnancy outcomes.

■ HERPES SIMPLEX VIRUS

Herpes simplex viruses (HSV) are enveloped double-stranded (ds)-DNA viruses of *Herpesviridae* family, which are transmitted across epithelial mucosal cells as well as through skin interruptions and migrate to nerve tissues where they persist latent.

Herpes simplex virus-1 predominantly seen in orofacial lesions and typically is found in the trigeminal ganglia, while HSV-2 is most commonly found in the lumbosacral ganglia. Both HSV-1 and HSV-2 can cause genital lesions. The overall seroprevalence of HSV among pregnant women is 72%.[1]

During pregnancy, HSV infection has been associated with spontaneous abortion, intrauterine growth restriction, preterm labor, and congenital and neonatal herpes infections.[2] The clinical management involves decreasing vertical transmission to the fetus, thereby decreasing the risk of neonatal herpes infection. The presence of antibodies to both HSV-1 and HSV-2 at the onset of pregnancy has the least risk of perinatal transmission. In contrast, primary genital HSV infection, late in pregnancy carries a 30–50% risk of neonatal infection, while early pregnancy infection carries a risk of <1%.[3] If primary HSV infection occurs during late pregnancy antibodies are not developed in time to suppress viral replication and shedding before labor. A total of 80–90%

of perinatal transmission occurs during labor and delivery.[4] The recurrent infections in pregnancy may also transmit to neonates. The symptom recurrence producing viral shedding at the onset of labor is associated with up to a 3% risk of neonatal herpes; both young age and recent infection are associated with increased viral shedding.[5,6] The asymptomatic viral shedding in recurrent disease at term has not been associated with neonatal disease.

Neonatal herpes infection is classified into three categories—localized skin, eye, and mouth (SEM); central nervous system (CNS) with or without SEM; and disseminated disease.[6-9] Infected newborns can present with significant neurologic deficits, blindness, seizures, and learning disabilities.

Suppressive antiviral therapy in the last month of pregnancy reduces the likelihood of asymptomatic viral shedding, clinical HSV recurrence, and cesarean delivery for recurrent lesions.[10-13] When lesions or prodromal symptoms are present at the onset of labor, cesarean section is recommended to minimize the risk of viral exposure to the infant, even if suppressive therapy has been used.[14]

Women with asymptomatic HSV in labor, invasive procedures should be avoided such as amniotomy, the use of fetal scalp electrodes,[15] and operative vaginal delivery.[16] This decreases fetal exposure to vaginal secretions containing the virus. Active management should be considered in these women when membranes rupture before the onset of labor.

When there is preterm premature rupture of the membranes (PPROM), the risks of prematurity must be weighed against the risks of HSV transmission, depending on the gestational age and clinical picture.

Diagnostic tests include maternal serum enzyme-linked immunosorbent assay (ELISA), immunoglobulin G (IgG), and immunoglobulin M (IgM) testing for HSV-1 and HSV-2, staining of smear (papanicolaou/Tzanck) from the fluid in the vesicle.

■ VARICELLA ZOSTER VIRUS

Varicella zoster virus is highly contagious, which causes varicella (chicken pox), is a consequence of primary infection and herpes zoster is due to reactivation of virus.

It is transmitted by respiratory droplets or by close contacts and characterized by widespread maculopapular to vesicular rash that starts on the face and trunk and then moves to the extremities. The incubation period is 15 days and can transmit the infection 2 days before and 5 days after the onset of the rash, until all the lesions have crusted.[17] After an initial episode of infection, the virus may persist latent in the dorsal root ganglia for years. The incidence of varicella in pregnancy is 0.7/1,000. Because varicella is mainly a disease of childhood, most women are immune before they become pregnant.[18]

The primary varicella infection during pregnancy is associated with significant maternal and fetal morbidity and mortality. The risk of congenital varicella syndrome ranges from 0.4–2% with maternal varicella infection during the first 20 weeks of gestation, and the risk is negligible after 20 weeks of gestation. Neonatal infection may occur in 10–20% of neonates whose mothers became acutely infected from 5 days before to 2 days after the delivery. Infants become symptomatic 5–10 days postpartum. Congenital varicella syndrome is characterized by limb hypoplasia, microcephaly, hydrocephaly, skin scarring, cataracts, chorioretinitis, intrauterine growth restriction, and mental retardation.[19] Development of this syndrome is thought to be a result of reactivation of the varicella virus in utero, as opposed to primary infection of the fetus.[20-22]

The risk of the congenital varicella syndrome is negligible with herpes zoster in pregnancy, because of IgG antibodies in the maternal blood prevent the virus from crossing the placenta and infecting the fetus.[23-26] Treatment for the pregnant woman targets decreasing maternal morbidity, as no treatment regimen has shown a decrease in the incidence of vertical transmission.

Diagnosis is done by clinical findings and detection of IgM or isolation of varicella virus by polymerase chain reaction (PCR).

■ CYTOMEGALOVIRUS

Cytomegalovirus (CMV) is a ds-DNA virus of member of the family of herpes virus. It is ubiquitous virus with variable clinical manifestations and the most common cause of congenital infection about 0.5-2% of all live births.[27] If this infection occurs during pregnancy, it can have detrimental effects on the pregnancy. Primary maternal infection carries 30-40% risk of transmission to neonate.

Maternal infection during the antepartum period is usually asymptomatic or may present with fever, fatigue, myalgias, rhinitis, pharyngitis, lymphadenopathy, and hepatosplenomegaly. Pregnancy may does not appear to affect the clinical severity of the infection.

Vertical transmission from the mother to the fetus can occur both primary and non-primary maternal infection. The maternal primary infection by the following mechanisms: transplacental or intrapartum via ingestion or aspiration of cervicovaginal secretions during delivery, postpartum via breastfeeding. Non-primary infection results from reactivation or reinfection with different strain.[28,29]

Cytomegalovirus primarily affects the ventricle, the organ of Corti and the neurons of the eighth cranial nerve, and cause of congenital hearing loss.[30] The rate of fetal transmission appears to increase with advancing gestation and the severity is inversely related to gestational age.

Most newborns of women with primary CMV infection and almost all newborns of women with non-primary infection in pregnancy are initially asymptomatic. A total of 10-15% of these initially asymptomatic newborns develop neurodevelopmental damage within the first 3 years of life.[31,32] Approximately 5-20% of newborns of mothers with primary CMV infection will have symptoms at birth.[33-35] The mortality rate is about 5%.

Diagnosis is done by detection of maternal anti-CMV IgG and IgM antibodies. Universal screening for pregnant women is not routinely recommended as the virus is ubiquitous.

■ RUBELLA

The rubella virus, an enveloped single-stranded (ss)-RNA virus, is a member of the family *Togaviridae*. It is transmitted by respiratory droplets and is primarily a mild disease in children. In adults, rubella is a self-limited disease characterized by rash, usually begins on the face and spreads to the trunk and extremities. The incubation period is 12-23 days. The infectious period is from 7 days before to 7-12 days after the onset of rash.[36] When maternal infection occurs in the first trimester, transmission rates are up to 50%, dropping to <1% after 12 weeks. High risk of birth defects occurs, if the infection occurs before 8 weeks.

Maternal rubella infection in pregnancy can cause spontaneous abortion, fetal infection, stillbirths or fetal growth restriction, and the congenital rubella syndrome (CRS). CRS characterized by heart defects, neurological defects, eye defects, sensorineural defects, hematological abnormality, hepatosplenomegaly, and diabetes. The risk of CRS depends on the gestational age at which maternal infection occurs.[37]

Diagnosis of primary maternal infection should be made by serologic tests. The diagnosis of fetal infection is done by detection of fetal serum IgM or viral culture of the amniotic fluid.

HUMAN IMMUNODEFICIENCY VIRUS

According to the Centers for Disease Control and Prevention (CDC), about 50,000 people get infected with human immunodeficiency virus (HIV) each year. About 80% of new cases in women are contracted through heterosexual intercourse, 20% by contaminated needles, and the remaining cases through blood products and maternal-child transmission.

The initial infection is asymptomatic, serological evidence occurs after 2–8 weeks up to 6 months. The most common clinical manifestations of the acute retroviral syndrome include fever, night sweats, lymphadenopathy, sore throat, rash, myalgia/arthralgia, headache, and recurrent infections such as herpes or candidiasis. Diagnosis is made with HIV immunoassay (ELISA or Western blot) and HIV viral RNA detection. In untreated cases, the levels of CD4 T cells decline and cause opportunistic infections lead to death. With antiretroviral treatment, life expectancy has increased significantly.

While the pregnancy does not affect disease course, HIV infection in pregnancy includes a risk of vertical transmission. This transmission may occur during intrauterine life, delivery, or breastfeeding. The greatest risk of transmission occurs with advanced maternal disease with high maternal HIV viral load. With no treatment, the risk of vertical transmission is as high as 25%, but with the implementation of universal antenatal HIV screening, counseling, maternal antiretroviral medication, and neonatal postexposure prophylaxis for newborns of women with HIV, delivery by cesarean section prior to onset of labor, and discouraging breastfeeding, the mother-to-infant transmission has decreased to <1%.[38] Intrapartum treatment with zidovudine reduces vertical transmission.

The hormonal status, the regulation of the mucosal environment in the female reproductive tract, and the morphological changes in the female reproductive tract associated with pregnancy play a critical role in the susceptibility to HIV.

HEPATITIS

Acute viral hepatitis is the most common cause of jaundice in pregnancy. The course of most viral infections is not affected by pregnancy.

Hepatitis A

Hepatitis A virus (HAV) infection is RNA virus, uncommonly diagnosed during pregnancy because of non-specific signs and symptoms. It is transmitted by the feco-oral route or through sexual contact.[39-41] The incidence of acute HAV infection in pregnancy is approximately 1:1,000 women. Vertical transmission of HAV during the pregnancy or puerperium is rare.[42-46]

Hepatitis B

Hepatitis B virus (HBV) is DNA virus, the most common form of chronic hepatitis around the world. Chronic carriers can continue to transmit the disease for many years before becoming symptomatic.[47] Chronic HBV infection leads to increased risk for chronic hepatic insufficiency, cirrhosis, and hepatocellular carcinoma. Transmission occurs by the exposure to contaminated blood products, body fluids, or sexual contact. HBV does not cross placenta, unless there is breach in the barrier. Acute HBV infection during pregnancy usually is mild and not associated with teratogenicity or mortality. Most neonatal infections are the result of contact with infected maternal blood and vaginal secretions during birth or acquired during breast feeding. A high maternal viral load is the most important risk factor for perinatal transmission. Delivery decisions should be made on the basis of obstetric indications.

Treatment is mainly supportive, with monitoring of liver biochemical tests and prothrombin time. Antiviral therapy is started unless the patient has acute liver failure or protracted severe hepatitis. Some patients occasionally will develop a hepatitis flare, liver biochemical tests should be monitored every trimester and postpartum.

Universal screening of all pregnant women allows for identification of Hepatitis B surface antigen positive women. Women found to be positive should also be screened for HIV and other forms of hepatitis such as hepatitis A and hepatitis C. Monitoring of liver biochemical tests and viral load help guide management and extent of disease. All infants of mothers with HBV should receive passive-active immunization with hepatitis B IgG and the hepatitis B vaccine within 12 hours of delivery.

Hepatitis C

The hepatitis C virus (HCV) is a ss-RNA virus, major cause of chronic hepatitis, cirrhosis, and hepatocellular carcinoma around the world.[48] Approximately 40% of patients infected with HCV recover completely and the rest become chronic carriers. The peak age of incidence of acute HCV is between 20-39 years.[49,50] Approximately 75% of asymptomatic patients are chronically infected.

Hepatitis C virus is transmitted parenterally, perinatally, and sexually. Risk of mother to child transmission is about 5%, rises to 15% for those with HIV and HCV.[51]

Women chronically infected with hepatitis C may have uneventful pregnancies. During pregnancy, pregnant women should be seen regularly by a gastroenterologist to monitor liver biochemical tests and viral load. During labor, invasive obstetric procedures and prolonged rupture of membranes should be avoided.[52] Cesarean delivery should be reserved for the usual obstetrical indications. Breastfeeding is not contraindicated.

Hepatitis E

Hepatitis E is caused by the hepatitis E virus (HEV). It is usually passed by feco-oral transmission through a contaminated water supply.[53] The infection is typically mild and self-limited without chronicity or clinical sequelae. The pregnant women in the second and third trimesters are mostly affected in epidemics. During pregnancy, the disease is more severe, the risk of postpartum haemorrhage (PPH) and maternal mortality occurs in 10-18% of patients in the third trimester. Premature deliveries, low birth weight (LBW), and high infant mortality of up to 33% are also observed.[54] The complications may include gestational hypertension, preeclampsia, proteinuria, edema, and kidney disease.[55]

INFLUENZA

The symptoms of influenza include cough, fever, malaise, rhinitis, myalgias, headache, chills, and sore throat and others include nausea and vomiting, otitis, and conjunctiva burning.

Pregnant women are at high risk for severe complications of influenza during seasonal influenza periods[56] and pandemics.[57-60]

Influenza viruses that infect humans are classified into three principal types (A, B, and C), of which types A and B are important causes of human disease. Types A and B are associated with seasonal epidemics, and only type A viruses have caused pandemics. Influenza A viruses are further classified on the basis of two surface proteins—hemagglutinin (H) and neuraminidase (N).

Pregnancy has been the highest risk factor for increased illness and death for both pandemic and seasonal influenza also at increased risk for influenza complications during seasonal influenza periods.[61] The pregnant women with underlying medical conditions, such as asthma are at increased risk.[62]

The effect of maternal influenza infection on the fetus is not well understood. Viremia is believed to occur infrequently in influenza,[63] and placental transmission of the virus also appears to be rare. The fetal effects are mostly, secondary to the maternal inflammatory response, rather than the result of a direct viral effect.[64]

The possible adverse pregnancy outcomes include increase in the defects of the CNS and other birth defects, spontaneous pregnancy loss, fetal death, and preterm delivery. The risk associated with influenza was reduced for women who received treatment with antipyretic medications and for those who had taken folic acid before and during early pregnancy.

There are associations between maternal influenza infection and childhood leukemia,[65] schizophrenia,[66] and Parkinson disease[67] as found in some studies. Even if the influenza virus does not have a direct effect on the fetus, fever that often accompanies influenza infection could have adverse effects. Factors that might decrease this risk include shorter fever duration,[68] use of fever-reducing medications,[68-70] and use of folic acid-containing supplements.[69] The vaccination is protective for both mother and fetus, especially for high-risk subpopulations, such as immunosuppressed pregnant women.

The CDC currently recommends influenza vaccine for all pregnant women in any trimester during flu season. The pregnant women with symptoms of influenza should be screened and treated immediately, especially those with comorbid medical conditions.

EBOLA AND LASSA FEVER

Ebola and Lassa viruses cause hemorrhagic fevers that have been reported mainly in Africa.[70]

Ebola virus disease is a rare but severe viral hemorrhagic fever that is caused by five different species of Ebola virus. The major outbreaks of Ebola hemorrhagic fever (EHF) occurred in Africa, especially in resource-constrained regions.

A major clinical manifestation was vaginal and uterine bleeding with 93% mortality within 10 days of illness onset,[71,72] and risk of preterm birth and abortion has also been reported in the different epidemics.[73]

Lassa fever or Lassa hemorrhagic fever (LHF) is an acute viral hemorrhagic fever caused by the Lassa virus, a member of arenavirus family of viruses and was first described in 1969 in the town of Lassa in Nigeria.[74,75] Lassa fever is endemic in eastern Sierra Leone where it is a major cause of mortality, especially in pregnant women.[76] The condition of the mother improved rapidly after evacuation of the uterus either by spontaneous abortion or normal delivery.

■ PARASITIC INFECTIONS

Parasitic infections affect tens of millions of pregnant women worldwide. These infections lead directly and indirectly to a spectrum of adverse maternal and fetal/placental effects. With the increase in global travel, healthcare providers will care for women who have recently moved from or travelled to areas where these infections are endemic.

The effect on maternal health and the developing fetus is dependent on the type of parasitic infection, the patient's natural immunity to that infection, and the parasite load.

The decision to treat a parasitic infection during pregnancy is based on knowledge of the associated morbidity and mortality, and the toxic effects of the antiparasitic drug. The pregnant woman should be informed of the risks of treating a parasitic disease during pregnancy. Delaying of treatment is appropriate when the infection does not cause an immediate threat to the mother or fetus.

Malaria

Malaria is one of the most prevalent and serious infectious diseases throughout the tropical and subtropical areas of the world. The common varieties encountered in India are *Plasmodium vivax* (*P. vivax*) and *Plasmodium falciparum* (*P. falciparum*). Malaria in pregnancy contributes to significant perinatal morbidity and mortality.

The Organism and Its Transmission

Malaria is caused by obligate intracellular protozoa of the genus *Plasmodium*. The four species known to infect humans are *P. vivax*, *Plasmodium ovale* (*P. ovale*), *Plasmodium malariae* (*P. malariae*), and *P. falciparum*. The disease is transmitted by the bite of an infected female anopheline mosquito, through transfusions, by blood contamination as a result of needle abuse, or congenitally. Following bite from an infected female anopheles mosquito, sporozoites are injected into human along with saliva.

Clinical Manifestations of Maternal Infection (Table 1)

The clinical presentation of malaria is dependent on host immunity and the infecting parasite. As the pregnancy is a state of immunosuppression, pregnant women are more susceptible to infection and its consequences. This effect is particularly apparent during the second half of pregnancy. The severity of the disease depends on the species, intensity of parasitemia,[77] extent of host resistance, speed of diagnosis and effective treatment. The severity of the disease is higher in primigravidae. Malaria is a leading cause of maternal mortality in many endemic regions.[78]

Symptoms of malaria in pregnancy may be nonspecific, and the condition often is misdiagnosed.[79,80] The anemia of pregnancy is potentiated during malarial infection secondary to hypersplenism, direct lysis of parasitized erythrocytes, and autoimmune hemolysis.[81] This rapid turnover of blood cells can produce serious folic acid deficiency and hypochromic microcytic iron deficiency anemia. In addition, placental function is so altered in heavy malarial infections that circulation, nutrients, and oxygen transport

TABLE 1: Treatment and chemoprophylaxis of malaria infections.

	Drug	Dosage*	Toxicity
P. vivax or P. ovale	Chloroquine phosphate followed by	600 mg orally followed by 300 mg 6 h, 24 h, and 48 h later	Chloroquine is not toxic during pregnancy at these doses. With prolonged use at higher doses, it has been associated with congenital defects, neonatal deafness, blindness, and central nervous system disturbances. Occasional gastrointestinal discomfort may be observed.
	Primaquine phosphate	30 mg orally daily for 14 days	Primaquine is contraindicated during pregnancy. Treatment with primaquine should be delayed until after delivery. It may cause hemolytic anemia in patients with glucose-6-phosphate dehydrogenase. Gastrointestinal discomfort may be observed. Primaquine is not required in treatment of congenital or transfusion malaria or *Plasmodium falciparum* (*P. falciparum*), *Plasmodium malariae* (*P. malariae*) infections
P. malariae	Chloroquine phosphate	600 mg orally followed by 300 mg 6 h, 24 h, and 48 h later	
P. falciparum uncomplicated	Quinine sulphate plus	600 mg orally three times/day for 7 days	
	Clindamycin	450 mg–three times/day for 7 days	
P. falciparum complicated Or Any species	Artesunate Or Quinidine gluconate plus	Artesunate intravenous (IV) 2.4 mg/kg at 0,12 and 24 h, then daily after. when patient is well, switched to oral Artesunate 2 mg/kg once daily Or Quinine-20 mg/kg loading dose infused over 4 h, followed by 10 mg/kg over 4 h every 8 h.	Recommended dosage of quinidine is not contraindicated in life-threatening chloroquine-resistant *P. falciparum* infection. Higher doses and prolonged use are contraindicated during pregnancy because of the association with abortion and hemolytic anemia. Arrhythmia, tinnitus, hypotension, nausea, abdominal pain, visual disturbance, and blood dyscrasia may be seen. Parenteral quinidine is limited due to associated cardiac arrhythmia
	Clindamycin OR	450 mg IV every 8 hours, when the patient is feeling well, switched to oral, for total of 7 days.	

Contd...

Contd...

	Drug	Dosage*	Toxicity
	Doxycycline	100 mg IV or PO every 12 h for 7 days	Not recommended during pregnancy because of effect on bone formation but may be used if benefit outweighs risks
Preventing relapse during pregnancy	Chloroquine phosphate followed by	300 mg orally once a week till delivery	
Preventing relapse after delivery	Primaquine phosphate	• 30 mg orally daily for 14 days for *vivax* • 15 mg orally once daily for 14 days for *ovale*	

to the fetus are markedly diminished.[82,83] The studies have shown a direct correlation between maternal malarial infection and second-trimester abortion, intrauterine death with macerated stillbirths, and fresh stillbirths due to intrapartum asphyxia.[84,85] The anemia produced by *P. falciparum* infection usually is seen after 20 weeks of pregnancy, and may induce congestive heart failure because of the reduced red cell mass.

The high fever associated with malaria also causes premature labor and delivery, and if infection is acquired before the 16th week, abortion may occur. In nonimmune women, malaria infection, if not treated immediately, may result in death of the fetus and occasionally of the mother.

Congenital Infection

Intrauterine transmission of malaria from mother to fetus occurs frequently, although the mechanism of transplacental passage of the parasite is unknown. The placenta acts as a major barrier to the malaria parasite and that its efficacy in blocking transmission is dependent on the mother's immune status.[86] Congenital infections are more likely to affect babies of non-immune mothers.

The placental sampling was more sensitive than maternal blood for detecting maternal infection, and more accurate in predicting fetal morbidity.[87] Direct penetration through chorionic villi, premature separation of the placenta, and physiologic transfusion of maternal red blood cells to the fetal circulation in utero or at the time of delivery have been postulated as mechanisms of transmission of congenital malaria. Other factors include passively transferred IgG, which has been postulated to be protected in utero and during the first few months of life. The onset of symptoms in congenital malaria typically occurs at 2–4 weeks of age, which is the estimated half-life of maternal IgG in the infant. Other factors that may protect the infant initially include fetal hemoglobin, abnormal hemoglobins that are resistant to malarial infection, the secretion of lymphokines or macrophage-derived toxic substances across the placenta to fetal circulation, and partial malaria chemotherapy during pregnancy.

Diagnosis

Diagnosis is based on clinical suspicion and confirmed by the finding of malaria parasites in Giemsa stained thick and thin blood smears, detection of PCR based plasmodium

DNA, fluorescent microscopy, and rapid malarial test.

After the diagnosis and speciation of malaria, treatment should be instituted immediately.

Although the antimalarial drugs are potentially toxic during pregnancy, the risk of not treating the infection in the pregnant mother is far greater. Chloroquine has not been found to have a harmful effect on the fetus when used in the recommended doses for malaria prophylaxis or treatment.

Entamoeba Histolytica Infection

Ten per cent of the world population and up to 80% in some tropical countries is infected with the intestinal protozoan *Entamoeba histolytica*.[88] Amebiosis is primarily is a disease of large intestine. The disease is transmitted by exposure to fecally contamination of food or water containing cyst form.

Clinical Manifestations

The symptoms may range from asymptomatic stage to fulminant bloody mucus diarrhea, intestinal perforation, peritonitis, and bleeding. The most common illness associated with amebic disease is colonic irritation characterized by colicky lower abdominal pain, with or without diarrhea. During pregnancy, amebic disease appears to be more frequently associated with acute exacerbations of the disease and with more prominent symptoms.[89-91] Infected pregnant women may have bloody, dysenteric stools with moderate abdominal pain and tenderness. The diarrhea is marked, the signs include fluid loss and electrolyte imbalance, which may adversely affect the pregnancy outcome[92] such as failure to gain weight, anemia, low birth weight, and intrauterine growth restriction (IUGR).[93]

The diagnosis of intestinal amebiasis is based on microscopic examination of fresh stool containing trophozoite and cyst. ELISA kits, PCR amplification rRNA genes for detection of species.

Therapy for amebiasis should be aimed at relief of symptoms; replacement of fluid, electrolytes, and blood; and eradication of the organism. Asymptomatic women who are known passers of *Entamoeba histolytica* (*E. histolytica*) cysts should have treatment delayed until after 14 weeks of gestation or until after delivery. Metronidazole 750 mg three times a day orally for 5-10 days may then be given.[94] An alternative drug is paromomycin 25-30 mg/kg/day in three divided doses for 7 days.[95] In patients with prominent symptomatic amebiasis of the intestine, metronidazole plus paromomycin should be given at the same doses.

The use of metronidazole alone for symptomatic intestinal disease will cure about 90% of patients. The addition of one of the luminal amebicides, such as paromomycin, will raise the cure rate to 100%.[96-98] In extraintestinal amebiasis, including hepatic abscess, metronidazole for 10 days is the drug of choice.

Giardia Lamblia Infection

Giardia lamblia (*G. lamblia*) is the leading protozoan cause of diarrhea in travelers and in waterborne outbreaks.[99,100] It is widely prevalent in tropics. *G. lamblia* is a multiflagellated protozoan with a trophozoite and a cyst stage. Infection is transmitted through ingestion of contaminated water or food containing *Giardia* cysts.

Clinical Manifestations

Symptomatic disease usually occurs 1-2 weeks after infection and is characterized by the sudden onset of watery, foul smelling diarrhea, abdominal distension, flatulence, nausea, anorexia, malabsorption, and abdominal cramps.

The adverse effects of *Giardia* infection on pregnancy are related to the associated diarrhea, fluid and electrolyte loss, anemia, vitamin deficiency and malabsorption, which may adversely affect the outcome of the pregnancy (IUGR and LBW). If a pregnant woman has associated dysgammaglobulinemia, giardiasis may be severe and more resistant to therapy.

Diagnosis

The diagnosis of giardiasis is based primarily on stool examination of cyst and trophozoite. A direct saline smear or preservation of the stool in formalin or PVA may aid in the identification of this organism. The Enterotest is a gelatin capsule containing a string that can be used to sample the duodenal contents for presence of specific anti *Giardia* IgG and IgM antibodies.[101]

Treatment

Pregnant women should receive therapy only if they are severely symptomatic because the infection may be self-limited in many persons. Tinidazole 500 mg twice daily for 3-5 days is recommended, metronidazole 250 mg thrice daily for 5 days. In pregnancy, a trial with paromomycin 10 mg/kg three times a day for 1 week is recommended.

TRICHOMONAS VAGINALIS INFECTION

Trichomonas vaginalis (*T. vaginalis*) is a pathogenic flagellated protozoan, exists in trophozoite stage in the human genitourinary tract. Transmitted primarily by sexual intercourse and causes vaginitis in women. The vaginal pH in trichomonal vaginitis usually is 5.5-7.0.[102] In women, *T. vaginalis* primarily infects the vaginal epithelium and less commonly, the endocervix, urethra, Bartholin's glands, and Skene's glands.

Clinical Manifestations

During pregnancy, infection with *T. vaginalis* commonly induces a prominent vaginal discharge. There is some evidence that growth of the parasite is enhanced in vitro by estrogens, and this may explain the severity of symptoms and tenacity of infection in colonized women during pregnancy or in those taking exogenous estrogens.

On physical examination, a purulent discharge may be present at the introitus and within the vagina; it may be characterized as a yellow-green homogeneous or frothy discharge. The vulva may be erythematous and edematous, and excoriations may be present. The vagina and cervix also may be erythematous, and small punctate hemorrhages may be present on the cervix (strawberry cervix).

There is conflicting information about the association of trichomonal vaginitis and puerperal fever and neonatal infection. There is little evidence that *T. vaginalis* is an invasive organism or that it produces amnionitis or endometritis. Between 2-17% of female infants born to infected mothers will have vaginal infection.[103] Neonatal vaginal epithelium is relatively mature as a result of the influence of maternal estrogen and is thus susceptible to *T. vaginalis* infection. Typically, these infections are asymptomatic, although a vaginal discharge may develop. Maternal estrogen is metabolized by 3-4 weeks of age, and vaginal epithelium returns to a prepubescent state that is relatively resistant to *T. vaginalis*.

The diagnosis of trichomonal infection is independent on the identification of *T. vaginalis* by wet-mount preparations, cultures, Papanicolaou smears, or special stains.

Metronidazole and other 5-nitroimidazoles, such as tinidazole and nimorazole, are recommended as standard therapy for trichomoniasis. The recommended dosage of metronidazole for initial treatment of trichomonal infection is 2 g orally as a single dose.[104]

Trypanosomiasis

Three species are pathogenic in humans, include *Trypanosoma gambiense* (West African trypanosomiasis), *T. rhodesiense* (East African trypanosomiasis), and *Trypanosoma cruzi* (*T. cruzi*) (Chagas' disease). African trypanosomiasis is transmitted by *Glossina* species (tsetse fly), and Chagas' disease is transmitted by reduviid bugs (*Triatoma species*).

All trypanosomes have the potential for transplacental transmission, with resulting intrauterine infection of the fetus during parasitemia. Infective *T. cruzi* may be found in breast milk and may infect the infant by direct inoculation or through the gastrointestinal tract.[105] African trypanosomiasis usually results in infertility, and may cause abortion, stillbirth, and premature labor when active or acquired during pregnancy. South American trypanosomiasis apparently has fewer adverse effects on fertility and pregnancy.

Diagnosis

Diagnosis of trypanosomiasis depends on demonstration of the organism in the peripheral blood, in tissue, or on serologic tests. All three species of trypanosomes may be demonstrated in the peripheral blood in the early phases of infection. In chronic disease, circulating trypanosomes are found less frequently, and elevated IgM and specific trypanosome antibody levels lead to definitive diagnosis.[106]

Treatment

For African trypanosomiasis, suramin is the most effective agent for non-CNS disease. After a 100–200-mg test dose, 1 g is given intravenously on the 1st, 3rd, 7th, 14th, and 21st days, for a total of 5 g. If CNS involved, an effective agent is melarsoprol (Mel B). Simultaneous treatment with steroids has been recommended to prevent the CNS toxicity associated with melarsoprol.

There is no satisfactory treatment for Chagas' disease, although nifurtimox 10 mg/kg/day for 3–4 months is an effective agent. Eflornithine, benznidazole, and γ-interferon have been used. These drugs are believed to be toxic during pregnancy, but usually trypanosomiasis is associated with infertility and abortion and, in severe cases, death of the patient. Thus, treatment with these drugs may be warranted. There are no drugs available for chemoprophylaxis, which are safe for use during pregnancy.[107]

Leishmaniasis

Leishmania are *obligate intracellular protozoa of which four species are known to infect humans. Leishmania donovani* (*L. donovani*) primarily infects the reticuloendothelial cells throughout the body. It causes the disease known as kala-azar, the major vector is the sandfly (*Phlebotomus*). *Leishmania tropica* (*L. tropica*) (Oriental sore) represents the classic form of cutaneous leishmaniasis. *Leishmania braziliensis* (*L. braziliensis*) and

Leishmania mexicana (L. mexicana) (New World leishmaniasis) induce a disease in which the patient has ulcers of the oral or nasal mucosa.

Clinical Manifestations

Visceral leishmaniasis: The visceral form of the disease has a prolonged incubation period with fever, which often consists of two daily spikes, may be abrupt or gradual in onset. Physical findings may include splenomegaly, lymphadenopathy, and hepatomegaly, with signs of portal hypotension and edema. Anemia and thrombocytopenia with hypergammaglobulin are frequently present and often are associated with bleeding. Most patients with visceral leishmaniasis are severely debilitated and infertile, although this form of leishmaniasis carries a potential risk of intrauterine fetal infection if pregnancy occurs during the early phase of the disease.[108,109] Congenital infection with leishmania has been associated with increased fetal wastage and almost always is associated with *L. donovoni* infection.

Diagnosis of visceral leishmaniasis is made by finding leishmanial organisms in stained preparations of the blood, bone marrow, lymph nodes, or material obtained by splenic puncture. Newer diagnostic modalities, which utilize PCR-based technology, are also being developed for the diagnosis of leishmaniasis.

Cutaneous leishmaniasis: The disease starts as a pruritic red papule at the site of inoculation. The lesion grows to an average diameter of 2 cm or more and tends to ulcerate 2–6 months after the bite of the vector.

Treatment: Cutaneous leishmaniasis is not known to carry serious risk to the mother or fetus, so treatment during pregnancy should be avoided and postponed until after delivery. However, patients with visceral leishmaniasis must be treated immediately regardless of pregnancy. Sodium antimony gluconate (Pentostam) is the drug of choice for all forms of leishmaniasis. For visceral leishmaniasis, the adult dose is 20 mg/kg/day intravenously or intramuscularly for 30 days. For cutaneous leishmaniasis, the dose is 0.6 g intramuscularly for 10 days. Patients who do not respond to antimonials should be treated with amphotericin B, 0.25–1 mg/kg intravenously daily or every other day for up to 8 weeks. The toxicity of antimonials during pregnancy is unclear.

INFECTION WITH INTESTINAL NEMATODES

Maternal infection with these intestinal roundworms usually is benign, except when there is a heavy worm burden.

Ascaris Lumbricoides

Ascaris lumbricoides (A. lumbricoides) is known as the giant roundworm of humans intestinal nematodes. About 25% of world population is infested with ascaris and it is mostly transmitted by ingestion of food contaminated with eggs of ascaris.

Clinical Manifestations

During the migratory phase of the larvae, the nematodes may cause pneumonia characterized by marked eosinophilia. This condition may be associated with fever, cough, wheezing, and migratory pulmonary infiltrates (Loeffler's syndrome). Adult worms may invade the female genital tract and cause tubo-ovarian abscess, pelvic pain, and menorrhagia. The adverse effects on fetus include LBW and preterm birth.

Diagnosis and Treatment

Diagnosis depends on the identification of characteristic eggs in the stool. Commonly, the recovery of an adult worm or identification of larvae in sputum or gastric aspirates may confirm the diagnosis. Chest X-ray shows patchy infiltration (Loeffler's syndrome).

Treatment of ascariasis should be withheld during pregnancy until after delivery because these infections usually are not associated with a significant risk to the mother or fetus. The drug of choice for treatment of intestinal infection in non-pregnant women is mebendazole 100 mg twice a day for 3 days. Albendazole 400 mg as a single dose is an alternative therapy. Albendazole/mebendazole should be avoided in the 1st trimester. Other alternative therapy includes pyrantel pamoate 10 mg/kg/day as single dose.

Hookworm

Human infection occurs with two species of hookworm, *Ancylostoma duodenale* and *Necator americanus*. Human infection is maintained by fecal contamination of the soil and ingestion of food containing larvae.

Clinical Manifestations

The major manifestations of the disease are dependent on the stage of infection and the number of invading parasites. Abdominal pain, diarrhea, and weight loss usually are noticed only in heavy infection with hookworm. The chronic manifestations of hookworm disease include iron deficiency anemia and hypoalbuminemia. During pregnancy, the main concern is iron deficiency anemia. If blood loss continues, potentiating the anemia of pregnancy and complications such as cardiac insufficiency and anasarca may develop. In pregnancy, management should be based on the degree of worm burden and the associated blood loss. The effects on the fetus are LBW, prematurity and increased mortality.

Diagnosis and Treatment

Diagnosis by direct microscopic examination of stool: Light to moderate worm infections during pregnancy can be managed with dietary and iron supplementation, and specific drug therapy can be withheld until after delivery. In pregnant women with a clinically high worm burden and significant anemia, therapy may be instituted with mebendazole, 100 mg orally twice a day for 3 days avoided in 1st trimester of pregnancy. Alternative therapy includes pyrantel pamoate 10 mg/kg orally as a single dose. Supportive therapy with replacement of iron, vitamins, and protein, and blood transfusion, if indicated.

Strongyloides Stercoralis

About 80 million people affected worldwide. It resides in the mucosa of the duodenum and jejunum.

Clinical Manifestations

Within the gastrointestinal tract, *Strongyloides* infection usually is asymptomatic, but may be associated with abdominal pain and tenderness in heavy infections, epigastric pain, tenderness, nausea, flatulence, vomiting, and diarrhea, iron deficiency anemia, malabsorption or protein-losing enteropathy. The respiratory symptoms include cough and breathlessness. Eosinophilia is a prominent feature of this infection. The effects on the fetus are LBW and IUGR.

Diagnosis and Treatment

Definitive diagnosis is done by finding of *Strongyloides stercoralis (S. stercoralis)* larvae in feces, duodenal fluid, jejunal biopsy, or sputum. Treatment consists of thiabendazole 25 mg/kg twice a day orally for 2–3 days. Albendazole 400 mg twice day for 3 days and ivermectin 200 µg/kg/day for 2 days are reasonable alternatives.

Because of the potential for dissemination, pregnant women with infection should be monitored carefully and treated if any complications are suspected. In asymptomatic disease treatment may be delayed till delivery.

Enterobius Vermicularis

About 300 million people infested worldwide. The predisposing factors are poor personal hygiene and oroperineal contact. Pinworm infection is one of the most common of all intestinal infections of humans. Pinworm infections are primarily asymptomatic and rarely cause complications in pregnancy. The symptoms are itching, pruritus ani, and pruritus vulvae. Occasionally, the migration of the parasite produces diseases, such as appendicitis, chronic salpingitis, vaginitis, or ulcerative lesions of the small and large bowel.[110]

Diagnosis and Treatment

Diagnosis is by direct microscopic examination of an adhesive cellophane tape pressed against the perianal region or swabs early in the morning. Therapy for pinworm infection during pregnancy should be postponed until after delivery.

Treatment consists of a single dose of mebendazole 100 mg orally that is repeated 2 weeks later. Alternative therapy includes pyrantel pamoate 10 mg/kg up to maximum 1 gm, or albendazole 400 mg orally in a single dose, which also should be repeated 2 weeks later.

Trichuris Trichiura (whip worm)

About 500–800 million people were affected worldwide. Most infections with *Trichuris trichiura (T. trichiura)* are asymptomatic, but may cause nausea, abdominal pain, and diarrhea have been associated with heavier infections. In severe infections with 800 or more worms, malnutrition, anemia or rectal prolapse may develop, often associated with secondary infection.

Diagnosis and Treatment

Diagnosis is based on fecal examination of ova. Therapy during pregnancy should be withheld until after delivery, at which time the patient may be treated with mebendazole 100 mg orally twice a day for 3 days. Pyrental palmoate 10 mg/kg up to maximum 1.0 gm can be recommended.

INFECTION WITH TISSUE-DWELLING NEMATODES

Tissue-dwelling nematodes are geographically widespread, particularly in the tropics, where they infect millions of people.

Trichinosis

Humans are infected by *Trichinella spiralis* organisms when they eat raw or inadequately cooked meat containing viable larvae.

Clinical Manifestations

Within the first week of infection, diarrhea, abdominal discomfort, and vomiting may become manifest. During the second week of infection, systemic symptoms such as fever, periorbital edema, subconjunctival hemorrhage, chemosis, myositis with pain and swelling, and weakness are common. There is no evidence that pregnancy exacerbates the clinical symptoms of trichinosis or the infection has an adverse effect on pregnancy.[111]

Diagnosis and Treatment

Diagnosis of trichinosis should be suspected in patients who have a history of recent consumption of poorly cooked meat and the clinical features. Definitive diagnosis is based on the finding of encysted larvae in a muscle biopsy specimen.

Treatment consists of mebendazole, 200-400 mg three times a day for 3 days, then 400-500 mg three times a day for 10 days. Steroids also have been recommended for severe symptoms. Symptomatic pregnant women should be treated.

Filariasis

The Organism and Its Life Cycle

In India 15 million people are affected. Bancroftian and Malayan filariases are similar clinical conditions that result from transmission of the filarial nematodes *Wuchereria bancrofti (W. bancrofti)* and *Brugia malayi (B. malayi)* by mosquitoes. *Onchocerca volvulus* and *Loa loa (L. loa)* are other filarial infections transmitted to humans by arthropod vectors. These infections may have adverse effects on maternal health, but in general do not have a specific effect on pregnancy or the neonate.

Clinical Manifestations

Wuchereria bancrofti and *B. malayi* infections are frequently asymptomatic. Symptoms are usually due to either acute inflammation or chronic lymphatic obstruction. Intermittent attacks of lymphangitis or lymphadenitis with fever, headache, backache, and nausea occasionally occur. In female patients, this process may affect the breast, vulva, and pelvic organs, leading to sexual difficulties and infertility. Elephantiasis of the vulva may obstruct labor and necessitate abdominal delivery. *L. loa* infection frequently is asymptomatic, but patients may have transient swelling or localized subcutaneous edema called *Calabar swellings*.

Diagnosis and Treatment

In filarial disease, diagnosis is based on clinical findings and finding of the parasite in the blood samples. Indirect fluorescence and ELISA tests can detect antibodies.

Treatment of *L. loa*, *W. bancrofti*, and *B. malayi* infection is by the use of diethylcarbamazine citrate, which is effective against microfilariae, but has little effect on adult worms. The recommended dosage is 50 mg orally on day 1, 50 mg three times a day on day 2, 100 mg three times a day on day 3, and 6 mg/kg/day in three doses on days 4 through 21. The recommended treatment for onchocerciasis is ivermectin 150 µg/kg orally once, repeated every 6-12 months. The ivermectin is well tolerated during pregnancy, with no major toxicities detected.[112] Because of the toxic effects of diethylcarbamazine during pregnancy, and it is recommended that therapy be delayed until after delivery unless symptoms require immediate treatment.

■ INFECTION WITH TREMATODES

Trematodes are parasitic flukes frequently found in humans and widely distributed throughout the world. Schistosomiasis has high rates of morbidity and mortality. Other flukes include *Clonorchis*, *Opisthorchis*, *Fasciolopsis*, *Fasciola*, and *Paragonimus*, which frequently infect the gastrointestinal tract or lung and often are associated with symptomatic disease.

Schistosomiasis

The three human blood flukes, *Schistosoma mansoni (S. mansoni), Schistosoma japonicum (S. japonicum),* and *Schistosoma haematobium (S. haematobium)*, infect >200 million people throughout the world.

Clinical Manifestations

Acute schistosomiasis is frequently associated with dermatitis or swimmers itch, which may be prominent 24 hours after penetration of the cercariae, which is characterized by the presence of a pruritic papular rash. *Katayama fever*, infections with *S. japonicum* initially presents with the acute onset of fever, chills, sweating, headache, and cough.

Chronic schistosomiasis frequently is asymptomatic. In patients with a heavy worm burden, prominent symptoms consist of fatigue and abdominal pain associated with intermittent diarrhea or dysentery and hepatosplenomegaly.

In *S. haematobium* infection, granulomatous reactions to the eggs located within the ureters and bladder may lead to obstruction of urinary flow or papillomatous irregularities of the bladder wall. It causes hematuria and dysuria, hepatosplenomegaly, bladder polyposis, and carcinoma.

The eggs of both *S. mansoni* and *S. haematobium* worms often are found in the reproductive organs of infected females lead to development of salpingitis, infertility, and ectopic pregnancies.[113] Similarly, lesions of the cervix cause abortion; vagina and vulva may cause dyspareunia and dystocia; schistosomiasis during pregnancy predisposes to malnutrition, proteinuria, recurrent UTI, anemia, and IUGR.

Diagnosis and Treatment

The diagnosis is made by the finding of schistosome eggs in feces, urine, vaginal discharge, or biopsy specimen of infected liver, rectum, or bladder tissue.

It is advisable to withhold treatment in pregnant women until after delivery because of possible toxicity to the fetus. For *S. haematobium* infection, praziquantel 40 mg/kg single dose is recommended. For *S. japonicum* infection, praziquantel 20 mg/kg three times a day for 1 day appears to be effective. For S. mansoni infection, praziquantel 20 mg/kg twice a day for 1 day is effective and oxamniquine 12–15 mg/kg as a single dose, contraindicated in pregnancy.

■ INFECTION WITH CESTODES

Tapeworms are highly prevalent in humans and their recurrence rates are high. The predisposing factors are consumption of raw or uncooked food. Four tapeworms primarily cause gastrointestinal infection: *Taenia saginata (T. saginata), Taenia solium (T. solium), Diphyllobothrium latum (D. latum)*, and *Hymenolepis nana (H. nana)*.

Clinical Manifestations

Large tapeworms are usually asymptomatic or may cause gastrointestinal symptoms such as nausea and diarrhea. The more prominent symptoms may be seen when humans are infected by worms in the larval stage known as *cysticercosis*. CNS involvement is common, and causes headache, papilledema, hemiparesis, decreased vision, and seizure, others are striated muscles and eyeballs.

Of the three tapeworms, *D. latum* causes severe effects on pregnancy. Large numbers of this worm can be present within the intestinal tract, and its ability to compete effectively for certain vitamins, such as vitamin B_{12}. Folate absorption may also be diminished by the presence of this tapeworm, and the two deficiencies may potentiate anemia of pregnancy. Symptoms may involve mild gastrointestinal discomfort, diarrhea or constipation, and symptoms of megaloblastic anemia.

Hymenolepis nana infection usually is asymptomatic or may induce mucosal irritation and with heavy infection may cause abdominal cramps, diarrhea, dizziness, and seizure. *Echinococcus granulosus* is associated with the development of hydatid cysts, primarily in the right lobe of the liver.

Diagnosis and Treatment

The diagnosis is done by finding eggs and proglottids in the feces. Diagnosis of cysticercosis is made by finding of small calcific densities on X-ray of the skull or extremities or identification of characteristic lesions by computed tomography (CT) or brain scan.

Treatment of intestinal tapeworms, including *T. saginata*, *T. solium*, and *D. latum*, is praziquantel 10–20 mg/kg in a single dose. Treatment of H. nana also is a single dose of praziquantel 25 mg/kg. Alternative therapy is niclosamide 2 g chewed thoroughly, then 1 g/day (two tablets) for 6 days. Albendazole 15 mg/kg/day for 8–28 days is recommended for cysticercosis. Treatment of cysticercosis or hydatid disease is based on surgical removal of the intact cyst if it is inducing obstructive symptoms.

REFERENCES

1. Xu F, Lee FK, Morrow RA, Sternberg MR, Luther KE, Dubin G, et al. Seroprevalence of herpes simplex virus type 1 in children in the United States. J Pediatr. 2007;151:374-7.
2. Brown ZA, Selke S, Zeh J, Kopelman J, Maslow A, Ashley RL, et al. The acquisition of herpes simplex virus during pregnancy. N Engl J Med. 1997;337:509-15.
3. Xu F, Sternberg MR, Kottiri BJ, McQuillan GM, Lee FK, Nahmias AJ, et al. Trends in herpes simplex virus type 1 and type 2 seroprevalence in the United States. Jama. 2006;296:964-73.
4. Enright AM, Prober CG. Neonatal herpes infection: Diagnosis, treatment and prevention. Semin Neonatol. 2002:7(4); 283-91.
5. Brown ZA, Wald A, Morrow RA, Selke S, Zeh J, Corey L. Effect of serologic status and cesarean delivery on transmission rates of herpes simplex virus from mother to infant. JAMA. 2003:286(2);203-9.
6. Brown ZA, Benedetti J, Selke S, Ashley R, Watts DH, Corey L. Asymptomatic maternal shedding of herpes simplex virus at the onset of labor: Relationship to preterm labor. Obstet Gynecol. 1996;87(4);483-8.
7. Kwon JY, Romero R, Mor G. New Insights into the Relationship between Viral Infection and Pregnancy Complications. Am J Reprod Immunol. 2014;71(5):387-90.
8. Gottlieb SL, Douglas JM, Schmid DS, Bolan G, Iatesta M, Malotte CK, et al. Seroprevalence and correlates of herpes simplex virus type 2 infection in five sexually transmitted-disease clinics. J Infect Dis. 2002;186(10): 1381-9.
9. Brown ZA, Gardella C, Wald A, Morrow RA, Corey L. Genital herpes complicating pregnancy. Obstet Gynecol. 2005;106(4): 845-56.
10. Sheffield JS, Hollier LM, Hill JB, Stuart GS, Wendel GD. Acyclovir prophylaxis to prevent herpes simplex virus recurrence at delivery: A systematic review. Obstet Gynecol. 2003;102(6):1396-1403.
11. Andrews WA, Kimberlin DF, Whitley R, Cliver S, Ramsey PS, Deeter R. Valacyclovir therapy to reduce recurrent genital herpes in pregnant women. Am J Obstet Gynecol. 2006;194(3):774-81.
12. Watts HD, Brown ZA, Money D, Selke S, Huang ML, Sacks SL, et al. A double-blind, randomized, placebo-controlled trial of acyclovir in late pregnancy for the reduction of herpes simplex virus shedding and cesarean delivery. Am J Obstet Gynecol. 2003;188(3):836-43.

13. Haun L, Kwan N, Hollier LM. Viral infections in pregnancy. Minerva Ginecol. 2007;59(2):159-74.
14. Xu F, Markowitz LE, Gottlieb SL, Berman SM. Seroprevalence of herpes simplex virus types 1 and 2 in pregnant women in the United States. Am J Obstet Gynecol. 2007; 196(1):43.e1-6.
15. Kimberlin DW, Lin CY, Jacobs RF, Powell DA, Frenkel LM, Gruber WC, et al. Natural history of neonatal herpes simplex virus infections in the acyclovir era. Pediatrics. 2001;108(2):223-9.
16. Kohelet D, Katz N, Sadan O, Somekh E. Herpes simplex virus infection after vacuum-assisted vaginally delivered infants of symptomatic mothers. J Perinatol. 2004; 24(3):147-9.
17. O'Boyle MKPD. Fetal infections. In: Diagnostic Imaging of Fetal Anomalies. Philadelphia: Lippincott Williams & Wilkins; 2003. pp. 745-76.
18. Gibbs RSSR. Maternal and fetal infectious disorders. In: RR Creasy RK (Ed). Maternal-Fetal Medicine. Philadelphia: WB Saunders; 1999. pp. 659-724.
19. ACOG Practice Bulletin. Perinatal Viral and Parasitic Infections. Number 20, September 2000. (Replaces educational bulletin number 177, February 1993). American College of Obstetrics and Gynecologists. Int J Gynaecol Obstet. 2002;76(1):95-107.
20. Chapman SJ . Varicella in pregnancy. Semin Perinatol. 1998;22(4):339-46.
21. Higa K, Dan K, Manabe H. Varicella-zoster virus infections during pregnancy: hypothesis concerning the mechanisms of congenital malformations. Obstet Gynecol. 1987;69(2):214-22.
22. Lamont RF, Sobel JD, Carrington D, Mazaki-Tovi S, Kusanovic JP, Vaisbuch E, et al. Varicella-zoster virus (chickenpox) infection in pregnancy. BJOG. 2011;118(10):1155-62.
23. Lamont RF. The role of infection in preterm labour and birth. Hosp Med. 2003; 64(11):644-7.
24. Lamont RF. Infection in the prediction and antibiotics in the prevention of spontaneous preterm labour and preterm birth. BJOG. 2003;110(Suppl 20):71-5.
25. Lamont RF, Nhan-Chang CL, Sobel JD, Workowski K, Conde-Agudelo A, Romero R. Treatment of abnormal vaginal flora in early pregnancy with clindamycin for the prevention of spontaneous preterm birth: a systematic review and metaanalysis. Am J Obstet Gynecol. 2011;205(3):177-90
26. Lamont RF, Sobel J, Mazaki-Tovi S, Kusanovic JP, Vaisbuch E, Kim SK, et al. Listeriosis in human pregnancy: a systematic review. J perinat med. 2011;39(3):227-36.
27. Syggelou A, Iacovidou N, Kloudas S, Christoni Z, Papaevangelou V. Congenital cytomegalovirus infection. Ann N Y Acad Sci. 2010;1205:144-7.
28. Ornoy A, Diav-Citrin O. Fetal effects of primary and secondary cytomegalovirus infection in pregnancy. Reprod Toxicol. 2006;21(4):399-409.
29. Kenneson A, Cannon MJ. Review and meta-analysis of the epidemiology of congenital cytomegalovirus (CMV) infection. Rev med virol. 2007;17(4):253-76.
30. McCarthy M, Auger D, Whittemore SR. Human cytomegalovirus causes productive infection and neuronal injury in differentiating fetal human central nervous system neuroepithelial precursor cells. J hum virol. 2000;3(4):215-28.
31. Boppana SB, Fowler KB, Britt WJ, Stagno S, Pass RF. Symptomatic congenital cytomegalovirus infection in infants born to mothers with preexisting immunity to cytomegalovirus. Pediatrics. 1999;104(1 Pt 1): 55-60.
32. Fowler KB, McCollister FP, Dahle AJ, Boppana S, Britt WJ, Pass RF. Progressive and fluctuating sensorineural hearing loss in children with asymptomatic congenital cytomegalovirus infection. J pediatr. 1997;130(4):624-30.
33. Yinon Y, Farine D, Yudin MH. Screening, diagnosis, and management of cytomegalovirus infection in pregnancy. Obstet gynecol surv. 2010;65(11):736-43.
34. Yinon Y, Kingdom JC, Odutayo A, Moineddin R, Drewlo S, Lai V, et al. Vascular dysfunction

in women with a history of preeclampsia and intrauterine growth restriction: insights into future vascular risk. Circulation. 2010;122(18):1846-53.
35. Istas AS, Demmler GJ, Dobbins JG, Stewart JA. Surveillance for congenital cytomegalovirus disease: a report from the National Congenital Cytomegalovirus Disease Registry. Clin Infect Dis. 1995;20(3):665-70.
36. Dontigny L, Arsenault MY, Biringer A, Clinical Practice Obstetrics Committee. Rubella in pregnancy. J Obstet Gynaecol Can. 2008;30(2):152-68.
37. Lee JY, Bowden DS. Rubella virus replication and links to teratogenicity. Clin microbiol rev. 2000;13(4):571-87.
38. Centers for Disease Control and Prevention (CDC). Epidemiology of HIV/AIDS–United States, 1981–2005. MMWR. 2006;55(21):589-92.
39. Fields BN, Knipe DM, Howley PM. Hepatitis A virus. In: Fields BN, Knipe DM, Howley PM, Chanock RM (Eds). Fields Virology, 3rd edition. New York: Lippincott-Raven Publishers; 1996. pp. 735-82.
40. Lemon SM. Type A viral hepatitis: epidemiology, diagnosis, and prevention. Clin Chem. 1997;43(8 Pt 2):1494-9.
41. Stapleton JT, Lemon SM. Hepatitis A and hepatitis E. In: JM Hoeprich PD, Ronald AR, (Eds). Infectious Diseases, 5th edition. Philadelphia: Lippincott Co; 1994. pp. 790-7.
42. Leikin E, Lysikiewicz A, Garry D, Tejani N. Intrauterine transmission of hepatitis A virus. Obstet Gynecol. 1996;88(4 Pt 2):690-1.
43. Erkan T, Kutlu T, Cullu F, Tümay GT. A case of vertical transmission of hepatitis A virus infection. Acta Paediatr. 1998;87(9):1008-9.
44. Renge RL, Dani VS, Chitambar SD, Arankalle VA. Vertical transmission of hepatitis A. Indian J Pediatr. 2002;69(6):535-41.
45. Duff P. Hepatitis in pregnancy. Semin Perinatol. 1998;22(4):277-83.
46. Duff P. Perinatal infectious disease. Semin Perinatol. 1998;22:241.
47. Ganem D, Schneider RJ. Hepadnaviridae: The Viruses and Their Replication. In: Knipe DM (Ed). Fields Virology, 4th edition. Philadelphia: Lippincott Williams & Wilkins; 2001. pp. 2923-69.
48. Maheshwari A, Ray S, Thuluvath PJ. Acute hepatitis C. Lancet. 2008;372(9635):321-32.
49. CDC. Recommendation for prevention and control of Hepatitis C virus. MMWR. 1998;47(RR19);1-39.
50. Bell BP, Mast EE, Terrault N, Hutin YJ. Prevention of hepatitis C in women. Emerg Infect Dis. 2004;10(11):2035-41.
51. Ward C, Tudor-Williams G, Cotzias T, Hargreaves S, Regan L, Foster GR. Prevalence of hepatitis C among pregnant women attending an inner London obstetric department: uptake and acceptability of named antenatal testing. Gut. 2000;47(2):277-80.
52. Mast EE, Hwang LY, Seto DS, Nolte FS, Nainan OV, Wurtzel H, et al. Risk factors for perinatal transmission of hepatitis C virus (HCV) and the natural history of HCV infection acquired in infancy. J Infect Dis. 2005;192(11):1880-9.
53. Naik SR, Aggarwal R, Salunke PN, Mehrotra NN. A large waterborne viral hepatitis E epidemic in Kanpur, India. Bull World Health Organ. 1992;70(5):597-604.
54. WHO. (2001). Introduction of hepatitis B vaccine into childhood immunization services: management guidelines, including information for health workers and parents. [online] Available from https://apps.who.int/iris/handle/10665/66957 [Last accessed November, 2022].
55. Patra S, Kumar A, Trivedi SS, Puri M, Sarin SK. Maternal and fetal outcomes in pregnant women with acute hepatitis E virus infection. Ann Intern Med. 2007;147(1):28-33.
56. Neuzil KM, Reed GW, Mitchel EF, Simonsen L, Griffin MR. Impact of influenza on acute cardiopulmonary hospitalizations in pregnant women. Am J Epidemiol. 1998;148(11):1094-102.
57. Harris JW. Influenza occurring in pregnant women. JAMA. 1919;72:978-80.
58. Nuzum JW, Pilot I, Stangl FH, Bonar BE. 1918 pandemic influenza and pneumonia in a large civilian hospital. IMJ Ill Med J. 1976;150(6):612-6.
59. Freeman DW, Barno A. Deaths from Asian influenza associated with pregnancy. Am J Obstet Gynecol. 1959;78:1172-7.

60. Hardy JM, Azarowicz EN, Mannini A, Medearis DN, Cooke RE. The effect of Asian influenza on the outcome of pregnancy, Baltimore, 1957–1958. Am J Public Health. 1961;51(8):1182-90.
61. Coffey VP, Jessop WH. Maternal influenza and congenital deformities. A follow-up study. Lancet. 1959;2(7109):935-8.
62. Cox S, Posner SF, McPheeters M, Jamieson DJ, Kourtis AP, Meikle S. Hospitalizations with respiratory illness among pregnant women during influenza season. Obstet Gynecol. 2006;107(6):1315-22.
63. Zou S. Potential impact of pandemic influenza on blood safety and availability. Transfus Med Rev. 2006;20(3):181-90.
64. Shi L, Tu N, Patterson PH. Maternal influenza infection is likely to alter fetal brain development indirectly: the virus is not detected in the fetus. Int J Dev Neurosci. 2005;23(2-3):299-305.
65. Kwan ML, Metayer C, Crouse V, Buffler PA. Maternal illness and drug/medication use during the period surrounding pregnancy and risk of childhood leukemia among offspring. Am J Epidemiol. 2007;165(1):27-35.
66. Ebert T, Kotler M. Prenatal exposure to influenza and the risk of subsequent development of schizophrenia. Isr Med Assoc J. 2005;7(1):35-43.
67. Takahashi M, Yamada T. A possible role of influenza A virus infection for Parkinson's disease. Adv Neurol. 2001;86:91-104.
68. Suarez L, Felkner M, Hendricks K. The effect of fever, febrile illnesses, and heat exposures on the risk of neural tube defects in a Texas-Mexico border population. Birth Defects Res A Clin Mol Teratol. 2004;70(10):815-24.
69. Shaw GM, Nelson V, Carmichael SL, Lammer EJ, Finnell RH, Rosenquist TH. Maternal periconceptional vitamins: interactions with selected factors and congenital anomalies? Epidemiology. 2002;13(6):625-30.
70. McCormick JB, Webb PA, Krebs JW, Johnson KM, Smith ES. A prospective study of the epidemiology and ecology of Lassa fever. J Infect Dis. 1987;155(3):437-44.
71. Bwaka MA, Bonnet MJ, Calain P, Colebunders R, De Roo A, Guimard Y, et al. Ebola hemorrhagic fever in Kikwit, Democratic Republic of the Congo: clinical observations in 103 patients. J Infect Dis. 1999;179(Suppl 1):S1-7.
72. Mupapa K, Mukundu W, Bwaka MA, Kipasa M, De Roo A, Kuvula K, et al. Ebola hemorrhagic fever and pregnancy. J Infect Dis. 1999;179(Suppl 1):S11-2.
73. Okware SI, Omaswa FG, Zaramba S, Opio A, Lutwama JJ, Kamugisha J, et al. An outbreak of Ebola in Uganda. Trop med int health. 2002;7(12):1068-75.
74. Johnson KM, McCormick JB, Webb PA, Smith ES, Elliott LH, King IJ. Clinical virology of Lassa fever in hospitalized patients. J Infect Dis. 1987;155(3):456-64.
75. McCormick JB, King IJ, Webb PA, Johnson KM, O'Sullivan R, Smith ES, et al. A case-control study of the clinical diagnosis and course of Lassa fever. J Infect Dis. 1987;155(3):445-55.
76. Brabin BJ. Epidemiology of infection in pregnancy. Rev infect dis. 1985;7(5):579-603.
77. McGregor IA: Epidemiology, malaria and pregnancy. Am J Trop Med Hyg. 1984;33(4):517-25.
78. Bray RS, Anderson MG. Falciparum malaria and pregnancy. Trans R Soc Trop Med Hyg. 1979;73(4):427-31.
79. Severe and complicated malaria. World Health Organization, Division of Control of Tropical Diseases. Trans R Soc Trop Med Hyg. 1990;84 Suppl 2:1-65.
80. Looareesuwan S, Phillips RE, White NG, Kietinun S, Karbwang J, Rackow C, et al. Quinine and severe falciparum malaria in late pregnancy. Lancet. 1985;2(8445):4-8.
81. Gilles HM, Lawson JB, Sibelas M, Voller A, Allan N. Malaria, anaemia and pregnancy. Ann Trop Med Parasitol. 1969;63(2):245-63.
82. Archibald HM. The influence of malarial infection of the placenta on the incidence of prematurity. Bull World Health Organ. 1956;15(3-5):842-5.
83. Aikawa M, Suzuki M, Gutierrez Y. Pathology of malaria. In: Kreier JP (Ed). Malaria, 2nd edition. New York: Academic Press; 1980. pp. 93-5.

84. Spitz AJW. Malaria infection of the placenta and its influence on the incidence of prematurity in Eastern Nigeria. Bull World Health Organ. 1959;21(2):242-4.
85. Jelliffe EFP. Low birth weight and malaria infection of the placenta. Bull World Health Organ. 1968;38(1):69-78.
86. Logie DE, McGregor IA: Acute malaria in newborn infants. Br Med J.1970;3:404-5.
87. Nyirjesy P, Kavasy T, Axelrod P, Fisher PR. Malaria during pregnancy: Neonatal morbidity and mortality and the efficacy of chloroquine prophylaxis. Clin Infect Dis. 1993;16(1):127-32.
88. Elsdon-Dew R. The epidemiology of amebiasis. Adv Parasitol. 1968;6:1-62.
89. Lewis EA, Antia AU. Amoebic colitis: Review of 295 cases. Trans R Soc Trop Med Hyg. 1969;63(5):633-8.
90. Rivera RA. Fatal postpartum amoebic colitis with trophozoites present in peritoneal fluid. Gastroenterology. 1972;62(2):314-7.
91. Abjoye AA: Fatal amoebic colitis in pregnancy and puerperium: a new clinico-pathological entity. J Trop Med Hyg. 1973;76(4):97-100.
92. Wagner VP, Smale LE, Lischke JH. Amebic abscess of the liver and spleen in pregnancy and puerperium. Obstet Gynecol. 1975;45(5):562-5.
93. David C. Infections in Obstetrics and Gynecology. Philadelphia: WB Saunders; 1980. pp. 86-9.
94. Kean BH. The treatment of amebiasis. JAMA. 1976;235(5):501.
95. Drugs for parasitic infections. Med Lett Drugs Ther. 1998;40(1017):1-12.
96. Griffin Jr FM. Failure of metronidazole to cure hepatic amebic abscess. N Engl J Med. 1973;288(26):1397.
97. Pittman FE, Pittman JC. Amebic liver abscess following metronidazole therapy for amebic colitis. Am J Trop Med Hyg. 1974;23(2):146-50.
98. Henn RM, Collin DB. Amebic abscess of the liver. JAMA. 1973;224(10):1394-5.
99. Brady PG, Wolfe JC. Waterborne giardiasis. Ann Intern Med. 1974;81(4):498-9.
100. Centers for Disease Control. Foodborne and Waterborne Disease Outbreaks. Annual Summary 1976. Atlanta: Centers for Disease Control; 1977.
101. Bezjak B: Evaluation of a new technique for sampling duodenal contents in parasitologic diagnosis. Am J Dig Dis. 1972;17(9):848-50.
102. Rein MF, Chapel TA. Trichomoniasis, candidiasis, and the minor venereal diseases. Clin Obstet Gynecol. 1975;18(1):73-88.
103. Al-Salihi FL, Curran JP, Wang J. Neonatal Trichomonas vaginalis: Report of 3 cases and review of the literature. Pediatrics. 1974;53(2):196-200.
104. Dykers JR. Single dose metronidazole for trichomonal vaginitis. N Engl J Med. 1975;293(1):23-4.
105. Lee RV. Parasitic infestations. In Burrow GN, Ferris TF (Eds). Medical Complications During Pregnancy. Philadelphia: WB Saunders; 1980. pp 438-63.
106. Greenwood BM, Whittle HC. Cerebrospinal fluid IgM in patients with sleeping sickness. Lancet. 1973;2(7828):525-7.
107. Barrett-Connor E. Chemoprophylaxis of amebiasis and African trypanosomiasis. Ann Intern Med. 1972;77:797-805.
108. Banerji D. Possible congenital infection in kala-azar. J Indian Med Assoc. 1955;24(11):433-5.
109. Low GC, Cook WE. A congenital case of kala-azar. Lancet.1926;211:1209.
110. Brooks TJ, Goetz CC, Plauche WC. Pelvic granuloma due to Enterobius vermicularis. JAMA. 1962;179(7):492-4.
111. Gould SE. Trichinosis in Man and Animals. Springfield, IL: Charles C Thomas; 1970.
112. Pacque M, Mupoz B, Poetschke L, Foose J, Greene BM, Taylor HR. Pregnancy outcome after inadvertent ivermectin treatment during community-based distribution. Lancet. 1990;336(8729):1486-9.
113. Cowper SG. A Synopsis of African Bilharziasis. London: HK Lewis; 1971.

Maternal Sepsis and its Management

Shazia Parveen, Ekta Tiwari, Shaheen Anjum

INTRODUCTION

Maternal sepsis is the third most common cause for maternal mortality after postpartum hemorrhage (PPH) and hypertensive disorders during pregnancy.[1] Around 11 women/1,000 live births had infections leading to near miss and mortality but in low- and middle-income groups 15 women/live births are affected. It may be a clinical manifestation of infections acquired in community or healthcare facilities. Healthcare-associated infections are often resistant to treatment leading to adverse outcomes.

According to the *Society of Critical Care Medicine (SCCM) sepsis* is defined as life-threatening organ dysfunction caused by dysregulated host response **(Fig. 1)**.[2]

Sepsis: Infection + systemic manifestations of infection.

Severe sepsis: Sepsis + sepsis-induced organ dysfunction/tissue hypoperfusion.

Septic shock: The persistence of hypoperfusion despite fluid resuscitation, it is a subset of sepsis in which particularly profound circulatory, cellular, and metabolic abnormalities are associated with a greater risk of mortality than with sepsis alone. Clinically they are identified by a vasopressor requirement to maintain mean arterial pressure of ≥65 mm Hg and serum lactate

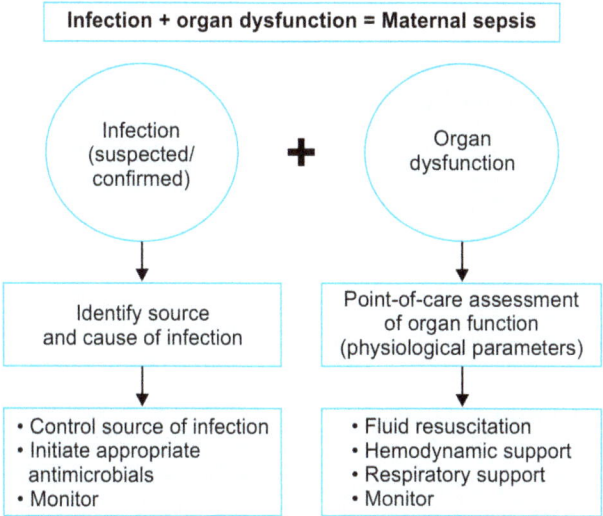

Fig. 1: Approach for implementation of the new WHO definition of maternal sepsis.

TABLE 1: Sequential Organ Failure Assessment (SOFA) score.

Organ system	SOFA score				
	0	1	2	3	4
PO_2/FiO_2 mm Hg	>400	<400	<300	<200	<100
Platelet count $10^3/\mu L$	>150	101–150	51–100	21–50	<20
Serum bilirubin mg%	<1.2	1.2–1.9	2–5.9	6–11.9	>12
Hypotension	None	MAP <70 mm Hg	Dopamine <5 µg/kg/min	Dopamine 5.1–15 or epinephrine ≤0.1 or epinephrine ≤0.1	Dopamine >15 epinephrine ≥0.1 or epinephrine ≥0.1
GCS	15	13–14	10–12	6–9	<6
Serum creatinine	<1.2	1.2–1.9	2–3.4	3.5–4.9	>5

(FiO_2: fraction of inspired oxygen; GCS: Glasgow Coma Scale; MAP: mean arterial pressure; PO_2: partial pressure of oxygen)

level >2 mmol/L (>18 mg%) in absence of hypovolemia. Sepsis is the primary cause of death from infection, especially if not recognized and treated promptly.[2]

According to the National Guidelines, sepsis and septic shock are the major causes of morbidity and mortality in the intensive care unit (ICU) patients worldwide.[3] Indian data shows a severe sepsis or septic shock incidence of 28% with a mortality of 18% in the adult ICU population. Early identification of sepsis and septic shock patients and appropriate management in the initial hours has seen a nearly 50% reduction in mortality during the last decade.

There is a mortality rate of 20-40% in case of severe sepsis and around 60% in case of septic shock.[4]

The SCCM task force has redefined sepsis as the Sequential Organ Failure Assessment (SOFA) scoring and its modified version quick SOFA (qSOFA) for easy identification of patients and their further management **(Tables 1 and 2)**.

A qSOFA score of ≥2 points indicates organ dysfunction and ICU admission.

TABLE 2: Quick Sequential Organ Failure Assessment (qSOFA) score.

qSOFA criteria	Points
Respiratory rate ≥22 breaths/min	1
Change in mental status	1
Systolic blood pressure ≤100 mm Hg	1

■ RISK FACTORS

- Obesity
- Diabetes/impaired glucose tolerance
- Anemia
- History of pelvic infection
- Septic abortion
- Postpartum endometritis
- Amniocentesis or any invasive prenatal procedure like chorionic villous sampling
- Cervical cerclage
- Prolonged rupture of membranes
- Impaired immunity/immunosuppressants
- Group B streptococcal infection in the previous baby or history of termination of pregnancy or miscarriage in the past 6 weeks[5,6]

- Impaired immune systems because of illness or drugs
- Invasive procedures during delivery (e.g., cesarean section, forceps delivery, and removal of retained products of conception)
- History of close contact with people with group A streptococcal infection, e.g., scarlet fever
- Infections other than obstetrics (pyelonephritis, cholecystitis, pneumonia, peritonitis, wound infection, and appendicular abscess).

PATHOGENESIS OF MATERNAL SEPSIS

Genital tract infections, especially ascending lower genital tract infections, are the most harmful as microorganisms can further disseminate and thus cause inflammation in form of cervicitis, endometritis, salpingitis or hydrosalpinx or pyosalpinx, tubo-ovarian abscesses or bacteremia that forms sepsis.[7]

Unacceptable health risks associated with intrauterine device (IUD) insertion in pelvic inflammatory disease (PID) patients and one more is toxic shock syndrome, rare life-threatening condition caused by toxins circulating in the bloodstream.

ETIOLOGY

Pelvic infections have three major sources of infection, i.e., endogenous microflora, intestinal flora, and sexual transmission.[7]

Three most common ways for spread of infection are as follows:
1. Migration of organism from the vagina into uterus traversing columnar epithelium
2. Via lymphatics
3. Ascending into the pregnant uterus and colonizing in amniotic fluid.

Most common route of Intraamniotic infection is ascent of endogenous flora of cervix and vagina.

Common pathogens involved:
- *Aerobic bacteria:* Group B beta-hemolytic Streptococcus, *Escherichia coli, S. aureus, Pseudomonas, Haemophilus influenzae, Klebsiella, Enterobacter*, etc.
- *Anaerobic bacteria: Clostridium* species, *Peptostreptococcus, Bacteroides* species, etc.
- *Others: Gardnerella vaginalis, Mycoplasma hominis, Ureaplasma urealyticum,* and *Chlamydia trachomatis*
  - *Clostridium perfringens* and *E. coli* are the most common pathogens in postnatal maternal sepsis cases.

DIAGNOSIS

Maternity modified systemic inflammatory response syndrome (SIRS) criteria for women, pregnant, and up to 42 days in the postnatal period:[8]
- Heart rate ≥100 beats/minute
- Respiratory rate ≥20 breathes/minute
- Temperature >38°C or <36°C
- White cell count >16.9 or <4 × 10⁹ cells/L or >10% immature bands
- Blood sugar level >7.7 mmol/L (in the nondiabetic)
- Acutely altered mental status
- Fetal heart rate >160 bpm.

MANAGEMENT OF SEPSIS

- *Surviving Sepsis Campaign (SSC) hour-1 bundle of care elements* **(Fig. 2)**:
  - Measure lactate level*
  - Obtain blood cultures before administering antibiotics
  - Administer broad-spectrum antibiotics
  - Begin rapid administration of 30 mL/kg crystalloid for hypotension or lactate level ≥ 4 mmol/L

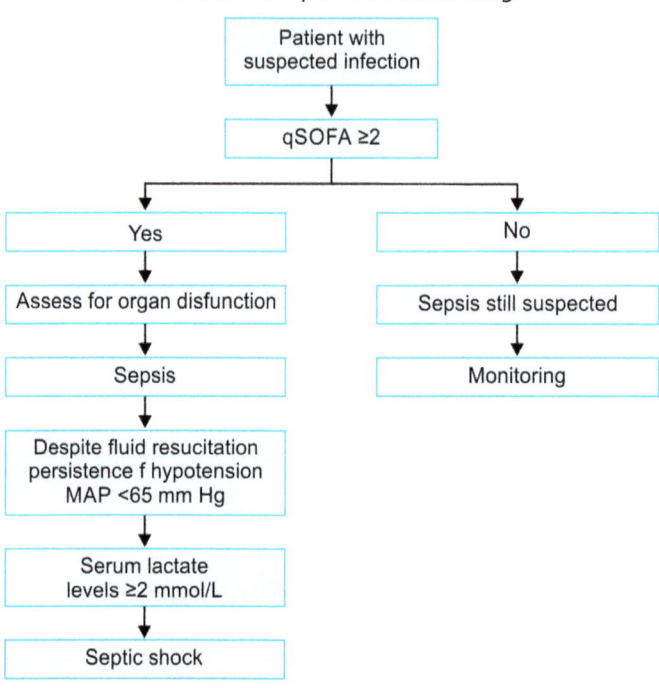

Flowchart 1: Septic shock monitoring.

(MAP: mean arterial pressure; qSOFA: quick sequential organ failure assessment)

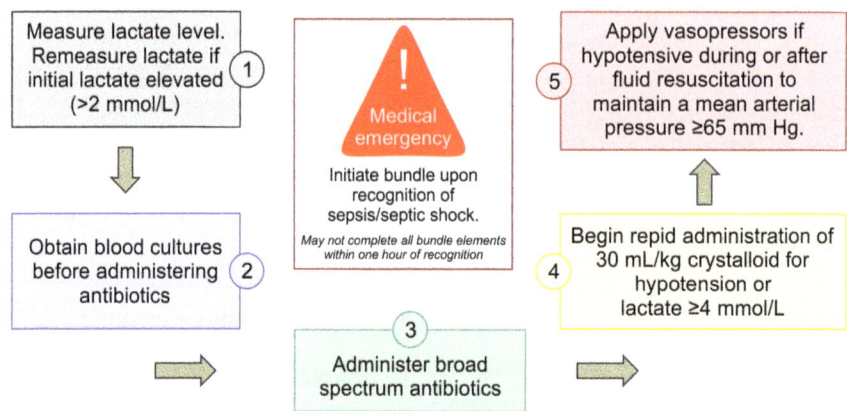

Fig. 2: Initial resuscitation of sepsis and septic shock 1-hour bundle.

- Apply vasopressors if hypotensive during or after fluid resuscitation to maintain mean arterial pressure (MAP) ≥65 mm Hg
- Remeasure lactate if initial lactate is elevated (>2 mmol/L) **(Flowchart 1)**.

The SSC 1-hour bundle is to improve the quality of patient care by early recognition of sepsis/septic shock and thus help in rapid diagnosis and immediate intervention.

- For critically ill patients with sepsis and septic shock, time is of the essence.
- Ideally these 1-hour bundle interventions should begin within the first hour of sepsis recognition but may not be necessarily completed in the first hour.
- Try to closely monitor the patient.

- Minimize time to treatment—sepsis and septic shock are medical emergencies.

ANTIMICROBIAL RECOMMENDATIONS

- Sepsis in pregnancy/after pregnancy:
  - Piperacillin-tazobactam 4.5 g IV 6 hourly
  - Cefoperazone + sulbactam 3 g IV 12 hourly
  - Methicillin-resistant *Staphylococcus aureus* (MRSA) cover with vancomycin/teicoplanin
- Septic abortion:
  - Empirical therapy:
    - Ampicillin 500 mg 6 hourly + metronidazole 500 IV 8 hourly
  - If previous partial antibiotic treatment then:
    - Piperacillin + tazobactam or cefoperazone + sulbactam after sending blood culture
- Salpingitis and tubo-ovarian abscess:
  - Ceftriaxone 250 mg IM/IV single dose
  - Ceftriaxone + metronidazole 500 BD for 14 days
  - Ceftriaxone + doxycycline 100 BD for 14 days
- Uncomplicated pyelonephritis:
  - Empirical therapy:
    - Amikacin 1 g OD IM/IV or
    - Gentamycin 7 mg/kg/day OD
  - Alternative regimen:
    - Piperacillin + tazobactam 4.5 g IV 6 hourly or
    - Cefoperazone + sulbactam 3 g IV 12 hourly or
    - Ertapenem 1 g IV OD
- Complicated pyelonephritis:
  - Empirical therapy:
    - Piperacillin + tazobactam 4.5 g IV 6 hourly or
    - Cefoperazone + sulbactam 3 g IV 12 hourly or
    - Amikacin 1 g OD IM/IV
  - Alternative regimen:
    - Imipenem 1 g IV 8 hourly or Meropenem 1 g IV 8 hourly
    - De escalate to ertapenam 1 g IVI OD if imipenem/Meropenem is initiated
    - If imipenem/meropenem initiated keep check of renal function
- Necrotizing fasciitis:
  - Empirical therapy:
    - Piperacillin + tazobactam 4.5 g IV 6 hourly or
    - Cefoperazone + sulbactam 3 g IV 12 hourly +
    - Clindamycin 600–900 mg IV 8 hourly
  - Alternative regimen:
    - Imipenem 1 g IV 8 hourly +
    - Clindamycin 600–900 mg IV TDS/linezolid 600 mg IV BD/daptomycin 6 mg/kg/day or
    - Ceftriaxone 2 g IV OD
- Secondary peritonitis, intra-abdominal abscess/gastrointestinal (GI) perforation:
  - Empirical therapy:
    - Piperacillin-tazobactam 4.5 g IV 8 hourly or cefoperazone-sulbactam 3 g IV 12 hourly
  - In sick patients:
    - Fluconazole IV 800 mg loading dose day 1 followed by 400 mg OD
  - Alternative regimen:
    - Imipenem 1 g IV 8 hourly or meropenem 1 g IV 8 hourly or doripenem 500 mg 8 hourly or ertapenem 1 g IV OD
- Community-acquired pneumonia:
  - Empirical therapy:
    - Amoxicillin clavulanate 1.2 g IV TDS or
    - Ceftriaxone 2 g IV OD for 5–7 days

- Alternative therapy:
  - Piperacillin-tazobactam 4.5 g IV 8 hourly or cefoperazone-sulbactam 3 g IV 12 hourly or
  - Imipenem 1 g IV 6 hourly
  - If MRSA add, linezolid 600 mg IV/oral 12 hourly
  - If atypical pneumonia—doxycycline 100 BD or azithromycin 500 OD
- Ventilator-associated pneumonia:
  - Beta-lactam-beta-lactamase inhibitor
  - Piperacillin/tazobactam + aminoglycoside (amikacin/gentamycin/tobramycin) or
  - Antipseudomonal fluoroquinolones (FQs) (cipro/levofloxacin)
  - For MRSA, vancomycin or linezolid
  - Second-line therapy—meropenem 60 mg/kg/day IV every 8 hourly and vancomycin 40 mg/kg/day IV every 6–8 hourly
  - Third-line therapy—colistin base 2.5–5 mg/kg/day IV every 6–12 hourly and vancomycin 40 mg/kg/day/IV every 6–8 hourly.

PREVENTION AND FUTURE STRATEGIES

Prevention of infection prevents sepsis.

The pillars of prevention of sepsis in obstetrics and gynecology are mainly hand hygiene, aseptic precaution during and after delivery, and preintervention adequate antibiotic coverage. These basic precautionary measures lead to a massive reduction in maternal morbidity and mortality because of sepsis.

It is well-said small step at a time adds on to huge change and success.

REFERENCES

1. Cheshire J, Dunlop C, Lissauer D. The Continuous Textbook of Women's Medicine, 1st edition. London, United Kingdom: The International Federation of Gynaecology and Obstetrics. 2021.
2. Evans L, Rhodes A, Alhazzani W, Antonelli M, Coopersmith CM, French C, et al. Surviving Sepsis Campaign: International Guidelines for Management of Sepsis and Septic Shock 2021. Crit Care Med. 2021;49:e1063-143.
3. Shields A, de Assis V, Halscott T. Top 10 Pearls for the Recognition, Evaluation, and Management of Maternal Sepsis. Obstet Gynecol. 2021;138(2):289-304.
4. HRP WHO. (2021). Statement on Maternal Sepsis. [online] Available from https://apps.who.int/iris/bitstream/handle/10665/254608/WHO-RHR-17.02-eng.pdf;jsessionid=789061A581D20963FF117471BF7777A9?sequence=1. [Last accessed November, 2022].
5. Royal College of Obstetricians and Gynaecologists. (2012). Sepsis in Pregnancy, Bacterial (Green-top Guideline No. 64a). [online] Available from https://www.rcog.org.uk/guidance/browse-all-guidance/green-top-guidelines/sepsis-in-pregnancy-bacterial-green-top-guideline-no-64a/. [Last accessed November, 2022].
6. Royal College of Obstetricians and Gynaecologists. (2012). Bacterial Sepsis following Pregnancy (Green-top Guideline No. 64b). [online] Available from https://www.rcog.org.uk/guidance/browse-all-guidance/green-top-guidelines/bacterial-sepsis-following-pregnancy-green-top-guideline-no-64b/. [Last accessed November, 2022].
7. Stud J, Tan SL, Chervenak FA. Current Progress in Obstetrics and Gynecology, 5th edition. India: TreeLife Media; 2019.
8. Department of Health. (2021). Sepsis Management for Adults (Including Maternity) (National Clinical Guideline No. 26). [online] Available from https://www.hse.ie/eng/about/who/cspd/ncps/sepsis/resources/national-clinical-guideline-no-26-sepsis-management-for-adults-including-maternity-2021.pdf. [Last accessed November, 2022].

Appendix

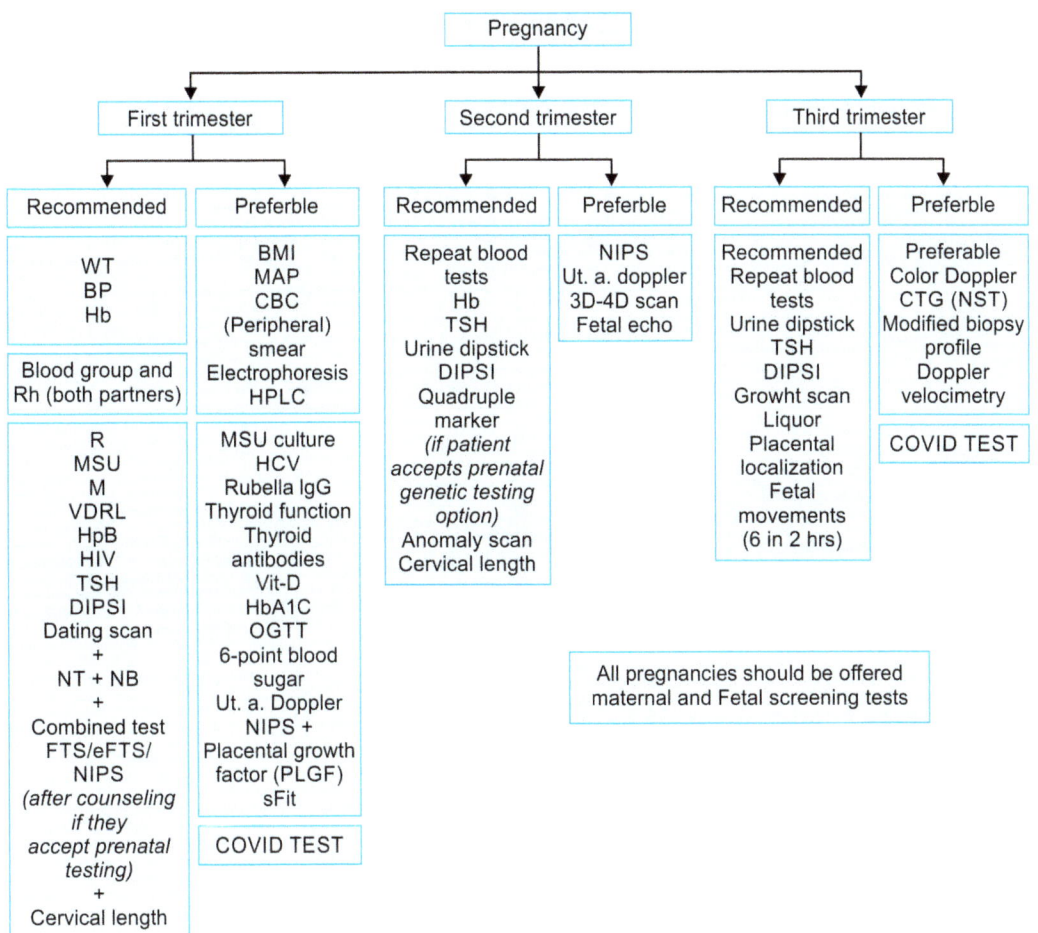

Appendix

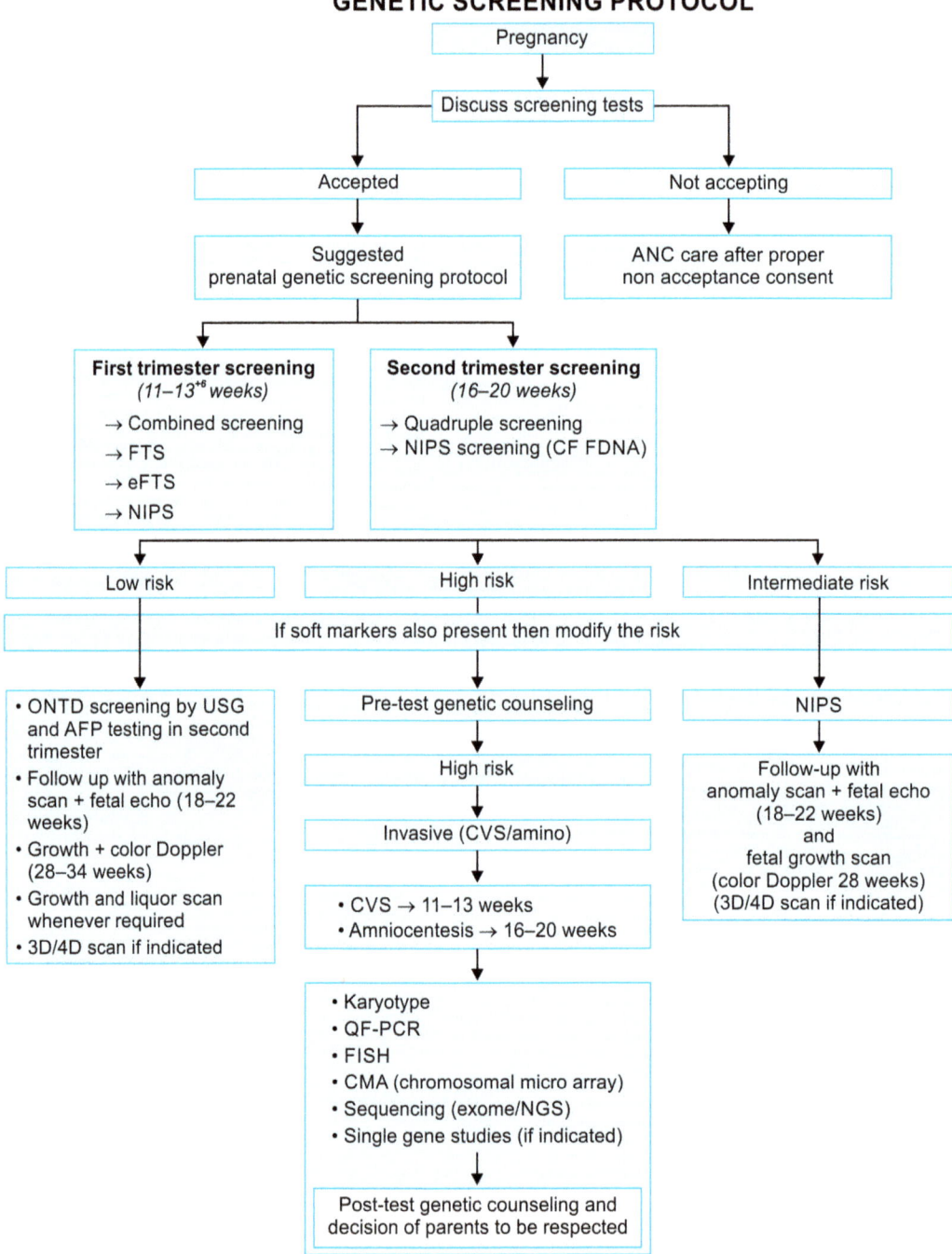

Index

Page numbers followed by b refer to box, f refer to figure, fc refer to flowchart, and t refer to table.

A

ABO blood group system 137, 149
Abortion 184
 incomplete 152
 septic 199
 spontaneous 161
Abruptio placentae 155, 156
Absolute neutrophil count 32
Acardius
 acephalus 133
 amorphous 133
 myelacephalus 133
Acid elution test 140, 141f
Acid-fast bacilli 72
Acidosis, metabolic 63
Acute asthmatic attack,
  management of 74
Acute fatty liver 62, 63, 66, 82, 96
 diagnosis of 64b
Acute kidney injury 114
 causes of 82t
 classification 81t
 network 81
 pregnancy-related 80
Acute leukemia 94
 treatment of 94
Acute lung injury, transfusion
  related 70, 76
Acute respiratory
 distress syndrome 68, 70, 75
 failure, causes of 68, 70t
Acute venous thromboembolism
  100
Acyclovir 18
Adhesive cellophane 187
African trypanosomiasis 184
Airways disease 70
Alanine transaminase 65, 114
Albendazole 187, 190
Albumin 61
Albuminuria 81
Albuterol 74
Alcohol 23
 use 5
Alkaline phosphatase 61
Alkaloids 108

Allopurinol 19
Alpha-fetoprotein 6, 61, 155
Alpha-globin 92
Alpha-thalassemia 92
Amantadine 18, 25
Ambulatory blood pressure
  monitoring 114
Amebiasis, therapy for 182
Amikacin 17
Aminoglycosides 17
Aminotransferases 63, 65
Amniocentesis 142f, 143f
Amniotic fluid 143f
 embolism 75, 77
Amoxicillin 16, 56
Amphotericin B 70
Ampicillin 16, 56
Analgesia 91, 101
Analgesics 20
Ancylostoma duodenale 186
Androgens 24
Anemia
 classification of 85
 diagnosis of 86, 87fc
 effect of 86, 86t
 hypochromic 91
 megaloblastic 89
 microangiopathic
  hemolytic 97
 physiological 85
 presence of 152
 severe 89
 symptoms of 93
Angiotensin-converting enzyme
  inhibitors 23
Antacid 20
Antepartum fetal surveillance 55
Antiallergics 20
Anti-C isoimmunization 149
Anticoagulation regimen 99
Anti-D dose 146
Antidepressants 20
Antidiabetics 20
Anti-E alloimmunization 149
Antiepileptic drugs 89
Antifibrinolytic plasminogen
  inhibitors 99

Antifungal agents 17
Antihypertensive 20
 therapy 119t
Antineoplastic agents 23
Antiphospholipid antibody
  syndrome 98, 162
Antipsychotics 20
Antithyroid
 antibodies 40
 drugs 20
Antitubercular drugs 18
Antivirals 25
Aortic stenosis 58
Arrhythmia 70
Arterial blood gas 82
Artesunate 19
Ascariasis, treatment of 186
Ascaris lumbricoides 185
Aspartate transaminase 65, 114
Aspiration 75, 154
Aspirin 99
 low-dose 99, 118
Assisted reproductive technology
  125, 155, 167, 168
 antenatal management of 169
Asthma 70, 72, 74
 risk factors of 73f
 severe 68
Asymptomatic bacteriuria 79
 screening of 84
Atrial fibrillation 58
Atypical hemolytic-uremic
  syndrome 98
Autoimmune diseases 5
Autoimmune thyroid disease 161
Azithromycin 16
Bacteria
 aerobic 197
 anaerobic 197

B

Bacteriuria, asymptomatic 79
Bartholin's glands 183
Beclomethasone 74
Bell's palsy 109
Benznidazole 184

Beta-blockers 46
Beta-human chorionic gonadotropin 151, 153, 154
Beta-thalassemia 91, 92
Bile acids 61
Biliary cirrhosis, primary 62
Bilirubin 65
Biophysical profile 134
Birth
    multiple 125
    trauma 32
    weight, low 177
Blood
    donation of 131
    glucose 36
    group, systems for 137
    pressure 114, 118
        diastolic 96, 114, 118
        measurement 114
        monitoring 114
    sugar
        fasting 33
        postprandial 33
    transfusion, indications for 89
Body mass index 31, 62
Bone marrow 185
Breastfeeding 24
Broad-spectrum antibiotics 102
Budd-Chiari syndrome 62
Budesonide 74
Burns 75

C

Calcium 120
Captopril 23
Carbenicillin 16
Carbimazole 47
Carbohydrates, complex 34
Cardiac disease 53, 54, 70
Cardiomyopathy, peripartum 57, 59, 59*b*
Cardiopulmonary transplantation 76
Cardiovascular issues 68
Cardiovascular risk 56*t*
    classification for 55
Carpal tunnel syndrome 109
Cataracts 174
Cefaclor 15
Cefadroxil 15
Cefazolin 15
Cefixime 15
Cefoperazone 15
Cefotaxime 15
Cefpirome 15
Ceftazidime 15
Ceftriaxone 15
Cefuroxime 15
Central nervous system 174
Cephalexin 15
Cephalosporins 15
Cerebral venous thrombosis 108
Cerebrovascular diseases 108
Cervical
    ectropion 151
    polyp 151
Cervicitis 151
Cesarean delivery 155
Cestodes 189
Chagas' disease 184
Chemotherapy 93
Chlamydia trachomatis 197
Chloramphenicol 16
Chloroquine 19
    phosphate 180, 181
Cholangitis, primary sclerosing 62
Cholestasis, intrahepatic 62, 66
Chorionic villous sampling 6, 135
Chorioretinitis 174
Chromosomal abnormality 164
    diagnosis for 6*fc*
Chronic kidney disease 79, 81, 82
    complications of 82*t*
Chronic lymphatic obstruction 188
Ciprofloxacin 17
Cirrhosis 62, 66
Clarithromycin 16
Clindamycin 16, 180
Clonorchis 188
Cloxacillin 16
Coagulation disorder 85, 98
Cocaine 23
Cold cough remedies 20
Collagen vascular diseases 79
Complete blood count 82
Compression neuropathies, postpartum 110, 110*t*
Conjoint twins 128*f*
Contraception 57
Control thyroid function 47
Cooley's anemia 92
Coomb's test 95
    direct 147*f*
    indirect 139*f*
Cord prolapse 128
Cordocentesis 142
Corticosteroids 24
    high-dose 95
Cough 71
Coumadin 102
Coumarin anticoagulants 23
Cromolyn sodium 74
Cutaneous leishmaniasis 185
Cyanosis 75
Cyclophosphamide 24
Cycloserine 18
Cystic fibrosis 76, 159
Cysticercosis, treatment of 190
Cytomegalovirus 109, 160, 162, 175

D

Deep venous thrombosis 100, 101, 109
    diagnosis of 101
    signs for 75
Dehydration 61
Dehydroepiandrosterone 163
Delivery
    management of 89
    mode of 37
    timing of 37
Deoxyribonucleic acid 125
Depression, respiratory 46
Desogestrel 57
Diabetes mellitus 29, 36, 160
    gestational 29-33, 33*fc*, 38, 108
    intrapartum care of 37
    types of 29
    uncontrolled 161
Diazepam 25
Dichorionic diamniotic 125
    twins, diagnosis of 128, 129
Diethylcarbamazine
    citrate 188
    toxic effects of 188
Diphyllobothrium latum 189
Discordant sex 129, 130
Disseminated intravascular coagulation 82, 96, 114
Dizziness 86
Doxycycline 181
D-penicillamine 25
Drugs
    abuse 156
    classification system 14*t*
    use 5
Dyspareunia 189
Dyspnea 54, 68, 70, 75, 77, 86, 101
    causes of 70*t*
    physiological 68
Dystocia 189

E

Early pregnancy
  bleeding in 151
  diagnosis for 151
Ebola 178
  hemorrhagic fever 178
  virus disease 178
Echinococcus granulosus 190
Echocardiogram 57, 59
Eclampsia 62, 64, 66
  syndrome 108
Ectopic pregnancy 151, 154
  management of 154b
Eculizumab 99
Edema, pulmonary 68, 75, 96
Eflornithine 184
Electrocardiography 57, 59
Elephantiasis 188
Elevated liver enzymes 64, 65
Enalapril 23
Endocervix 183
Endocrine diseases 27
Enoxaparin 100
Entamoeba histolytica infection 182
Enterobacter 197
Enterobius vermicularis 187
Enzyme-linked immunosorbent
  assay 163, 174
Epstein-Barr virus 109
Ergonovine 74
Ertapenem 16
Erythroblastosis fetalis 139
Estimated delivery date 6
Estrogen, maternal 183
Ethambutol 18, 72
Ethionamide 18
Exercise 119

F

Famcyclovir 18
Fasciola 188
Fasciolopsis 188
Fatigue 86
Fatty liver, acute 62, 63, 66, 82, 96
Febuxostat 19
Ferrous fumarate 88
Ferrous gluconate 88
Ferrous sulfate 88
Fetal
  assessment, invasive
    tests for 141
  blood sampling 144
  bradycardia 156
  cardiac activity 134
  complications 127, 133
  growth restriction 4
  hyperbilirubinemia 139
  screening
    investigations for 8
    protocol 4fc
  thyroid gland 41
Feticide 132
Fetomaternal hemorrhage 138
  incidence of 137
Fetoscopic laser occlusion 132
Fetus 85
  delivery of 77
  papyraceus 127f
Filarial disease 188
Filariasis 188
Fine-needle aspiration 48
Fluconazole 17, 25
Fluoroquinolones 17
Fluticasone 74
Folate deficiency 89, 90t
Folic acid antagonist 23
Follicle stimulating hormone 125
Free thyroxine 163
Fresh frozen plasma 99
Fromoterol 74
Fungal pneumonia 70

G

Gallstones 62
Gamma-glutamyl transferase 63
Gancyclovir 18
Gardnerella vaginalis 197
Gastric acid aspiration 76
Gastrointestinal infection 189
Genetic 90
  counseling 169
  factors 117
  testing 3
Genital tract infections 197
Gentamicin 17, 56
Gestational diabetes mellitus
    29-33, 33fc, 38, 108
  development of 30
  history of 29
  management of 34
  prevention of 31
  screening for 31
  testing for 32fc
Gestational sac 152
  number of 129, 130
Gestational transient
    thyrotoxicosis 44, 45
Gestational trophoblastic
    disease 46
Giardia infection, adverse
    effects of 183
Giardia lamblia 182
  infection 182
Giardiasis, diagnosis of 183
Giemsa stained 181
Glanzmann's thrombasthenia 95
Glasgow coma scale 196
Glomerular filtration rate 79, 81
Glomerulonephritis 79
Glucose
  homeostasis, abnormal 29
  intolerance 29
  monitoring 36
  tolerance, impaired 33
Glyburide 35
Granulomatous reactions 189
Graves' disease 46
Graves' hyperthyroidism 161
Griseofulvin 18
Guillain-Barré syndrome 109

H

Haemophilus influenzae 68
Hashimoto thyroiditis 42
Headache 86, 106, 189
  causes of 106
  classification of 107fc
  primary 106
Heart
  disease 57f
    signs for 53, 54
    symptoms of 53, 54
    valvular 58, 58b
  failure 44
    classification of 55t
    functional classification
      of 55
  rate 59
HELLP
  classification of 65t
  syndrome 62, 94, 113, 120
  diagnosis of 64
Hemagglutinin 178
Hematological disorder 85
Hematoma, subcapsular 64
Hemiparesis 189
Hemoglobin 61, 91, 151
  A1C 163
  H 92
  quantitative disorders of 91
  thalassemic 91

Hemoglobinopathy 90
　classification of 91*b*
Hemolysis 64, 141
　absence of 65
　disease 139
Hemolytic uremic syndrome 94
Hemorrhage 99
　antepartum 82
　atonic postpartum 127
　intraparenchymal 64
　intraventricular 168
　postpartum 167, 195
　transplacental 149
Hepatic diseases 61, 66
　classification of 61, 62*t*
Hepatic rupture 64
Hepatitis 176
　A 176
　autoimmune 62
　B 92, 177
　　vaccine 177
　　virus infection 177
　C 92, 177
　E 177
　　virus 177
　viral 62
Hepatotoxicity, drug-induced 62
Herpes
　infection, neonatal 174
　simplex virus 160, 162, 173
Hodgkin's lymphoma 93
Homan's sign 101
Hookworm 186
Hormonal dysfunction 92
Hormone 24
Human chorionic gonadotropin 6, 40, 45
Human immunodeficiency virus 5, 92, 162, 176
Human leukocyte antigens 116
Human teratogens 23*t*
Hydatid
　cysts, development of 190
　disease 190
Hydrops fetalis 139
Hydroxycarbamide 91
Hymenolepis nana 189
　infection 190
Hyperammonemia 63
Hyperandrogenemia 161
Hyperemesis gravidarum 44, 45, 61, 62, 66
Hyperglycemia 126
Hyperhomocysteinemia 161
Hyperinsulinemia 161

Hyperpigmentation, postinflammatory 4
Hyperprolactinemia 161
　transient 162
Hypertension
　chronic 82, 156
　gestational 82, 177
　management, severe 120, 121*f*
　portal 66
　pregnancy-induced 91
　systolic 108
Hypertensive disorders 113, 161
　classification of 113*fc*, 115*t*
　pathology of 117, 117*f*
　prevention of 118*t*
　types of 114*t*
Hyperthyroidism 44, 48
　familial gestational 45
　moderate 45
　subclinical 44
　trophoblastic 45
Hyperuricemia, drugs used for 19
Hyperventilation 77
Hypoalbuminemia 63
Hypoglycemia 46
　neonatal 32
　risk of 35
　signs for 37
Hypothesis 116
Hypothyroidism 42, 48
　congenital 42
　effect of 42
　management of 43*fc*
　primary 42
　secondary 42
　subclinical 42
　treatment for 43
Hypothyroxinemia, maternal 42
Hypovolemia, symptoms of 151
Hypoxemia 76
Immune thrombocytopenia 94, 95
　treatment of 95

I

Immunoglobulin 152
　G 163
　low levels of 139
　M 163
Immunological factors 116, 117*fc*, 162
In utero events, sequence of 139, 140*f*

Infections 94, 171, 173, 185, 187-189
　neonatal 174
　parasitic 179
　spread of 197
　treatment of 91
　viral 173
Infertility, rate of 92
Influenza 178
　symptoms of 178
　viruses 178
Inspired oxygen, fraction of 196
Insulin 34
　resistance 161
　role of 34
　supplementation 35
Intensive care unit 77, 82, 109
Interlocking twins 128*f*
Interstitial lung diseases 76
Intertwin membrane 129, 130
Intestinal nematodes 185
Intestinal tapeworms, treatment of 190
Intramuscular injections 88
Intrauterine
　blood transfusion 144, 147*f*
　contraceptive devices 57, 197
　death 4, 80
　growth restriction 174, 182
　transfusion 144
Intravenous immune globulin 109
Invasive mechanical ventilation 77
Iodine 41
　deficiency 42
Ipratropium 74
Iron
　amount of 88*t*
　deficiency anemia, management of 86
　dextran complex 88
　preparations 88*t*
　sucrose complex 89
Ischemic tissue 98
Isoimmunization 137
Isoniazid 18, 72
Isotretinoin 24
Itraconazole 17, 25

K

Kala-azar 184
Kanamycin 17

Kell antigen system 149
Ketoconazole 17
Ketosis 61
Kidney
  disease 5, 81
    chronic 79, 81, 82
    end-stage 81
  function
    loss of 81
    tests 82
  injury, acute 114
  insufficiency, acute 79
  solitary 83
  ureters, and urinary bladder 82
Kyphoscoliosis 77

L

Labetalol 119
Labor 55
  management of third
    stage of 89
Lactate dehydrogenase 65
Lactation difficulties 127
Lambda sign 129
Lassa fever 178
Late pregnancy 155t
  bleeding in 154
Laxatives 20
Leflunomide 25
Left ventricular ejection fraction
  56, 58
Leishmania 184
  braziliensis 184
  donovani 184
  mexicana 185
Leptospira 162
Leukemia 93
  acute 94
    lymphocytic 93
    myelogenous 93
  chronic 93
    myelogenous 93
Leukotriene
  agents 74
  receptor antagonists 74
Levalbuterol 74
Levofloxacin 17
Linezolid 17
Lipoprotein, low-density 59
Lisinopril 23
Lithium 24
Liver
  disease 61
    pre-existing 66

pregnancy-specific 66t
  types of 61
  dysfunction, severity of 97
Loeffler's syndrome 185, 186
Long-acting injectable
  progesterone 57
Low platelets 65
  count syndrome 64
Lower respiratory tract infections,
  drugs used for 21
Lower segment cesarean
  section 156
Low-molecular-weight heparin
  58, 59, 91
Lung diseases, restrictive 76
Luteal phase defect 162
Lymph nodes 185

M

Macrolides 16
Malaria 179
  congenital 181
  infections
    chemoprophylaxis of 180t
    treatment of 180t
  symptoms of 179
Malignancy 151
Maternal infection
  clinical manifestations of 179
  primary 176
Maternal influenza infection 178
Maternal sepsis 195, 195f
  pathogenesis of 197
Mean arterial pressure 4f
Mebendazole 187, 188
Medroxyprogesterone 57
Mefloquine 19
Megaloblastic anemia 89
  sign of 90t
  symptoms of 90t
Mental retardation 174
Meralgia paresthetica 110
Mercury manometer 114
Meropenem 16
Metformin 35
  dosage for 35
Methicillin 16
Methimazole 25, 47
  maternal usage of 47
Methotrexate 154
Methyldopa 119
Methylergonovine 74
Methylmercury 24
Metoprolol 46, 47

Metronidazole 182, 184
  use of 182
Mezlocillin 16
Miconazole 17
Middle cerebral artery 142-144
Migraine 107
Miscarriage 151, 161
Misoprostol 24
Mitral stenosis 58
Monochorionic diamniotic
  pregnancy 125
Monochorionic monoamniotic
  pregnancy 125
Moxifloxacin 17
Multifetal pregnancy reduction
  134, 134f
Myasthenia gravis 110
Mycoplasma hominis 197

N

Nasal intubation 77
Nausea 97
Necator americanus 186
Necrotizing enterocolitis 168
Necrotizing fasciitis 199
Nedocromil 74
Neisseria gonorrhoeae 162
Neonatal herpes infection 174
  risk of 173
Neonatal infection 174
  risk of 173
Neonatal intensive care unit
  80, 167
Nephrectomy 83
Nephropathy, diabetic 83
Neural tube defects 6fc
Neurologic dysfunction 97
Neurological diseases 106
Neurological disorders 106, 110
Neuromuscular disorders,
  hereditary 76
Neuropathy, classification
  of 109fc
Neutropenia 94
Niclosamide 190
Nifedipine 119
Nine square thyroid
  evaluation 41f
Nitrofurantoin 16
Non-Hodgkin's lymphoma 93
Noninvasive test 142
Noninvasive ventilation 77
Non-selective technique 132
Norfloxacin 17

Normal maternal glucose metabolism 30
Nuchal translucency 6

O

Obesity 5
Obstetric disorder 76
Ofloxacin 17
Oligoamnios 131
Operative deliveries 161, 167
Opisthorchis 188
Oral antidiabetic medications 35
Oral contraceptive pills 125
Oral corticosteroid 74
Oral glucose tolerance test 30, 33, 163
Oral hypoglycemic agents 35
Oral iron 88
Orthopnea 54
Oxygen, partial pressure of 196

P

Pain, abdominal 97
Palpitations 86
Papilledema 189
Paragonimus 188
Parenchymal disease, pulmonary 77
Parenteral iron treatment 88
　indication for 88b
Paromomycin 183
Paroxysmal nocturnal hemoglobinuria 99
Partner's vasectomy 57
Peak systolic
　velocimetry 142, 143f
　velocity 144
Pelvic
　infection 102, 197
　inflammatory disease 197
Percutaneous umbilical blood sampling 142
Perinatal death 32
Peritonitis, secondary 199
Phlebotomus 184
Piperacillin 16
Placenta 85
　previa 155, 156
Placental abruption 155
Placental masses, number of 129, 130
Placental transfer 21
Placentation, abnormal 155

Plasma
　glucose, fasting 33
　volume 53
Plasmapheresis 46
Plasmodium
　falciparum 179
　malariae 179
　ovale 179
　vivax 179
Platelet
　disorders 94
　storage pool disorder 96
Pneumonia 68
　bacterial 68
　community-acquired 199
　ventilator-associated 200
Pneumothorax 68
Polycystic ovarian syndrome 160, 161, 167
Polycythemia, signs for 38
Polyhydramnios 126, 131
Polymerase chain reaction 163
Posterior reversible encephalopathy syndrome 108
Postpartum anti-D dose 145
Post-thyroidectomy 42
Potassium iodine solution 47
Praziquantel 190
Prednisone 95
Preeclampsia 62, 64, 66, 76, 96, 167
　increased risk of 118
　syndrome 108
Pregnancy 71f, 74, 152
　bleeding in 151
　disorders of 108
　early 151
　ectopic 151, 154
　hematological changes during 86t
　high-risk 3
　late 155t
　medical termination of 72
　molar 151, 152
　multiple 125, 168
　normal
　　physiological changes of 61
　　signs of 54t
　　symptoms of 54t
　physiological changes in 53
　related acute kidney injury 80
　　management of 81, 82t
Rh
　incompatible 145fc
　negative 146fc

　situations, high-risk 5
　specific liver disease, management of 66
　symptoms of 77
Preterm
　birth 167
　labor 126, 128, 161
Primaquine 19
　phosphate 180, 181
Progesterone 152
　supplementation 151
Progestin
　androgenic 24
　only pills 57
Prophylactic anticoagulation 99, 101
Propranolol 47
Proteinuria 116
Psychiatric medications 24
Puerperium, management of 89
Pulmonary artery pressure 58
Pulmonary disease 68
Pulmonary embolism 68, 101
　treatment of 102
Pyelonephritis 83, 199
Pyrazinamide 18, 72
Pyridoxine 72
Pyrimethamine 89

Q

Quick sequential organ failure assessment score 196t
Quinidine gluconate plus 180
Quinine 19
　sulphate plus 180
Quintero staging system 131

R

Radionuclide cardiac imaging 54
Red blood cells 85, 137
Regurgitant lesions 58, 58b
Relaxation strategies 106
Renal disease 81, 83t, 96
　end-stage 79
　management of 83t
Renal disorders 79
Renal dysfunction 63
Renal physiology 79, 79t
Renal plasma flow 79
Renal replacement therapy 82
Respiratory disease 68
Respiratory distress syndrome 75, 168
Rh factor inheritance probability, description of 138f

Rh isoimmunization 137, 143
  epidemiology of 137
  etiology of 137
  pathophysiology of 140*f*
Rhesus system 137
Rheumatic heart disease 53, 56
Ribavirin 25
Rifabutin 18
Rifampicin 18, 72
Rosette test 140, 141*f*
Rubella 175
  infection, maternal 176
  virus 162

S

Salmeterol 74
Salpingitis 199
  development of 189
Schistosoma
  haematobium 189
  japonicum 189
Schistosomiasis 189
Scleroderma 98
Sclerosis, multiple 110
Seizure 189
Selective serotonin reuptake
    inhibitors 24
Sensitization, severity of 140
Sepsis 62, 198*f*
  management of 197
  prevention of 200
  severe 195
Septic pelvic thrombophlebitis
    102
Septic shock 195, 198*f*
  monitoring 198*fc*
Septostomy 132
Sequential organ failure
    assessment score 196*t*
Serum albumin 79
Serum thyroid binding
    globulin 40
Sex chromosomal
    aberrations 168
Sexually transmitted infections 4
Shock, septic 195, 198*f*
Shoulder dystocia 32
Sickle cell
  anemia 90, 159
  disease 90
    management of 91
Single embryo transfer 125
Single fertilized ovum 125
Single fetal demise 128, 133

Singleton assisted reproductive
    technology 168
Spectrophotometric charts
    141, 143*f*
Sputum 71
Staphylococcus aureus 68
Streptococcus pneumoniae 68
Streptomycin 17, 18
Stroke 108
  hemorrhagic 108
  recurrence, risk of 108
  volume 53
Strongyloides
  infection 186
  stercoralis 186
Succinylcholine 109
Sulfonamides 16
Suppressive antiviral therapy 174
Syncope 54
Synthesize iodothyronines 41
Systemic lupus erythematosus 83,
    95, 162

T

Tachycardia 75, 102
Tachypnea 75, 102
Taenia
  saginata 189
  solium 189
Tapeworm 189
Teratogenic drugs 21, 23, 25
Teratogenicity 21
Teratogens 13
Tetracycline 16, 24
Thalassemia 91
Theophylline 74
Thionamide 46
  intolerance 47
Thrombocythemia 99
  essential 99
Thrombocytopenia 94, 95,
    96, 97
  gestational 94
  hereditary 94
  inherited 95
  severe 96
Thrombocytosis 99
Thromboembolic disease 100
Thromboembolism
  high risk for 101
  pulmonary 75
Thrombophilia
  acquired 99, 164
  inherited 100

Thrombophilic disorders 99
Thrombophlebitis, superficial 100
Thrombotic microangiopathies
    96, 97
Thrombotic thrombocytopenic
    purpura 94
Thyroid
  adaptation 40
  antibody 161
  cancer 48, 49
  disease 5
  disorder 40, 161
  function 40, 41
    assessment of 40
    tests 41*t*, 47
  hormone 44
    functions of 40
    synthesis 46
  nodule 48, 49
  peroxidase antibodies 43
  stimulating hormone 43, 161
  storm 44
Thyroidectomy 46, 161
Thyroiditis, postpartum 48
Thyrotoxicosis, factitious 45
Thyrotropin receptor antibody 47
Thyroxine 43
Tigecycline 17
Tinidazole 183
Tiredness 54
Tissue dwelling nematodes 187
Tobramycin 17
Togaviridae 175
TORCH infections 173
Toxic adenoma 45, 46
Toxic multinodular goiter 45, 46
Toxoplasma gondii 162
Transaminases 61
Transesophageal
    echocardiography 54
Transient ischemic attacks 108
Trematodes 188
Treponema 162
  pallidum 162
Triamcinolone 74
Trichinella spiralis 187
Trichinosis 187
Trichomonal infection, diagnosis
    of 184
Trichomonas vaginalis
    infection 183
Trichuris trichiura 187
Triiodothyronine 163
Trimethoprim 89
Trypanosoma gambiense 184

Trypanosomiasis 184
  diagnosis of 184
Tuberculosis 71, 72
  drug-resistant 72, 72*fc*, 73
  drug-sensitive 72, 73
  management of 73*t*
  modes of transmission of 71*f*
  multidrug-resistant 72
Tubo-ovarian abscess 199
Twin
  classification of 126*f*
  delivery of second of 130
  gestations, antenatal examination of 135
  peak 129
  twin transfusion syndrome 130, 168

U

Ultrasonography 7, 152
Ultrasound, abdominal 62
Unfractionated heparin 58, 100
Upper respiratory tract infections, drugs used for 21
Ureaplasma urealyticum 197
Urethra 183
Urinary tract infection 79, 80
  drugs used for 20
Urolithiasis 83

Uterine 4*f*
  bleeding, excessive 152
  curettage 154
  rupture 155
Uteroplacental trauma 155
Uterus, rupture of 155

V

Vaginal bleeding 151, 154
  risk factors for 155*t*
  signs for 155
  symptoms for 155
Vaginal epithelium 183
Vaginitis 151
Valproate 23
Valvular disease, anticoagulation for 58, 58*b*
Vancomycin 16, 56
Variceal bleeding 66
Varicella infection, primary 174
Varicella zoster virus 174
Vasa previa 155, 156
Vascular anastomoses, laser ablation of 132
Vasculitis 98
Vena cava, inferior 102
Venous thromboembolism 70, 127
Ventilatory management 77
Viral pneumonia 68, 69
Virchow's triad 100

Visceral leishmaniasis 185
  diagnosis of 185
Visual disturbances 96
Vitamin
  B12 189
  C 118
  E 118
Vomiting 97, 152
von Willebrand factor 97

W

Warfarin 23
Weakness 86
West African trypanosomiasis 184
Whip worm 187
White blood cell disorders 93
Wilson's disease 62
Worsening asthma 68
Wuchereria bancrofti 188

Y

Yolk sac 152

Z

Zafirlukast 74
Ziehl-Neelsen stain 72
Zika 109
  infection 5
Zileuton 74

www.ingramcontent.com/pod-product-compliance
Ingram Content Group UK Ltd.
Pitfield, Milton Keynes, MK11 3LW, UK
UKHW052202140425
457402UK00003B/24